HANDBOOK OF
Clinical Nutrition

D0201960

HANDBOOK OF
Clinical Nutrition

Fourth Edition

Douglas C. Heimburger, MD, MS
Professor
Division of Clinical Nutrition and Dietetics
Departments of Nutrition Sciences and Medicine
University of Alabama at Birmingham
Birmingham, Alabama

Jamy D. Ard, MD
Assistant Professor
Division of Clinical Nutrition and Dietetics
Departments of Nutrition Sciences and Medicine
University of Alabama at Birmingham
Birmingham, Alabama

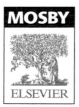

MOSBY

ELSEVIER

MOSBY
ELSEVIER

1600 John F. Kennedy Boulevard
Suite 1800
Philadelphia, PA 19103-2899

HANDBOOK OF CLINICAL NUTRITION, 4/e   ISBN-13: 978-0-323-03952-9
Copyright © 2006, 1997, 1989, 1981 by   ISBN-10: 0-323-03952-9
Mosby Inc. All rights reserved.

Notice

Knowledge and best practice in this field are constantly changing. As new
research and experience broaden our knowledge, changes in practice, treatment
and drug therapy may become necessary or appropriate. Readers are advised
to check the most current information provided (i) on procedures featured or
(ii) by the manufacturer of each product to be administered, to verify the
recommended dose or formula, the method and duration of administration, and
contraindications. It is the responsibility of the practitioner, relying on their own
experience and knowledge of the patient, to make diagnoses, to determine dosages
and the best treatment for each individual patient, and to take all appropriate
safety precautions. To the fullest extent of the law, neither the Publisher nor the
Editors assume any liability for any injury and/or damage to persons or property
arising out of or related to any use of the material contained in this book.

Library of Congress Cataloging-in-Publication Data

Heimburger, Douglas C.
        Handbook of clinical nutrition / Douglas C. Heimburger, Jamy D. Ard.—4th ed.
          p. ; cm.
        ISBN 0-323-03952-9
        1. Diet therapy—Handbooks, manuals, etc. I. Heimburger, Douglas C. II. Ard, Jamy D.
III. Title.
        [DNLM: 1. Diet Therapy—Handbooks. 2. Nutrition—Handbooks. WB 39 H467h 2006]
RM217.2.H45 2006
615.8'54—dc22

                                                                        2005054010

Acquisitions Editor: Jim Merrit
Editorial Assistant: Nicole DiCicco
Project Manager: David Saltzberg

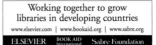

Working together to grow
libraries in developing countries
www.elsevier.com | www.bookaid.org | www.sabre.org
ELSEVIER   BOOK AID International   Sabre Foundation

Printed in the United States of America

Last digit is the print number: 9   8   7   6   5   4   3   2   1

List of Co-Authors

Jaime Aranda-Michel, MD
Division of Gastroenterology,
Hepatology, and Transplantation,
Mayo Clinic, Jacksonville, Florida

Jamy D. Ard, MD
Assistant Professor, Division of
Clinical Nutrition and Dietetics,
Departments of Nutrition
Sciences and Medicine,
University of Alabama at
Birmingham, Birmingham,
Alabama

Joseph E. Baggott, PhD
Assistant Professor of Nutrition
Sciences, University of Alabama
at Birmingham, Birmingham,
Alabama

Reinaldo Figueroa, MD
Nemours Children's Clinic
Arnold Palmer Hospital,
Orlando, Florida

Frank A. Franklin, Jr., MD, PhD
Professor, Division of Pediatric
Gastroenterology and Nutrition,
Departments of Pediatrics and
Nutrition Sciences, University of
Alabama at Birmingham,
Birmingham, Alabama

W. Timothy Garvey, MD
Professor and Chair, Department
of Nutrition Sciences, University
of Alabama at Birmingham,
Birmingham, Alabama

Douglas C. Heimburger, MD, MS
Professor, Division of Clinical
Nutrition and Dietetics,
Departments of Nutrition
Sciences and Medicine,
University of Alabama at
Birmingham, Birmingham,
Alabama

Gabriel Ionescu, MD
Fellow, Division of
Gastroenterology, Department of
Medicine, St. Luke's-Roosevelt
Hospital, Columbia University
College of Physicians and
Surgeons, New York, New York

Elizabeth M. Kitchin, MS, RD
Assistant Professor, Division of
Clinical Nutrition and Dietetics,
Department of Nutrition
Sciences, University of Alabama
at Birmingham, Birmingham,
Alabama

Donald P. Kotler, MD
Professor, Division of
Gastroenterology, Department
of Medicine, St. Luke's-Roosevelt
Hospital, Columbia University
College of Physicians and
Surgeons, New York, New York

Cristina Lara-Castro, MD, PhD
Postdoctoral Fellow, Department
of Nutrition Sciences, University
of Alabama at Birmingham,
Birmingham, Alabama

Christopher D. Lorish, PhD
Associate Professor of Education in Medicine, University of Alabama at Birmingham, Birmingham, Alabama

Jeffrey Mechanick, MD
Associate Professor and Director, Metabolic Support, Mt. Sinai School of Medicine, New York, New York

Sarah L. Morgan, MD, MS, RD
Professor and Director, Division of Clinical Nutrition and Dietetics, Departments of Nutrition Sciences and Medicine, University of Alabama at Birmingham, Birmingham, Alabama

Abdullah Mubarak, MD
Fellow, Hepatology and Liver Transplantation, Mayo Clinic, Jacksonville, Florida

Laura E. Newton, MA, RD
Instructor, Division of Clinical Nutrition and Dietetics, Department of Nutrition Sciences, University of Alabama at Birmingham, Birmingham, Alabama

Christine S. Ritchie, MD
Associate Professor, Division of Gerontology and Geriatric Medicine, Department of Medicine, University of Alabama at Birmingham, Birmingham-Atlanta VA Geriatric Research Education and Clinical Center (GRECC), Birmingham, Alabama

James M. Shikany, DrPH, PA-C
Assistant Professor, Division of Preventive Medicine, Department of Medicine, University of Alabama at Birmingham, Birmingham, Alabama

Bonnie A. Spear, PhD
Associate Professor, Department of Pediatrics, University of Alabama at Birmingham, Birmingham, Alabama

Glen Thompson, PharmD
Director, Department of Pharmacy, Cooper Green Hospital, Birmingham, Alabama

Janet D. Tisdale, MPH, RD, CDE
Senior Nutritionist, Obstetric Complications Clinic, Department of Obstetrics and Gynecology, University of Alabama at Birmingham, Birmingham, Alabama

This volume is dedicated to the memory of Roland L. Weinsier, MD, DrPH. The first edition of the *Handbook of Clinical Nutrition* was one of Roland's early contributions to national and international medical nutrition education, and he encouraged and coauthored the second and third editions. He is remembered as a humble and effective leader among nutrition scientists, educators, clinicians, and administrators, a mentor and role model to many, and a kind and generous friend. His passions and influence endure through the impact of this and other publications, the lives of the patients he helped, the research that is being carried on by the many outstanding scientists he trained and inspired, and the nationally recognized educational programs he established at the University of Alabama at Birmingham and elsewhere.

Preface

In 1977, Drs. Roland Weinsier and Charles Butterworth wrote the first version of the *Handbook of Clinical Nutrition*. That version was published locally in response to requests from medical students, residents, and dietitians for a pocket-sized nutrition manual in a ready-reference format. It came at a time when nutrition support services were just beginning to appear and little practical information or guidance was available for members of the health care team who were interested in providing nutritional support for hospitalized patients.

Subsequent editions of the *Handbook* were published in 1981, 1989, and 1997. The second edition encompassed the rapid expansion of information on nutritional support of the acutely ill patient that occurred in the 1980s. The third edition was updated to inform clinicians of the many medical-nutrition advances of the 1990s and to expand the emphasis on health promotion and preventive nutrition services. This fourth edition continues that trend, as evidence on the influence of nutrition on disease risk and health outcomes has become increasingly sophisticated and robust. All sections of the book have been updated to incorporate new concepts, references, and for the first time, online resources. This edition also contains new chapters on:

- Counseling for lifestyle change, to make implementation of dietary change practical and accessible
- Complementary and alternative nutritional therapies, to address the increasing interest of the lay public and the expanding evidence base in this area
- Metabolic syndrome, to integrate this increasingly prevalent syndrome into the context of dietary habits and nutritional interventions

We hope that once again physicians, nurses, dietitians, pharmacists, and other health care practitioners will find the *Handbook of Clinical Nutrition* valuable in strengthening their ability to provide effective health care and to prevent disease through nutritional and lifestyle interventions.

Douglas C. Heimburger, MD, MS
Jamy D. Ard, MD

Introduction

For some time the American public has shown a significant interest in the relationships between nutrition and health. The media continually fuel this interest, overwhelming consumers with books, articles, testimonials, advertisements, and infomercials proclaiming the health advantages of certain foods and diets while denouncing others as life-threatening. The Internet has become a major source of information for many and can provide sound advice, but its immunity to quality control often produces misinformation. The scientific community and media have often reversed advice previously given on health issues, prompting many persons to become either wary or cynical of medical science. Time-honored associations between what is consumed and a person's physical health, such as the association of certain foods with a stomachache or of a hearty meal with a sense of well-being, have made many individuals susceptible to questionable health claims, whereas apparent scientific inconsistencies and rising skepticism have led others to justify maintaining unhealthy habits. Some assume that an ounce of nutritional prevention must be worth more than a pound of cure, and others opine that scientists don't know what they're talking about.

Unfortunately, physicians are too often unprepared or ill-equipped to provide guidance to their patients. The stock phrase, "Before going on this or any other diet, seek the advice of your physician," is often a device to protect commercial interests rather than the public. Nevertheless, many individuals prefer to receive information about nutrition from their doctors and tend to trust the validity of their advice more than when it comes from other sources.

We live in a time during which remarkable scientific progress is being made in our understanding of nutrient requirements and the interactions between diet and health. With the development of new laboratory methods, electronic devices, computers, and radioisotopes, a person's nutritional status can be assessed more rapidly and accurately than ever before. It is also possible to meet nutritional requirements of patients for indefinite periods, even when they have lost virtually the entire gastrointestinal tract. Considerable progress is also being made in understanding nutrient metabolism in specific disease states. The role of nutrition in the etiology and management of obesity, heart disease, cancer, diabetes, and other leading causes of morbidity and death is being studied intensively. We believe that nutrition promises to be an increasingly important component of the health care armamentarium in the years ahead.

Public demand coupled with rapid advances in nutrition science and biomedical technology has increased the pressure on medical professionals to learn about and incorporate nutrition into their practices. A well-informed community of health care professionals who can perform nutritional assessments and provide effective nutritional counseling and support is needed. To be effective, these professionals must have essential information and practical references at their fingertips and at the patient's bedside in well-organized and indexed formats. This compact volume is intended to meet this need for a wide range of practitioners. It is our hope that by equipping health care professionals with the tools needed to deliver nutritional care, this book will contribute to the welfare of healthy persons and patients alike.

Contents

PART I

Nutrition for Health Maintenance

Health Promotion and Disease Prevention

JAMY D. ARD, MD

Nutrition and Disease Prevention

Nutrition plays a central role in health by virtue of the simple fact that everyone must eat as a matter of survival. The complexity arises when the choice of foods and accompanying nutrients leads to either health benefits or detrimental effects. The impact of nutrition on altering risk for disease is generally slow and only gradually evident after lengthy exposure to a given dietary pattern. However, because we all must eat, changing detrimental eating patterns to healthier patterns can have a significant impact on preventable disease risk factors for the individual and the population at large.

In the United States, many preventable deaths from problems such as heart disease and cancer occur in individuals with moderate risk. If a relatively small reduction in risk for a disease occurred in this group, there would be major benefits for the population at large. These benefits occur because of sheer volume: There are large numbers of people with moderate risk, whereas those with the highest risk make up a much smaller proportion of the population. Even making great risk reductions for this smaller high-risk group is less powerful than making small risk reductions in the larger group. For example, modifying diets to reduce coronary heart disease (CHD) in the general population is thought to be worthwhile because most deaths occur not among those at high risk due to high serum cholesterol levels, but in people who have only moderate elevations in serum cholesterol (i.e., 200 to 240 mg/dL). Therefore, from the nutrition perspective, much of disease prevention is about making small and important changes in the diets of as many people as possible.

A lower level of impact at the individual level for population-targeted nutrition interventions is to be expected because of the numerous factors that can modify the nutrition-disease risk relationship. Genetics, environment, and physical activity are all examples of factors that can modify the effect of nutrition on disease risk at the individual level. Although genetic factors can affect individual susceptibility, they appear to account for only a small part of the observed variation in disease incidence among populations, as exemplified by the tendency of immigrants to acquire the disease rates of their adoptive countries. More attention is being given to the impact of the local environment and its ability to influence dietary patterns through enhancing availability of various food sources and types. A major challenge for each individual is to consume a total energy intake that is matched to energy expenditure. Energy expenditure via leisure time physical activity is an important component of overall energy balance. As health care providers, we must consider these factors as we attempt to supplement dietary recommendations for the general population with more sophisticated, individually based dietary interventions in the attempt to achieve optimal disease risk reduction.

Trends in Diet and Disease

At the turn of the 20th century, the leading causes of death were infectious diseases, and curing them would have reduced death rates. Today, most of the leading causes of death in Western countries are strongly influenced by lifestyle, and medical resources are mainly invested in treating diseases associated with specific lifestyles. Heart disease, cancer, and stroke account for two thirds of all deaths in the United States. One third will die from CHD before age 65, and many others will be disabled by these illnesses and their complications.

Changes in eating patterns parallel these disease trends. In lieu of the high-fiber, low-fat foods once consumed as the basis of our diet, refined starches, sweets, saturated fats, and salt comprise a major share of today's typical American diet. Table 1–1 lists 8 of the top 15 causes of death in the United States that are strongly influenced by nutrition. As the table shows, five are strongly linked with dietary habits and three are associated with alcohol abuse. The table also details the many dietary contributions to obesity, atherosclerosis, osteoporosis, diverticular disease, and neural tube defects, which cause significant morbidity and indirect mortality.

Traditionally, the goal and measure of success of our health care system has been to increase life expectancy, regardless of well-being or quality of life. However, reducing morbidity—that is, improving quality of life and maximizing the period of good health—may be a more important goal. The *Dietary Guidelines for Americans 2005,*[1] on which this chapter is focused, attempts to provide evidence-based recommendations for diet and physical activity that, if adopted, may lead to achievement of a higher quality of life and optimal health.

Current Dietary Habits in the United States

Since the publication of previous *Dietary Guidelines for Americans* in 1995 and 2000, public awareness of dietary intake has increased substantially. This heightened awareness is likely fueled by a constant stream of media coverage related to the increased prevalence of obesity in the United States and our growing obsession with fad diets. The attention has also been associated with changes in nutrition labeling practices and promotion of the United States Department of Agriculture/Department of Health and Human Services (USDA/DHHS) MyPyramid, a pictorial depiction of how American diets should be structured (Fig. 1–1). Certainly, food manufacturers and producers are aware of the public's increased health consciousness and have launched promotional efforts to tout the beneficial effects of their food products.

Table 1–1	DIETARY INFLUENCES ON THE MAJOR CAUSES OF DEATH AND MORBIDITY IN THE UNITED STATES	
Cause of Death or Morbidity	Factors Associated with Decreased Risk	Factors Associated with Increased Risk
Death		
Heart diseases	Intake of complex carbohydrates, particular fatty acids (e.g., monounsaturated, polyunsaturated, and ω-3 fatty acids from fish), soluble fiber, polyphenols, soy proteins, antioxidants (vitamins E, C; β-carotene, selenium), folic acid, moderate alcohol	Intake of saturated fat, cholesterol; excess calories, sodium, abdominal distribution of body fat
Cancer	Intake of fruits and vegetables (for β-carotene, vitamins A, C, D, and E, folic acid, calcium, selenium, phytochemicals), fiber	Intake of excess calories, fat, alcohol, red meat, salt- and nitrite-preserved meats; possibly grilled meats; abdominal distribution of body fat
Cerebrovascular diseases	Intake of potassium, calcium, ω-3 fatty acids	Sodium, alcohol consumption (as with hypertension)
Accidents		Excess alcohol consumption

Diabetes mellitus	Fiber intake	Intake of excess calories, fat, alcohol; abdominal distribution of body fat
Suicide		Excess alcohol consumption
Chronic liver disease and cirrhosis		Excess alcohol consumption
Hypertension and hypertensive renal disease	Intake of fruits and vegetables, potassium, calcium, magnesium, ω-3 fatty acids	Intake of sodium, alcohol, excess calories, total and saturated fat; abdominal distribution of body fat
Morbidity		
Obesity		Intake of excess calories and fat
Osteoporosis	Intake of calcium, vitamin D, vitamin K	Intake of excess of vitamin A, sodium, protein
Diverticular disease, constipation	Fiber intake	
Neural tube defects	Folic acid intake	

Anatomy of MyPyramid

One size doesn't fit all

USDA's new MyPyramid symbolizes a personalized approach to healthy eating and physical activity. The symbol has been designed to be simple. It has been developed to remind consumers to make healthy food choices and to be active every day. The different parts of the symbol are described below.

Activity

Activity is represented by the steps and the person climbing them, as a reminder of the importance of daily physical activity.

Moderation

Moderation is represented by the narrowing of each food group from bottom to top. The wider base stands for foods with little or no solid fats or added sugars. These should be selected more often. The narrower top area stands for foods containing more added sugars and solid fats. The more active you are, the more of these foods can fit into your diet.

Personalization

Personalization is shown by the person on the steps, the slogan, and the URL. Find the kinds and amounts of food to eat each day at MyPyramid.gov.

Proportionality

Proportionality is shown by the different widths of the food group bands. The widths suggest how much food a person should choose from each group. The widths are just a general guide, not exact proportions. Check the Web site for how much is right for you.

Variety

Variety is symbolized by the 6 color bands representing the 5 food groups of the Pyramid and oils. This illustrates that foods from all groups are needed each day for good health.

Gradual Improvement

Gradual improvement is encouraged by the slogan. It suggests that individuals can benefit from taking small steps to improve their diet and lifestyle each day.

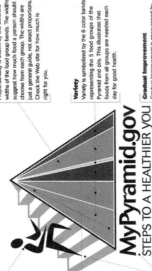

MyPyramid.gov
STEPS TO A HEALTHIER YOU

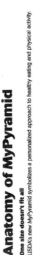

U.S. Department of Agriculture
Center for Nutrition Policy and Promotion
April 2005 CNPP-16

USDA is an equal opportunity provider and employer.

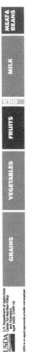

| GRAINS | VEGETABLES | FRUITS | MILK | MEAT & BEANS |

Figure 1-1. USDA/DHHS Food Guide Pyramid (www.MyPyramid.gov).

In spite of the increased awareness, numerous dietary surveys of the population reveal multiple areas for improvement in current dietary patterns. Surveys suggest that people in higher education and income brackets have been more responsive to public health recommendations. Intake of total fat has declined to 34% and 32% of calories for men and women, respectively[2] Fruit and vegetable intake is less than optimal, with a major portion of vegetable intake obtained from white potatoes, typically fried, and a significant portion of fruit intake obtained from juices and other beverages. In addition, fiber intake is less than recommended, partially because of less than optimal fruit and vegetable intake. The low fiber intake is also a result of higher than recommended consumption of refined grain products such as white bread, pasta, and rice. These products displace the higher fiber alternatives. Consumption of added sugar (sugars and syrups that are added to foods during processing or preparation or at the table) is also on the rise as sweetened beverages and desserts are more common in schools, offices, and homes. The intake of milk and dairy products has declined over time as well, particularly among children and adolescents, being replaced primarily by carbonated beverages and fruit-flavored drinks.[3] Another trend involves increased frequency of meals consumed outside the home. As time pressures increase and commercially prepared foods are more available, palatable, and affordable, the proportion of the population consuming meals away from home has grown dramatically. The odds of eating out at least one or more times per week were 40% higher from 1999 to 2000 relative to 1987.[4] The reported number of commercially prepared meals consumed per week is positively related to energy intake; persons who eat out more frequently consume higher amounts of total energy.[4] In addition, the portion sizes that are available in restaurants have increased, particularly for many entrée and dessert items.

The challenge for the panel convened to develop the newest national dietary guidelines was to move the population from this current dietary pattern to an overall eating pattern that is associated with lower disease risk and promotes optimal health.

Eating for Optimum Health

There have been at least seven reports of *Dietary Guidelines for Americans* published in recent years, and many more reports of national dietary guidelines outside of the United States. It is noteworthy that there is close agreement on the general recommendations made in these reports, which enhances their credibility. The most widely publicized guidelines are those embodied in the USDA/DHHS MyPyramid (see Fig. 1–1), a graphic that prioritizes food groups in terms of their importance to health. In 2005, MyPyramid underwent a significant change to reflect new scientific evidence related to optimal eating patterns. Many of the major messages from the new guidelines are consistent with previous versions; however, because many Americans experienced difficulty in applying previous guidelines to their daily routine while receiving apparently conflicting information on a regular basis about the types of nutrients to consume, significant effort has been invested in increasing the personalization of MyPyramid and translating the latest scientific findings into dietary guidance. Another major change was to include physical activity recommendations as a key part of MyPyramid and *Dietary Guidelines*. The complete "Key Recommendations" for the general population from the 2005 *Dietary Guidelines* are shown Box 1–1.

The nine major messages of the *Dietary Guidelines for Americans 2005* are summarized below.

Dietary Guidelines

Consume a Variety of Foods within and among the Basic Food Groups While Staying within Energy Needs

Consuming a variety of foods provides the opportunity to achieve recommended nutrient intakes. As previously mentioned, the goal of achieving recommended nutrient intakes is to prevent chronic disease, a change in focus

BOX 1–1 *Dietary Guidelines for American 2005:*
Key Recommendations for the General Population[1]

Adequate Nutrients within Calorie Needs

Consume a variety of nutrient-dense foods and beverages
within and among the basic food groups while choosing
foods that limit the intake of saturated and *trans* fats,
cholesterol, added sugars, salt and alcohol.

Meet recommended intakes within energy needs by
adopting a balanced eating pattern, such as the United
States Department of Agriculture (USDA) Food Guide or the
Dietary Approaches to Stop Hypertension (DASH)
Eating Plan.

Weight Management

To maintain body weight in a healthy range, balance calories
from and beverages with calories expended.

To prevent gradual weight gain over time, make small
decreases in food and beverage calories and increase
physical activity.

Physical Activity

Engage in regular physical activity and reduce sedentary
activities to promote health, psychological well-being, and
a healthy body weight.

- To reduce the risk of chronic disease in adulthood: Engage in
  at least 30 minutes of moderate-intensity physical activity,
  above usual activity, at work or home on most days of
  the week.
- For most people, greater health benefits can be obtained by
  engaging in physical activity of more vigorous intensity or
  longer duration.
- To help manage body weight and prevent gradual, unhealthy
  body weight gain in adulthood: Engage in approximately
  60 minutes of moderate- to vigorous-intensity activity on
  most days of the week while not exceeding caloric intake
  requirements.
- To sustain weight loss in adulthood: Participate in at least
  60 to 90 minutes of daily moderate-intensity physical activity
  while not exceeding caloric intake requirements. Some people
  may need to consult with a health care provider before
  participating in this level of activity.

Achieve physical fitness by including cardiovascular conditioning,
stretching exercises for flexibility, and resistance exercise or
calisthenics for muscle strength and endurance.

Box continued on following page

BOX 1–1 *Dietary Guidelines for American 2005:* Key Recommendations for the General Population[1] *(Continued)*

Food Groups to Encourage

Consume a sufficient amount of fruits and vegetables while staying within energy needs. Two cups of fruit and $2^1/_2$ cups of vegetables per day are recommended for a 2000-calorie intake, with higher or lower amounts depending on the calorie level.

Choose a variety of fruits and vegetables each day. In particular, select from all five vegetable subgroups (dark green, orange, legumes, starchy vegetables, and other vegetables) several times a week.

Consume 3 or more ounce-equivalents of whole grain products per day, with the rest of the recommended grains coming from enriched or whole grain products. In general, at least half the grains should come from whole grains.

Consume 3 cups per day of fat-free or low-fat milk or equivalent milk products.

Fats

Consume less than 10% of calories from saturated fatty acids and less than 300 mg/day of cholesterol, and keep *trans* fatty acid consumption as low as possible.

Keep total fat intake between 20% and 35% of calories, with most fats coming from sources of polyunsaturated and monounsaturated fatty acids, such as fish, nuts, and vegetable oils.

When selecting and preparing meat, poultry, dry beans, and milk or milk products, make choices that are lean, low-fat, or fat-free.

Limit intake of fats and oils high in saturated and/or *trans* fatty acids, and choose products low in such fats and oils.

Carbohydrates

Choose fiber-rich fruits, vegetables, and whole grains often.

Choose and prepare foods and beverages with few added sugars or caloric sweeteners, such as amounts suggested by the USDA Food Guide and the DASH Eating Plan.

Reduce the incidence of dental caries by practicing good oral hygiene and consuming sugar- and starch-containing foods and beverages less frequently.

Sodium and Potassium

Consume less than 2300 mg (approximately 1 teaspoon of salt) of sodium per day.

BOX 1–1   *Dietary Guidelines for American 2005:* Key
Recommendations for the General Population[1] *(Continued)*

Choose and prepare foods with little salt. At the same time,
consume potassium-rich foods, such as fruits and vegetables.

Alcoholic Beverages

Those who choose to drink alcoholic beverages should do so
sensibly and in moderation—defined as the consumption of
up to one drink per day for women and up to two drinks per
day for men.

Alcoholic beverages should not be consumed by some
individuals, including those who cannot restrict their alcohol
intake, women of childbearing age who may become
pregnant, pregnant and lactating women, children and
adolescents, individuals taking medications that can interact
with alcohol, and those with specific medical conditions.

Alcoholic beverages should be avoided by individuals engaging
in activities that require attention, skill, or coordination, such
as driving or operating machinery.

Food Safety

To avoid microbial foodborne illness:

* Clean hands, food contact surfaces, and fruits and vegetables.
  Meat and poultry should not be washed or rinsed.
* Separate raw, cooked, and ready-to-eat foods while
  shopping, preparing, or storing foods.
* Cook foods to a safe temperature to kill microorganisms.
* Chill (refrigerate) perishable food promptly and defrost
  foods properly.
* Avoid raw (unpasteurized) milk or any products made from
  unpasteurized milk, raw or partially cooked eggs or foods
  containing raw eggs, raw or undercooked meat and poultry,
  unpasteurized juices, and raw sprouts.

---

from the earliest guidelines that focused on preventing
deficiencies of various nutrients. The basic food groups
include fruits; vegetables; grains; milk, yogurt, and
cheese; and meat, poultry, fish, dry beans, eggs, and nuts.
The Dietary Guidelines Advisory Committee specifically
noted however, that additional efforts are still warranted
to promote higher dietary intakes of vitamin E, calcium,
magnesium, potassium, and fiber by children and adults

and higher intakes of vitamins A and C by adults. The probability of nutritional adequacy for these nutrients was less than 60% for adult men and women, and the mean intake for potassium and fiber was less than adequate in all age groups.

While achieving adequate nutrition using a variety of foods is the main thrust of this first recommendation, *Dietary Guidelines* reminds us that particular attention should be paid to maintaining an energy-balanced state by matching caloric intake to energy expenditure. Consuming a large variety of foods has been associated with higher energy intake.[5] To manage caloric intake, we are advised to limit intake of foods that have low nutritive value, such as added sugars, solid fats, and alcoholic beverages. Foods that are high in these components are typically energy-dense and have few essential nutrients that play a role in disease prevention. In addition, the strategy of substituting nutrient-rich foods for those that are nutrient-poor and calorically dense improves the nutrient profile and reduces caloric intake.

For several population subgroups, *Dietary Guidelines* delineates a few special nutrient recommendations. First, adolescent females and women of childbearing age are encouraged to increase dietary intake of iron-rich foods and maintain a folic acid intake of 400 micrograms per day. The recommendations for increased iron and folic acid intake for this group are targeted at reducing the incidence of iron deficiency and neural tube defects, respectively. Second, a substantial proportion of the population over the age of 50 has a reduced capacity to absorb vitamin B_{12} in its naturally occurring food-bound form. However, the crystalline form of vitamin B_{12} can be readily absorbed, and it is recommended that individuals over the age of 50 meet their recommended daily allowance of vitamin B_{12} by consuming foods fortified with B_{12} or by taking vitamin B_{12} supplements. Finally, the committee recommends that individuals at high risk for low levels of vitamin D, including the elderly, persons with dark skin, and persons exposed to little UVB radiation, obtain extra vitamin D from vitamin D-fortified foods and/or supplements that contain vitamin D.

Control Calorie Intake to Manage Body Weight

The management of body weight appears early in the set of major recommendations as a result of the increasing prevalence of obesity in the United States. Significant attention has been devoted to altering the proportions of carbohydrates, fats, and proteins in the diet as a way to control weight. However, the emphasis of this second recommendation is that total energy intake, from any combination of energy sources, is a primary determinant of body weight. To maintain one's body weight, energy intake must be matched with energy expenditure. To lose weight, an energy deficit must be created by either reducing caloric intake or increasing energy expenditure with physical activity, or a combination of the two.

Because a majority of the population is considered overweight (body mass index [BMI] ≥ 25 kg/m^2) and nearly one third is obese (BMI ≥ 30 kg/m^2), much of the emphasis for this recommendation is directed toward preventing further weight gain and promoting weight loss. An essential key to limiting weight gain or losing weight via calorie restriction is to reduce one's intake of added sugars, solid fats, and alcohol. As noted in the first recommendation, these items are calorically dense and provide few essential nutrients. Another key factor is to consume foods that are low in energy density, such as fruits and vegetables. Limiting portion sizes, particularly of foods that are high in energy density, is another recommended strategy for managing body weight.

Be Physically Active Every Day

The enhanced emphasis on physical activity and its relationship to diet and disease prevention and health promotion is evident by the inclusion of a figure to represent activity on MyPyramid (a person climbing steps on the side of the pyramid; see Fig. 1–1). In general, the *Dietary Guidelines* call for moderate physical activity for at least 30 minutes per day on most days of the week to promote fitness and reduce the risk of chronic health conditions such as obesity, hypertension, diabetes, and CHD. Moderate-intensity physical activity, which expends 3 to 5 metabolic equivalents or METs (1 MET involves consumption of 3.5 mL oxygen/kg/min), is achieved by walking at a brisk pace of 3 to 4 mph, bicycling on level ground, light swimming, gardening, or mowing a lawn. The same benefits may be achieved by participating in vigorous physical activity 20 minutes per day, three days of the week. Vigorous physical activity expends 6 or more METs and is achieved by jogging, running, aerobic dancing, competitive sports, heavy yard or construction work, brisk swimming, or fast bicycling. It should be emphasized, particularly to patients with differing levels of physical fitness, that the primary determinant of the impact of physical activity on health outcomes is the total volume of physical activity rather than its intensity alone. Therefore, most individuals can achieve significant health benefits using moderate physical activity, as long as its duration is sufficient.

Additional outcomes of interest include prevention of unhealthy weight gain and avoidance of weight regain following weight loss. Based on a report from the Institute of Medicine in 2002 cited in *Dietary Guidelines,* most adults need up to 60 minutes of moderate to vigorous physical activity on most days to prevent unhealthy weight gain.[6] For those who previously lost weight and are trying to avoid weight regain, the recommendation is to participate in 60 to 90 minutes of moderate physical activity daily.

Increase Daily Intake of Fruits and Vegetables, Whole Grains, and Nonfat or Low-fat Milk and Milk Products

For many Americans, the intake of the food groups in this set of recommendations is well below recommended levels. For this reason, *Dietary Guidelines* groups them together. The other rationale for grouping them together is that they form the basis of a dietary pattern that has been shown to have multiple positive effects on disease risk factors. This dietary pattern, known as Dietary Approaches to Stop Hypertension (DASH), is detailed in Chapter 19. The *Dietary Guidelines* also review evidence for the roles of each of the food groups in disease prevention and treatment.

As noted previously, fruit and vegetable intake is less than optimal in the United States, resulting in lower than desirable levels of fiber, vitamins, minerals, and phytonutrient intakes. The range of intake recommended for fruits and vegetables on a daily basis is $2\frac{1}{2}$ to $6\frac{1}{2}$ cups, depending on an individual's energy needs. The goal for persons who require 2000 calories per day to maintain their weight is to consume $4\frac{1}{2}$ cups of fruits and vegetables daily. Daily consumption should be from a variety of fruits and vegetables, ranging from citrus and other fruits to dark green leafy and bright orange vegetables. Scientific evidence demonstrates that increased consumption of fruits and vegetables is important for reducing risk for cardiovascular disease, cancer, and diabetes. Diets high in fruits and vegetables have also been associated with maintenance of body weight, successful weight loss, and long-term maintenance of weight loss.[7]

The emphasis on whole grain intake is related to two factors: (1) Whole grains are an important source of energy and 14 nutrients including fiber; (2) Inclusion of whole grains in the diet will likely displace refined grains that are less nutrient-dense. Similar to the impact of fruits and vegetables, diets high in whole grains reduce the risk of cardiovascular disease and Type 2 diabetes. Whole grain intake is also associated with successful weight control. *Dietary Guidelines* recommends daily intake of at least three 1-ounce equivalents of whole grain foods, preferably instead of refined grains.

Nonfat and low-fat milk and other milk products are key sources of calcium, magnesium, potassium, and vitamin D. The milk food group is key for achieving and maintaining peak bone mass and preventing osteoporosis. Milk and other dairy products have also been associated with lower levels of insulin resistance in several population studies. There is growing interest in the role of milk in regulating body weight and enhancing weight loss. It was the committee's opinion that the current evidence did not support a definitive effect of milk group consumption on weight loss. However, studies do show that consumption of the milk group is not associated with weight gain. The recommended level of intake is 3 cups of milk or equivalent milk products per day, preferably nonfat or low-fat products such as skim milk and yogurt.

Choose Fats Wisely for Good Health

Dietary Guidelines provides specific instruction regarding types of dietary fat and their relationships to CHD. While low fat intake (less than 20% of calories) often results in weight reduction because of low total energy intake, the combination of low fat and high carbohydrate intake, particularly from refined grain sources, can elevate serum triglycerides and depress high-density lipoprotein (HDL) cholesterol levels. On the other hand, high fat intakes of more than 35% of calories are associated with obesity and CHD because of high energy intake and increased saturated fat intake, respectively. Therefore, total fat intake between 20% and 35% of calories is recommended for all Americans 18 years and older. For children aged 2 and 3, the lower limit of fat intake is 30%, while for children aged 4 to 18, the lower limit is 25% of calories.

The primary objective for this recommendation is to reduce the risk of CHD, which involves lowering low-density lipoprotein (LDL) cholesterol. This can be achieved by keeping dietary intake of saturated fat below 10% of calories, *trans* fat below 1% of calories, and cholesterol below 300 mg per day, by limiting intake of animal fat, partially hydrogenated vegetable oils, and eggs and organ meats, respectively. In addition to these recommendations, consuming monounsaturated fatty acids (MUFA) and polyunsaturated fatty acids (PUFA) can be beneficial for CHD risk. Diets that substitute MUFA for saturated fat reduce LDL cholesterol. Fatty fishes such as salmon, tuna, and lake trout are high in PUFA (known as n-3 fatty acids), and intake of 2 servings per week of fatty fish is associated with decreased risk of sudden cardiac death. More details on dietary fats and CHD risk are provided in Chapter 20.

Choose Carbohydrates Wisely for Good Health

While fat intake has garnered much of the public's attention since the early 1980s, in recent years significant thought has been shifted toward carbohydrates. This has produced a variety of misconceptions regarding the effects of carbohydrates, resulting in a large number of people trying to avoid carbohydrates altogether. In most instances, restricting carbohydrates leads to lower energy intake, simply because of decreased food intake; however, this dietary pattern is not sustainable for most individuals. Carbohydrates, when chosen properly, are an important part of a healthful diet and serve as a key energy source for the body.

Because maintaining fiber intake is important for promoting healthy laxation and reducing the risk of Type 2 diabetes and CHD, *Dietary Guidelines* recommends that carbohydrate choices be rich in fiber. The recommended amount of dietary fiber (14 g per 1000 calories) can be achieved within the acceptable carbohydrate range of 45% to 65% of calories per day by choosing foods from the fruit, vegetable, and grain groups that are high in fiber while avoiding excessive intake of refined grains and added sugars. Whole fruits are preferred over fruit juice. Added sugars may increase the palatability of food but they add little nutrition other than energy. Prospective studies in multiple populations have shown that added sugar intake, particularly in sweetened beverages, is associated with weight gain over time. The objective of reducing added sugars is to lower total energy intake, enabling individuals to meet their nutrient requirements by using more nutrient dense foods and not exceeding the calorie level required to maintain their weight.

Choose and Prepare Foods with Little Salt

In the United States, the median daily sodium intakes for men and women aged 31 to 50 are 4300 mg and 2900 mg, respectively—well above the committee's recommendation of 2300 mg per day. *Dietary Guidelines* recommends this as the upper limit of sodium intake for the general population primarily because of the direct relationship between sodium intake and blood pressure. The use of the upper limit is intended to protect special populations that may be more sensitive to the hypertensive effects of sodium (African Americans, middle-aged and older individuals, and persons with hypertension, diabetes, or kidney disease), but may be unaware of their sensitivity. Lowering sodium intake can be difficult in a food environment where sodium is ubiquitous in food processing. In addition to limiting added salt in food preparation and at the table, useful strategies include limiting the use of prepared sauces, broths and soups, salty snack foods, and canned foods. The preference for high sodium intake is a learned behavior that individuals can modify relatively easily to increase acceptance of lower-sodium foods.

If You Drink Alcoholic Beverages, Do So in Moderation

From 1999 to 2001, 60% of the U.S. adult population reported drinking alcoholic beverages, with 95% having moderate consumption, or less than one to two drinks per day. Several studies have shown that moderate alcohol intake is associated with a lower risk of CHD (see Chapter 20). However, it is not recommended that nondrinkers start consuming alcohol to lower their risk of CHD because excessive drinking poses significant health risks that offset any potential advantages. This is particularly true for young adults because alcohol intake has not been associated with any health benefits in this age group; on the contrary, it is associated with increased risk of traumatic injury and death. It should be clear that abstention is an important option for all individuals, particularly for those who have difficulty restricting their drinking to moderate levels, individuals with specific medical conditions, women who may become pregnant or who are pregnant, and women who are breastfeeding.

Keep Food Safe to Eat

Foodborne illnesses are responsible for a number of hospitalizations and deaths each year in the United States. *Salmonella*, *Listeria*, and *Toxoplasma* are responsible for more than 75% of the 5000 annual deaths related to foodborne diseases. These illnesses can be prevented with the use of proper food safety techniques. Basic food safety recommendations include: (1) cleaning hands, contact surfaces, and fruits and vegetables; (2) separating raw, cooked, and ready-to-eat foods during food preparation and storage; (3) cooking foods to a safe temperature; (4) refrigerating perishable foods properly; and (5) avoiding higher-risk foods, particularly for the very young, pregnant women, the elderly, and immunocompromised persons.

Summary of the Dietary Guidelines

Experimental data and lessons derived from populations with low rates of chronic diseases, such as atherosclerosis, obesity, diabetes, and cancer, point strongly to several common dietary factors that should form the foundation for our daily eating patterns. As compiled in the *Dietary Guidelines for Americans 2005,* fruits, vegetables, and whole grains constitute the basis of a healthful diet; reduced-fat milk and milk products are also key components. Maintaining adequate intakes of these food groups will ensure high levels of key nutrients such as fiber, vitamins C, A, and E, potassium, magnesium, and calcium. Other foods should be added with the goal of limiting chronic disease risk (primary prevention) or treating known risk factors and disease (secondary prevention). Therefore, choices for dietary fats should emphasize MUFA and PUFA while limiting intake of saturated and *trans* fatty acids and cholesterol. Limiting added sugars helps to avoid weight gain from excessive calories and reduces risk for Type 2 diabetes. Matching energy expenditure to energy intake is a key factor in modifying disease risk and should be the final consideration in the dietary pattern. Maintaining a physically active lifestyle, at work and at leisure, has an independent health benefit in addition to assisting with weight management.

While *Dietary Guidelines for Americans 2005* provides recommendations for general health promotion and disease prevention, it is helpful to understand the relationship between these guidelines and others that

Table 1–2	DIETARY GUIDELINES PROMULGATED BY NATIONAL ORGANIZATION*

	Organization				
	United States Department of Agriculture and Department of Health and Human Services *Dietary Guidelines for Americans 2005*	**National Cholesterol Education Panel ATP III Therapeutic Lifestyle Change (TLC) Diet (2002)**	**National High Blood Pressure Education Program/ Joint National Committee 7 Dietary Approaches to Stop Hypertension (DASH, 2003)**	**American Diabetes Association (2004)**	**American Cancer Society (2002)**
Indication or objective	General health promotion and disease prevention	Elevated cholesterol/heart disease prevention	Pre-hypertension and hypertension	Diabetes	Cancer prevention
Nutrient/Food Group					
Total energy	Adequate energy intake to maintain a healthy weight		Reduce energy intake to lose weight if overweight	Reduced energy intake and modest weight loss can improve glycemia and insulin resistance	Choose foods that help maintain a healthful weight
Fruits/ Vegetables	2 cups of fruit and 2½ cups of		8-10 servings per day		≥5 servings per day

vegetables per 2003 calories per day

Meat		2 servings or less per day; limit red meat intake	Limit consumption of red meats, especially those high in fat and processed
Dairy	2–3 servings per day of low-fat dairy	2–3 servings per day of low-fat dairy	
Grains	3 or more ounce-equivalents of whole grain products	7–8 servings of whole grains and whole grains products	Choose whole grains in preference to refined grains
Fat	20%–35% of daily energy intake	Less than 27% of daily energy intake	
Saturated fats	Less than 10% of daily energy intake	Less than 7% of daily energy intake	Less than 10% of daily energy intake; those with LDL cholesterol ≥100 may benefit from lowering saturated fat to <7%.

Table continued on following page

Table 1-2 DIETARY GUIDELINES PROMULGATED BY NATIONAL ORGANIZATION* (Continued)

Polyunsaturated fats	Up to 10% of daily energy intake	Up to 10% of daily energy intake	Up to 10% of daily energy intake	Up to 10% of daily energy intake
Monounsaturated fats	10%–20% of daily energy intake	Up to 20% of daily energy intake	Up to 20% of daily energy intake	15%–20% of daily energy intake; combination of MUFA and carbohydrates should equal to 60%–70% of total energy intake
Trans fats	Less than 1% of daily energy intake	Intake should be kept low		Intake should be minimized
Cholesterol	Less than 300 mg per day	Less than 200 mg per day	150 mg per day	Less than 300 mg per day; those with LDL cholesterol ≥100 may benefit from lowering cholesterol intake to 200 mg per day
Carbohydrates	45%–65% of daily energy intake	50%–60% of daily energy intake	55% of daily energy intake	Total amount of carbohydrate is more important than the source or type
Sugar	Limit added sugars			Sucrose and sucrose-containing foods

Protein	Approximately 15% of daily energy intake	18% of daily energy intake	do not need to be restricted 10%–20% if renal function is normal	
Alcohol	Up to 2 drinks per day for men and up to 1 drink per day for women; persons in special circumstances (e.g., pregnancy, history of alcoholism) should abstain	Less than 2 drinks per day for men and less than 1 drink per day for women	If individuals choose to drink, limit to 2 drinks per day for men and 1 drink per day for women	For people who drink, limit to 2 drinks per day for men and 1 drink per day for women
Sodium	Up to 2300 mg per day	Less than 2400 mg per day	Less than 2400 mg per day	
Potassium		4700 mg per day		
Calcium		1200 mg per day	1000–1500 mg per day	
Magnesium		500 mg per day		

*For further detail, refer to the Web sites listed in this chapter and the contents of the respective disease-specific chapters.
LDL, low-density lipoprotein; MUFA, monounsaturated fatty acids.

are recommended by various national health organizations. Summaries of the key features of dietary guidelines promulgated by national organizations for preventing and/or managing major chronic diseases are shown in Table 1-2. There is significant convergence among the various guidelines, and there are no significant conflicts or discrepancies. Each disease indication, however, may require specific attention to particular aspects of the respective diet to target isolated risk factors or metabolic pathways.

Application

It is the responsibility of health care providers to take population-based science and apply it to a variety of individuals, each with a different set of characteristics and circumstances. Nowhere is this more true than in nutrition. Assessment of individual disease risk and dietary intake is the starting point for tailoring dietary advice based on recommended guidelines. Because much of nutrition is related to behavior (food preparation, food choices, physical activity, etc.), simply understanding and imparting the facts of nutrition may lead to less than optimal implementation. The keys to reaching individuals at moderate risk for chronic disease are related to understanding their perspectives on disease risk and providing clear, consistent health messages that are supported by the guidelines. The *Handbook of Clinical Nutrition* attempts to provide some of the basic nutrition knowledge and skills to enable health practitioners to be successful at promoting health and preventing and treating diseases.

REFERENCES

1. U.S. DHSS/USDA: Dietary Guidelines for Americans 2005. Washington, DC, G.P.O., 2005; available at http://www.healthierus.gov/dietaryguidelines/.
2. Thompson FE, Midthune D, Subar AF, et al: Dietary intake estimates in the National Health Interview Survey, 2000: Methodology, results, and interpretation. J Am Diet Assoc 105:352–363, quiz 487, 2005.
3. Cavadini C, Siega-Riz AM, Popkin BM, et al: US adolescent food intake trends from 1965 to 1996. Arch Dis Child 83:18–24, 2000.

4. Kant AK, Graubard BI: Eating out in America, 1987–2000: Trends and nutritional correlates. Prev Med 38:243–249, 2004.
5. McCrory MA, Fuss PJ, McCallum JE, et al: Dietary variety within food groups: Association with energy intake and body fatness in men and women. Am J Clin Nutr 69:440–447, 1999.
6. Food and Nutrition Board, Institute of Medicine: Dietary Reference Intakes for Energy, Carbohydrate, Fiber, Fat, Fatty Acids, Cholesterol, Protein, and Amino Acids (Macronutrients). Washington, DC, Institute of Medicine, National Academy Press, 2002; available at www.nap.edu/books/0309085373/html/index.html.
7. Rolls BJ, Ello-Martin JA, Tohill BC, et al: What can intervention studies tell us about the relationship between fruit and vegetable consumption and weight management? Nutr Rev 62:1–17, 2004.

WEB SITES

American Cancer Society, http://www.cancer.org
American College of Sports Medicine, http://www.acsm.org/
American Diabetes Association, http://www.diabetes.org
American Heart Association, http://www.americanheart.org
National Cholesterol Education Program, http://www.nhlbi.nih.gov/about/ncep/index.htm
National High Blood Pressure Education Program, http://www.nhlbi.nih.gov/ guidelines/hypertension/
Nutrition Data.com, http://www.nutritiondata.com
U.S. DHSS/USDA *Dietary Guidelines for Americans 2005*, http://www.healthierus.gov/dietaryguidelines/ (will be revised in 2010)
U.S. DHSS/USDA MyPyramid, www.MyPyramid.gov

2

Counseling for Lifestyle Change

FRANK A. FRANKLIN, JR., MD •
CHRISTOPHER D. LORISH, PhD

This chapter presents ideas and a practical strategy for working effectively with patients who put themselves at risk for serious health problems by making poor lifestyle choices, such as consuming too many calories, practicing adverse dietary patterns, not exercising, smoking, and abusing alcohol or drugs.

Many patients come to the physician with complaints often associated with their lifestyle choices that put them at greater risk for preventable mortality or more serious medical conditions. Clinicians have the challenge of intervening effectively with these patients. Remaining silent about the patient's behavior until treatable symptoms occur only enables the patient's detrimental behavior through tacit approval. Other choices are available. Physicians can refer the patient to a local psychologist or dietitian or community weight/alcohol/tobacco management program. When referral is not an option, it is incumbent upon the physician and office staff to provide adequate behavior change counseling.

Through its *Put Prevention into Practice* program, the federal Agency for Healthcare Research and Quality seeks to assist health care practitioners in delivering appropriate clinical preventive services.[1] *Put Prevention into Practice* outlines steps to create an office-based system for delivering preventive services. Many practical tools for creating forms and other documents are included to minimize the burden on clinicians and office staff. While this office system approach to prevention provides useful tools, it does not completely address how physicians and office staff can successfully discuss prevention issues such as dietary habits and activity with patients during office visits. A helpful and widely used framework, the "5A's" protocol, is discussed below. There are at least three necessary, though not sufficient, conditions that should be present to promote change in the patient's unhealthy behavior.

Necessary Conditions for Productive Behavioral Counseling

Knowledge

For an unhealthy habit to change, the burden of being informed lies both with the clinician and the patient. Clinicians must know about the mechanisms of and treatments for poor lifestyle habits, as well as available community resources for addressing problems, such as abuse of tobacco, illicit drugs, or alcohol. They must also be ready with practical solutions to common barriers patients face when attempting changes. Texts and journals are sources for proven treatments, while listening to patients may be the source of understanding the common barriers to and facilitators of change. More importantly, to be both time efficient and effective, clinicians need to know and understand an approach to discussing these topics, such as the 5A's. Studies indicate that one commonly used method—telling a patient to change an unhealthy habit in a clear, succinct, and strong way—results in less than 10% of smokers quitting, a rate that many clinicians may find too low to sustain their efforts.

Patients' knowledge deficits need to be addressed if they are to implement and maintain behavior change, and focused teaching by clinic staff at each visit keeps the learning manageable. If patients are expected to change using clinically proven approaches, they need to be given a sufficiently detailed plan. In addition, it is useful to inform patients about the short- and long-term health consequences that are more likely if their behavior does not change. This approach might also motivate patients if they can be assisted in verbalizing how any health or psychosocial consequences might negatively affect valued aspects of their lives such as work, family, religious beliefs, leisure, finances, or appearance.

Motivation

Patients must decide to refrain from unhealthy behaviors and adopt healthier ones. The clinician's goal is to try to influence a patient's choices before serious medical consequences ensue. Just informing patients about health risks, while necessary, is usually not sufficient for a decision to change. The risks are easily minimized by a variety of rationalizations. Table 2–1 summarizes a different strategy for promoting the patient's decision to change.

Patients who are not thinking about changing are precontemplative. They can be encouraged to become contemplative, the next stage before making a decision, by thinking about important consequences of their behavior. If the patient responds "yes" or "maybe" to a question about readiness, the clinician can conclude that the patient is at least thinking about change for some reason yet to be revealed. Discussing important consequences with the patient next may cause him or her to decide to change during that office visit. If that occurs, a beginning plan for changing the unhealthy habit can be made. If not, the adverse behavior can be discussed with the patient at a later visit.

Motivational reflection is the technique used to promote the patient's decision to change. The strategy is to help the patient identify—likely over several visits—all the important present and future consequences of changing or continuing the habit. To apply this strategy successfully, the patient must feel that the clinician genuinely cares about them, has a sincere interest in understanding their perspective, and is "on their side." The clinician's success criterion for such a discussion is to have the patient leave the office thinking more deeply about the important things at stake. Table 2–2 shows how a physician might initiate and follow up on this motivational reflection process.

Table 2-1	ADDRESSING THE PATIENT'S MOTIVATION	
Task	Method	Purpose
1. Determine the patient's readiness to change.	Ask "Have you thought about losing weight in the last month?"	If the patient is not thinking about changing, he is not ready for a solution. Go to 2.
2. Facilitate the patient's understanding of important consequences of changing and not changing. Use the Motivational Reflection technique.	Ask, "Can you think how losing weight might improve your appearance, finances, relationships, ability to work and do fun stuff?"	You are helping the patient identify the things in her life important enough to cause a decision to change.
3. Give a strong, clear message that you believe the patient needs to change.	Say, "For all the reasons you just told me, as your doctor I encourage you strongly to change."	In addition to the intrinsic motivation developed in 2, you are using your social influence to encourage a change.

Table 2–2	PROMOTING THE DECISION TO CHANGE
More Helpful	**Ask the patient to identify positive consequences** that would occur if the adverse behavior is changed (specifically related to work, family and leisure activities, finances, appearance, health, religion).
	Ask the patient to identify important negative consequences if the adverse behavior continues.
	Ask the patient what good things would result if each positive consequence occurred.
Less Helpful	**Assume the patient will not change and remain silent.**
	Tell the patient the reasons he or she has to change.
	Try to frighten the patient into changing by discussing only the worst outcomes.

Even people who make changes find that maintaining them is challenging. In addition to addressing barriers, two other support mechanisms are useful. First, the clinician should attempt to involve the patient in a community weight, tobacco, or alcohol control program that will provide information, encouragement, and accountability. The clinician should also monitor the patient's progress and provide encouragement, praise, and accountability at follow-up visits. Using a patient log of adherence to the plan and follow-up visits or telephone calls from office staff to discuss the patient's problems and progress indicate both that the clinician is interested in the patient's success and holds the patient accountable to following the plan.

Addressing Barriers to Change

Even motivated, informed patients encounter barriers to starting or continuing plans to change their dietary habits and activity patterns. When this occurs, two common barriers need to be explored. First, there may be one or more powerful antecedent conditions that provoke the unhealthy behaviors and for which the patient sees no alternatives. For example, patients often eat, drink, and smoke to self-medicate for negative feelings such as stress, boredom, anxiety, and depression. A long-distance truck driver may eat or smoke in response to boredom or fatigue from driving. If the patient has no alternative plan to deal with those feelings, the unhealthy behavior will continue until a plan for coping differently is developed and practiced. Asking what is the "worst thing" or "worst fear" about changing often allows patients to verbalize what keeps them stuck.

The second barrier is that some physical, social, financial, emotional, environmental, or time problem prevents or decreases the patient's ability to carry out the plan. For example, a patient commits to a modest walking program but does not start because the weather is too hot, he or she lacks comfortable shoes or feels embarrassed. Making a point to ask about and assist patients in developing their own solutions for these barriers should increase their chances of successfully making changes and preventing relapses.

Enabling Conditions for Successful Appointments

Responding to Patient Resistance

Whether or not a patient asks for help, advice giving characterizes most patient-physician appointments. Recognizing the patient's ambivalence about behavior change is critical to minimizing resistance. When the physician initiates a discussion of an unhealthy lifestyle behavior, the patient may respond with verbal and/or nonverbal resistance to discussing the issue. The clinician's response to the patient's resistance influences whether the rest of the visit moves the patient closer to deciding to change.

Resistance (i.e., a negative judgment made by the patient about discussing an issue like weight control) manifests itself in a variety of behaviors (e.g., patient silence, eyes shifting down or away, "yes, but" excuses, or quickly made insincere and nonspecific promises to do something about the behavior). If the clinician ignores these resistance signals and tells the patient what to do, the patient is commonly less interested in discussing the topic at future visits, and the clinician may give up the power struggle by becoming silent about the issue.

To respond more effectively to a patient's resistance, it is useful to understand its sources. Resistance is often the result of guilt about the behavior, perceived lack of autonomy, a sense of hopelessness about the ability to change the behavior, or the perception that the physician will preach, nag, or exhort the patient to do something he or she is not ready to do. Resistance is reduced when the patient feels in control of the decision making. Table 2–3 lists helpful responses to patient resistance.

Patient-Centered vs. Physician-Centered Counseling

The adoption of a patient-centered approach requires working with the patient as a partner in solving a problem rather than diagnosing and telling the patient what to do. Clinicians can be more patient-centered by adopting a

Table 2–3	RESPONSES TO PATIENT RESISTANCE
More Helpful	**Acknowledge** that you sense the patient's reluctance to discuss the topic.
	Reassure the patient that you will not nag, preach, judge, or tell him or her what to do.
	Ask permission to discuss the topic, after acknowledging and reassuring. If the answer is "no," do not proceed.
	If a tentative "yes" is given, proceed and avoid preaching, judging, or telling the patient what to do.
	Keep the patient in control of the decision making by asking permission and offering options.
	End the conversation at any time if resistance increases.
Less Helpful	**Don't notice,** ignore, or exert pressure to overcome the patient's resistance.
	Tell the patient what habit has to be changed.
	Give specific instructions about how to change a harmful behavior without assessing the behavior or soliciting the patient's ideas.

position of genuine curiosity about the patient's readiness to change, about what would motivate the patient to change, and about what the patient knows about how to change. Patient-centered interactions use targeted questions in each of those areas, careful listening to the patient's responses, and negotiation of a plan if the patient is ready. This patient-physician interaction that addresses the patient's needs and individually tailors the information to the patient is more satisfying to both, is more effective, and eliminates the rote and routine that promotes physician burn-out. Awareness of the necessary and enabling conditions for change allows the clinician to enter into a more effective exchange with the patient. The 5A's protocol is a useful approach that addresses these conditions.

The 5A's Brief Behavioral Counseling Protocol

While parts of the 5A's protocol can be completed in 90 seconds or less, the longest version—taking approximately 15 minutes—will be developed here with suggestions of how to use different components. The concepts implicit in the protocol can be useful both for working with patients on initially changing unhealthy habits and for addressing poor adherence to established treatments. The features of the 5A's are outlined by the U.S. Public Health Service in the context of smoking cessation;[2] examples of 5A's counseling are available on the Internet.[3] Table 2–4 summarizes the protocol. A shorter version of the 5A's involves asking the patient if he is ready to make a change, probing motivating consequences, and negotiating a beginning plan if ready.

To provide a context for the application of the 5A's listed below, assume that Mr. Smith, a 42-year-old male who has been your patient for the last 10 years, comes to your office complaining of right shoulder pain. You have noted his steady weight gain over the 10 years but have not addressed it and he has seemed unconcerned. You note that he appears even heavier and smells of tobacco. Mr. Smith mentions neither his weight nor smoking to you. You first address his complaint, and then you address his weight.

Table 2–4	THE 5A'S BRIEF BEHAVIORAL COUNSELING PROTOCOL FOR DIET AND PHYSICAL ACTIVITY*
5A's Step	**Counseling Script**
1. Address issue	Mr/Ms. _____, I would like to discuss your _____ with you today. Would that be ok?
2. Assess and Motivate	*Recent attempts* Have you tried to _____ in the past 3 months? **If "yes," ask:** What did you do? What problems did you have? What did you do that was successful? Why did you stop? *Readiness to change* Have you thought about trying to _____ in the last month? **If "no," do motivation and exit.** *Motivation to change* Mr/Ms. _____, what activity now, or in the future, would you miss if you were to become ill? What is the worst thing about missing that? What other activities would you hate to miss? What is the worst thing about missing them? What good things (relationships, work, leisure and other activities) might happen in your life if you change your _____?
3. Advise	As your physician, it is important that you _____ for all the reasons you just told me and for other important medical reasons.
4. Assist	What high-fat, fried, sugary foods could you eat less of tomorrow? Ask only if answer is "yes" to Readiness to Change question. **Negotiate goal(s) and specifics—how much, how often, what size, etc.,** to achieve goal. **Educate briefly** about recommended behavior change (e.g., diet, exercise, smoking cessation) or health risks. **Request** patient to keep a log for review at next session. **Assess barriers:** What could keep you from starting this program and continuing until our next visit?
5. Arrange follow-up	I will see you in _____ weeks to see how you are progressing.

*Support provided by the UAB Nutrition Academic Award, Frank Franklin MD, PhD, Principal Investigator.

Step 1—Address the Issue

Purpose: Shift the patient's attention to a behavioral issue and address any resistance the patient shows to discussing the issue.

Method: To accomplish this dual purpose, ask the patient's permission to discuss the topic, acknowledge any discomfort the patient shows about discussing the topic, reassure the patient that you will not lecture or tell him what to do, and, finally, ask permission again to discuss the issue if the initial response involved resistance in order to keep the patient in control of the decision making.

Say something like the following: "I would like to talk to you about your weight. I really think it is important to your health. Could we spend a few minutes doing that?"

Additional Points: If the response is "no," end the discussion. If it is a tentative "yes," avoid preaching, being judgmental, invoking guilt, or telling the patient what to do when the patient is not receptive.

Step 2—Assess and Motivate

Task 1—Recent Prior Attempts

Purpose: Information about whether and how the patient has recently tried to change is useful during plan negotiation—to avoid methods that have not worked, refine ones that have, identify areas of patient confusion or ignorance about changing, and note whether the patient feels demoralized about changing. This is often the place in the discussion where you ask the patient to give a history of typical foods and quantities consumed during the day and where the foods are eaten.

Method: Say something like: "Have you tried to change *your diet* in the last 3 months?" If "yes," ask, "What did you do? Are you still doing it? How well is it working? Why did you stop, if you have?" Then, ask about the patient's typical diet by asking something like, "What is the first thing you ate yesterday and how much? What is the next thing and how much?" Repeat until an entire 24-hour period is covered.

Additional Points: If time is short, you could omit Task 1; it is possible to negotiate a plan in Step 4 without having this information. A risk in omitting Task 1 is that you may encourage the patient to change using a method that he has already tried without success.

Task 2—Assess Readiness to Change

Purpose: The answer to the first question in Table 2–1 determines the task on which you will spend the rest of your time. A "no" answer indicates that the patient is probably not actively thinking about his behavior as a problem that requires change. Your time is best spent facilitating the patient's decision to change by inquiring about important consequences. A "yes" response probably indicates that the patient believes he has a problem behavior that may need changing but is not yet committed to doing anything. With this type of patient, you have a good chance of negotiating an initial plan for behavior change, but only if you are able to move the patient from thinking about the problem to action.

Method: Say something like, "I am curious, Mr. Smith, have you thought about changing your diet or activity to lose weight in the last (30 days/next 30 days/now)?"

Additional Points: A briefer version of the 5A's protocol could begin with this question if you have data on the patient's BMI, smoking status, or alcohol use. It is important to include the time frame to determine whether the patient is thinking about changing now.

Task 3—Influence the Decision to Change

Purpose: By asking the patient to discuss current and future important consequences, you are helping him determine whether the consequences of his current behavior are more important than potential consequences of altering the behavior. If the patient has verbalized what is at stake and still is reluctant to change, he is likely being influenced by powerful positive physical, emotional, or social reasons for engaging in the habit that would need to be identified and alternatives found.

Method: In addition to the phrasing in Table 2-4, you can say something like, "I would like us to think a bit about some consequences for a minute. I am curious. Can you think what good (or bad) things might happen to your health, your relationships, your job, your leisure activities, finances, appearance, religious beliefs (cueing with these general areas will promote a response) now and in the future if you do or do not reduce your weight?" To promote more thinking about what would happen, follow up with something like, "What would be the best thing about that?" or "What would that mean?" or "If that happened, what good would come from it?" The more consequences Mr. Smith thinks about in this visit, the greater the likelihood he will decide to change, allowing you to negotiate a plan.

Additional Points: If you only have 2 minutes to spend with a patient to discuss a harmful habit, this motivational reflection will be the most powerful thing you can do to influence the patient to make a decision to change sooner rather than later. You are working—likely over many visits—to help the patient make the decision to change sooner rather than later.

Step 3—Advising the Patient

Purpose: In this step, you attempt to affect the patient's decision to change by using whatever social influence you have developed by giving a clear, strong, succinct message about what you think the patient should do. Your message will have more effect if it is said with genuine concern and conviction.

Method: You can say something like, "As your physician, for all the reasons you have told me and for some important health reasons we may talk about, it is important for you to *lose weight*... (silence). Could we talk about how you could improve your diet or activity to do that?" If the patient is precontemplative, finish with "I sense that you are not ready to do anything now, but when you are, I am ready to help you." Then, educate briefly about a health consequence or treatment option. If the patient is contemplative, ask whether the patient is ready to discuss options for changing the habit.

Additional Points: In some very brief versions of the 5A's, the advice statement comes first, followed by the readiness to change question and negotiating a plan if the patient is ready.

Step 4—Assist the Patient

Task 1—Negotiate a Plan

Purpose: Get the patient to initiate behavior change by negotiating as many dietary and activity changes as he is willing to make. Because the patient is most likely to adhere to behavior changes he suggests, this is accomplished by asking him what he is willing to change. To carry out this strategy, ask the patient about unhealthy foods that could be avoided, healthy foods that could be added, or types of physical activity that could be increased. If the patient does not know what to do, then suggest some small, simple changes and ask which ones the patient is willing to try and implement permanently. Deciding among options keeps the patient in control of the decision making and reduces resistance. It is useful to teach the patient simple principles of managing energy intake and increasing physical activity to create negative energy balance, and of promoting increased intake of healthy foods such as fruits and vegetables. During future visits, address barriers or problems the patient encountered in starting or following the plan and negotiate additional changes, moving gradually to a plan, possibly with explicit goals, that reflects a more optimal pattern of diet and activity.

Method: Say something like, "I am curious. What food or foods would you be willing to give up or even eat less of—especially high-fat, fried, or sugary foods (cues the patient to think of the problematic foods)—to help you lose weight?" Try to negotiate a bit more by educating about the weight-loss process—decreased calories and increased activity—and ask something like, "Is there any activity you would be willing to do more of—like walking—to help you burn more calories and lose weight faster?" Keep asking the patient if there is any other food or activity until he indicates there are no more. Be sure to negotiate the plan details—what, how often, how much—and write them down for the patient as both a reminder and as his "contract" with you.

Task 2—Identify and Address Barriers

Purpose: Physical, economic, social, environmental, or psychological barriers can cause even well-intentioned patients to fall short of their goals for behavior change. It is likely that these barriers are real threats and not resistance-caused excuses. The strategy is to ask the patient to identify what barriers would cause him not to start the plan. If the patient identifies a barrier, before offering your advice, ask whether he has a solution, thereby fostering his problem-solving capability. If there are no good solutions, you may have to change the plan or delay it. Barriers that arise later can be addressed at a follow-up visit.

Method: After negotiating a plan, ask if there are any barriers or reasons that the plan could not start the next day or week and what problems the patient anticipates in following the plan once it is started. You can say something like, "Can you think of anything that would keep you from starting this plan tomorrow or continuing it once you started?" Because the clinician does not likely have enough time to address more than one barrier or to schedule frequent visits, it is worthwhile to encourage the patient to participate in community support programs that may be important to the patient's success. Finally, ask the patient to complete an activity log of the negotiated plan. The log for diet and activity is simply checking off that they have done what they agreed with you to do on the days they agreed, or recording dietary intake and physical activity. Research indicates that persons who use logs are more successful in following their plans, probably because logs serve as both a reminder and an accountability mechanism. To enhance patient accountability and relapse prevention, remind the patient that the dietary and activity log will be reviewed at the next visit to identify solutions to any of the patient's problems.

Step 5—Arrange Follow-up

Purpose: In addition to following up on the medical problem, the return visit serves as an accountability mechanism that provides time to review the log form and a means to negotiate more changes and solve problems the patient had following the initial plan. Follow-up also reinforces to the patient a serious commitment by the physician to assist with these difficult changes. If no plan was negotiated and only consequences were discussed, do not underestimate the power of motivational reflection to influence the patient's thinking and move him closer to a decision to change.

Harmful habits can be changed, but patients may relapse to their bad habits. Because there is no intervention that ensures that a patient's new habits will be sustained, it is useful to think of these problems as chronic conditions that will need continuous monitoring and intervention. The best practice is to remain persistent, positive, and patient-centered while addressing the patient's knowledge deficits, motivations, barriers, and resistance. The 5A's protocol provides a method for systematically addressing each issue.

REFERENCES AND WEBSITES

1. Agency for Healthcare Research and Quality: Put Prevention into Practice. Rockville, Md, U.S. DHSS; http://www.ahrq.gov/clinic/ppipix.htm.

2. Pi-Sunyer F, Becker D, Bouchard D, et al.: Treating Tobacco Use and Dependence—Clinician's Packet. A How-To Guide for Implementing the Public Health Service Clinical Practice Guideline. U.S. DHSS; http://www.surgeongeneral.gov/tobacco/clinpack.html.
3. Fiore M, Bailey W, Cohen S, et al.: Diet and Activity Counseling: A Contemplative Patient. University of Alabama School of Medicine; http://strweb.lhl.uab.edu/PRG016/Module01/Unit02/.

SUGGESTED READING

Rollnick S, Mason P, Butler C: Health Behavior Change: A Guide for Practitioners. Edinburgh, Churchill Livingstone, 2000.

3

Nutrients: Metabolism, Requirements, and Sources

DOUGLAS C. HEIMBURGER, MD

The current U.S. and Canadian guidelines for desirable intakes of macronutrients and micronutrients were developed by the Food and Nutrition Board, Institute of Medicine, who published Dietary Reference Intakes (DRIs) in a series of volumes beginning in 1997.[1-6] Like the 1989 report on Recommended Dietary Allowances (RDAs), the DRIs are reference values that apply to the healthy general population. Unlike earlier reports that included only RDAs, the DRIs also contain Estimated Average Requirements (EARs), Adequate Intakes (AIs), and Tolerable Upper Intake Levels (ULs). The EAR is the nutrient intake estimated to meet the requirement as defined by a specific indicator in 50% of individuals. The EAR serves as a basis for establishing an RDA for the nutrient if sufficient data exist to set it at two standard deviations above the EAR. This makes the RDA the estimated daily nutrient intake sufficient to meet the requirements of 97% to 98% of individuals. The AI is nutrient intake that appears to sustain a defined nutritional state; it exceeds the EAR, and in some cases the RDA, for the nutrient. The UL is the maximum level of intake that is unlikely to incur a risk of adverse health effects; it is established when sufficient data are available.

Whereas previous versions of the RDAs focused on dietary intakes required to prevent deficiencies, the DRI volumes recommend levels of intake that not only prevent deficiencies but may also promote long-term health and disease prevention. The expansion in focus from deficiency prevention to health promotion and

44

disease prevention is based on substantial evidence related to nutritional risks for heart disease, cancer, obesity, osteoporosis, congenital neural tube defects, and other conditions. This broadened scope is most relevant for antioxidant nutrients, energy, lipids, cholesterol, dietary fiber, calcium, and folate. For example, as the prevalence of obesity has increased, more specific recommendations for energy intake are required. The DRIs for energy are expressed as Estimated Energy Requirements (EERs) and are derived using formulas specific to various categories of weight, height, age, gender, and physical activity level with a view toward achieving and maintaining appropriate body weights (Box 3–1).

BOX 3–1   Estimated Energy Requirements (EER) for Adults*

Men 19 years and older
EER = 662−9.53 × Age [y] + PA (15.91 × Weight [kg] + 539.6 Height [m])
Women 19 years and older
EER = 354−6.91 × Age [y] + PA (9.36 × Weight [kg] + 726 × Height [m])
Where PA is a physical activity coefficient based on physical activity level (PAL), and PAL is the ratio of total energy expenditure (TEE) divided by basal energy expenditure (BEE) over 24 hours.
PA = 1.00 if PAL is estimated to be ≥1.0 and <1.4 (Sedentary)
PA = 1.11 if PAL is estimated to be ≥1.4 and <1.6 (Low Active)
PA = 1.25 if PAL is estimated to be ≥1.6 and <1.9 (Active)
PA = 1.48 if PAL is estimated to be ≥1.9 and <2.5 (Very Active)

---

*For additional information on EER and its components, including equations for children, see Chapter 5 of Source 5.
From Food and Nutrition Board, Institute of Medicine: Dietary Reference Intakes for Energy, Carbohydrate, Fiber, Fat, Fatty Acids, Cholesterol, Protein, and Amino Acids (Macronutrients). Washington, DC, Institute of Medicine, National Academy Press, 2002.

This chapter contains basic information about nutri-ents, in tabular form. The tables are far from exhaustive, but provide a quick reference to important facts about each of the major nutrients. Information on human nutrient requirements and food sources from the DRIs is provided in Tables 3–1 through 3–5. The tables detail the functions, body stores, deficiencies, associated signs and symptoms, treatment indications, and potential toxicities of the nutrients.

The reader should consult the References and Suggested Readings at the end of the chapter or the National Academy Press DRI website (http://www.nap.edu/) for additional information.

Table 3–6 details the functions, body stores, deficien-cies, associated signs and symptoms, treatment indica-tions, and potential toxicities of the nutrients.

Vitamin Supplements

With billions of dollars being spent annually on vitamin and mineral supplements in the United States, their appropriate use is an important issue. Reasons cited for supplement use include health enhancement, disease prevention, prophylaxis against the stresses of daily living, restoration of vigor and energy, and prevention or cure of a variety of conditions ranging from the common cold and premenstrual syndrome to arthritis, depression, and cancer. Many of these reasons for using supplements are unfounded. While vitamin deficiencies cause a variety of signs and symptoms (Table 3–5), it does not follow that vitamin deficiency is a frequent cause of those symptoms in the United States, or that nutrient supplements will improve those symptoms when they result from other causes.

Vitamin Toxicities

Most vitamins act as cofactors in biochemical reactions and are required in minute quantities supplied by a varied diet. When dose levels far exceed the body's

Text continued on p. 115.

Table 3-1 DIETARY REFERENCE INTAKES: ELECTROLYTES AND WATER

Nutrient	Function	Life Stage Group	AI	UL	Selected Food Sources	Adverse Effects of Excessive Consumption	Special Considerations
			(g/d)	(g/d)			
Sodium	Maintains fluid volume outside of cells and thus normal cell function.	Infants			Processed foods to which sodium chloride (salt)/benzoate/ phosphate have been added; salted meats, cold cuts; nuts, cold cuts; margarine; butter; salt added to foods in cooking or at the table. Salt is ~40% sodium by weight.	Hypertension; increased risk of cardio-vascular disease and stroke.	The AI is set based on being able to obtain a nutritionally adequate diet for and other nutrients to meet the needs for sweat losses for individuals engaged in recommended levels of physical activity. Individuals engaged in activity at higher levels or in humid climates resulting
		0–6 mo	0.12	ND			
		7–12 mo	0.37	ND			
		Children					
		1–3 y	1.0	1.5			
		4–8 y	1.2	1.9			
		Males					
		9–13 y	1.5	2.2			
		14–18 y	1.5	2.3			
		19–30 y	1.5	2.3			
		31–50 y	1.5	2.3			
		51–70 y	1.3	2.3			
		>70 y	1.2	2.3			

Table continued on following page

Table 3-1 DIETARY REFERENCE INTAKES: ELECTROLYTES AND WATER *(Continued)*

Nutrient	Function	Life Stage Group	AI	UL	Selected Food Sources	Adverse Effects of Excessive Consumption	Special Considerations
		Females					in excessive sweat may need more than the AI. The UL applies to apparently healthy individuals without hypertension; it thus may be too high for individuals who already have hypertension or who are under the care of a health care professional.
		9–13 y	1.5	2.2			
		14–18 y	1.5	2.3			
		19–30 y	1.5	2.3			
		31–50 y	1.5	2.3			
		51–70 y	1.3	2.3			
		>70 y	1.2	2.3			
		Pregnancy					
		14–18 y	1.5	2.3			
		19–50 y	1.5	2.3			
		Lactation					
		14–18 y	1.5	2.3			
		19–50 y	1.5	2.3			
Chloride	With sodium, maintains fluid volume outside of cells and thus normal cell function.	Infants			See above; about 60% by weight of salt.	In concert with sodium, results in hypertension.	Chloride is lost usually with sodium in sweat, as well as in vomiting and diarrhea. The AI and UL are
		0–6 mo	0.18	ND			
		7–12 mo	0.57	ND			
		Children					
		1–3 y	1.5	2.3			

equimolar in amount to sodium since most of sodium in diet comes as sodium chloride (salt).

4–8 y	1.9	2.9
Males		
9–13 y	2.3	3.4
14–18 y	2.3	3.6
19–30 y	2.3	3.6
31–50 y	2.3	3.6
51–70 y	2.0	3.6
>70 y	1.8	3.6
Females		
9–13 y	2.3	3.4
14–18 y	2.3	3.6
19–30 y	2.3	3.6
31–50 y	2.3	3.6
51–70 y	2.0	3.6
>70 y	1.8	3.6
Pregnancy		
14–18 y	2.3	3.6
19–50 y	2.3	3.6
Lactation		
14–18 y	2.3	3.6
19–50 y	2.3	3.6

Table continued on following page

Table 3–1	DIETARY REFERENCE INTAKES: ELECTROLYTES AND WATER *(Continued)*						
Nutrient	Function	Life Stage Group	AI	UL	Selected Food Sources	Adverse Effects of Excessive Consumption	Special Considerations
Potassium	Maintains fluid volume inside/outside of cells and thus normal cell function; acts to blunt the rise of blood pressure in response to excess sodium intake, and decrease markers of bone turnover and recurrence of kidney stones.	Infants 0–6 mo 7–12 mo Children 1–3 y 4–8 y Males 9–13 y 14–18 y 19–30 y 31–50 y 51–70 y >70 y Females 9–13 y 14–18 y 19–30 y 31–50 y	0.4 0.7 3.0 3.8 4.5 4.7 4.7 4.7 4.7 4.7 4.5 4.7 4.7 4.7	No UL	Fruits and vegetables; dried peas; dairy products; meats and nuts.	None documented from food alone; however, potassium from supplements or salt substitutes can result in hyperkalemia and possibly sudden death if excess is consumed by individuals with chronic renal insufficiency (kidney disease) or diabetes.	Individuals taking drugs for cardiovascular disease such as ACE inhibitors, ARBs (angiontensin receptor blockers), or potassium sparing diuretics should be careful not to consume supplements containing potassium and may need to consume less than the AI for potassium.

		(L/d)		
	51–70 y	4.7		
	>70 y	4.7		
	Pregnancy			
	14–18 y	4.7		
	19–50 y	4.7		
	Lactation			
	14–18 y	5.1		
	19–50 y	5.1		
Water			No UL	All beverages, including water, as well as moisture in foods (high moisture foods include watermelon, meats, soups, etc.).
Maintains homeostasis in the body and allows for transport of nutrients to cells and removal and excretion of waste products of metabolism.	Infants		No UL because normally functioning kidneys can handle more than 0.7 L (24 oz) of fluid per hour; symptoms of water intoxication include hyponatremia, which can result in heart failure and	Recommended intakes for water are based on median intakes of generally healthy individuals who are adequately hydrated; individuals can be adequately hydrated at levels below as well as above the AIs provided. The AIs provided are for total water in temperate climates.
	0–6 mo	0.7		
	7–12 mo	0.8		
	Children			
	1–3 y	1.3		
	4–8 y	1.7		
	Males			
	9–13 y	2.4		
	14–18 y	3.3		
	19–30 y	3.7		
	31–50 y	3.7		
	51–70 y	3.7		
	>70 y	3.7		

Table continued on following page

Table 3–1	DIETARY REFERENCE INTAKES: ELECTROLYTES AND WATER (Continued)					
Nutrient	Function	Life Stage Group	AI	UL	Selected Food Sources	Adverse Effects of Excessive Consumption	Special Considerations
		Females				rhabdomyolosis (skeletal muscle tissue injury) which can lead to kidney failure.	All sources can contribute to total water needs: beverages (including tea, coffee, juices, sodas, and drinking water) and moisture found in foods.
		9–13 y	2.1				
		14–18 y	2.3				
		19–30 y	2.7				
		31–50 y	2.7				
		51–70 y	2.7				Moisture in food accounts for about 20% of total water intake. Thirst and consumption of beverages at meals are adequate to maintain hydration.
		>70 y	2.7				
		Pregnancy					
		14–18 y	3.0				
		19–50 y	3.0				
		Lactation					
		14–18 y	3.8				
		19–50 y	3.8				
Inorganic sulfate	Required for biosynthesis of 3'-phospho-adenosine-	Infants 0–6 mo 7–12 mo	No recommended intake was set because	No UL	Dried fruit (dates, raisins, dried apples), soy flour,	Osmotic diarrhea was observed in areas where water supply	

5'-phosphate (PAPS), which provides sulfate when sulfur-containing compounds are needed such as chondroitin sulfate and cerebroside sulfate.

Children
1–3 y
4–8 y

Males
9–13 y
14–18 y
19–30 y
31–50 y
51–70 y
>70 y

Females
9–13 y
14–18 y
19–30 y
31–50 y
51–70 y
>70 y

Pregnancy
14–18 y
19–50 y

adequate sulfate is available from dietary inorganic sulfate from water and foods, and from sources of organic sulfate, such as glutathione and the sulfur amino acids, methionine and cysteine. Metabolic breakdown of the recommended intake for protein

fruit juices, coconut milk, red and white wine, bread, as well as meats that are high in sulfur amino acids.

had high levels; odor and off taste usually limit intake, and thus no UL was set.

Table continued on following page

Table 3-1 DIETARY REFERENCE INTAKES: ELECTROLYTES AND WATER (Continued)

Nutrient	Function	Life Stage Group	AI	UL	Selected Food Sources	Adverse Effects of Excessive Consumption	Special Considerations
		Lactation 14–18 y 19–50 y	and sulfur amino acids should provide adequate inorganic sulfate for synthesis of required sulfur-containing compounds.				

Adequate Intakes (AIs) may be used as a goal for individual intake. For healthy breastfed infants, the AI is the mean intake. The AI for other life stage and gender groups is believed to cover the needs of all individuals in the group, but lack of data prevents being able to specify with confidence the percentage of individuals covered by this intake; therefore, no Recommended Dietary Allowance (RDA) was set. UL, the maximum level of daily nutrient intake that is likely to pose no risk of adverse effects. Unless otherwise specified, the UL represents total intake from food, water, and supplements. Due to lack of suitable data, ULs could not be established for potassium, water, and inorganic sulfate. In the absence of ULs, extra caution may be warranted in consuming levels above recommended intakes. ND, not determinable due to lack of data of adverse effects in this age group and concern with regard to lack of ability to handle excess amounts. Source of intake should be from food only to prevent high levels of intake.

Source: Refs. 1–6. These reports may be accessed via www.nap.edu. Copyright 2004 by The National Academies. All rights reserved. Published with permission.

Table 3-2	DIETARY REFERENCE INTAKES: ELEMENTS						
Nutrient	Function	Life Stage Group	RDA/AI*	UL	Selected Food Sources	Adverse Effects of Excessive Consumption	Special Considerations
Arsenic	No biological function in humans although animal data indicate a requirement	Infants 0–6 mo 7–12 mo	ND ND	ND ND	Dairy products, meat, poultry, fish, grains and cereal	No data on the possible adverse effects of organic arsenic compounds in food were found. Inorganic arsenic is a known toxic substance.	None
		Children 1–3 y 4–8 y	ND ND	ND ND			
		Males 9–13 y 14–18 y 19–30 y 31–50 y 51–70 y >70 y	ND ND ND ND ND ND	ND ND ND ND ND ND		Although the UL was not determined for arsenic, there is no justification for adding arsenic to food or supplements.	
		Females 9–13 y 14–18 y	ND ND	ND ND			

Table continued on following page

Table 3–2	DIETARY REFERENCE INTAKES: ELEMENTS *(Continued)*						
Nutrient	Function	Life Stage Group	RDA/AI*	UL	Selected Food Sources	Adverse Effects of Excessive Consumption	Special Considerations
		19–30 y	ND	ND			
		31–50 y	ND	ND			
		51–70 y	ND	ND			
		>70 y	ND	ND			
		Pregnancy					
		≤18 y	ND	ND			
		9–30 y	ND	ND			
		31–50 y	ND	ND			
		Lactation					
		≤18 y	ND	ND			
		19–30 y	ND	ND			
		31–50 y	ND	ND			
				(mg/d)			
Boron	No clear biological function in humans	Infants			Fruit-based beverages and products, potatoes,	Reproductive and developmental effects as observed in animal studies	None
		0–6 mo	ND	ND			
		7–12 mo	ND	ND			

although animal data indicate a functional role

			legumes, milk, avocado, peanut butter, peanuts
Children			
1–3 y	ND	3	
4–8 y	ND	6	
Males			
9–13 y	ND	11	
14–18 y	ND	17	
19–30 y	ND	20	
31–50 y	ND	20	
51–70 y	ND	20	
>70 y	ND	20	
Females			
9–13 y	ND	11	
14–18 y	ND	17	
19–30 y	ND	20	
31–50 y	ND	20	
51–70 y	ND	20	
>70 y	ND	20	
Pregnancy			
≤18 y	ND	17	
19–30 y	ND	20	
31–50 y	ND	20	

Table continued on following page

Table 3–2	DIETARY REFERENCE INTAKES: ELEMENTS *(Continued)*						
Nutrient	Function	Life Stage Group	RDA/AI*	UL	Selected Food Sources	Adverse Effects of Excessive Consumption	Special Considerations
		Lactation					
		≤18 y	ND	17			
		19–30 y	ND	20			
		31–50 y	ND	20			
			(mg/d)	*(mg/d)*			
Calcium	Essential role in blood clotting, muscle contraction, nerve transmission, and bone and tooth formation	Infants			Milk, cheese, yogurt, corn tortillas, calcium-set tofu, Chinese cabbage, kale, broccoli	Kidney stones, hypercalcemia, milk alkali syndrome, renal insufficiency	Amenorrheic women (exercise- or anorexia nervosa–induced) have reduced net calcium absorption.
		0–6 mo	210*	ND			
		7–12 mo	270*	ND			
		Children					There are no consistent data to support that a high-protein intake increases calcium requirement.
		1–3 y	500*	2500			
		4–8 y	800*	2500			
		Males					
		9–13 y	1300*	2500			
		14–18 y	1300*	2500			
		19–30 y	1000*	2500			
		31–50 y	1000*	2500			
		51–70 y	1200*	2500			
		>70 y	1200*	2500			

Females			
9–13 y	1300*	2500	
14–18 y	1300*	2500	
19–30 y	1000*	2500	
31–50 y	1000*	2500	
51–70 y	1200*	2500	
>70 y	1200*	2500	
Pregnancy			
≤18 y	1300*	2500	
19–30 y	1000*	2500	
31–50 y	1000*	2500	
Lactation			
≤18 y	1300*	2500	
19–30 y	1000*	2500	
31–50 y	1000*	2500	

		($\mu g/d$)				
Chromium	Helps to maintain normal blood glucose levels.				Some cereals, meats, poultry, fish, beer	Chronic renal failure	None
	Infants						
	0–6 mo	0.2*	ND				
	7–12 mo	5.5*	ND				
	Children						
	1–3 y	11*	ND				
	4–8 y	15*	ND				

Table continued on following page

Table 3-2	DIETARY REFERENCE INTAKES: ELEMENTS (Continued)					
Nutrient	Function	Life Stage Group	RDA/AI*	UL	Selected Food Sources	Adverse Effects of Excessive Consumption	Special Considerations

		Males				
		9–13 y	25*	ND		
		14–18 y	35*	ND		
		19–30 y	35*	ND		
		31–50 y	35*	ND		
		51–70 y	30*	ND		
		>70 y	30*	ND		
		Females				
		9–13 y	21*	ND		
		14–18 y	24*	ND		
		19–30 y	25*	ND		
		31–50 y	25*	ND		
		51–70 y	20*	ND		
		>70 y	20*	ND		
		Pregnancy				
		≤18 y	29*	ND		
		19–30 y	30*	ND		
		31–50 y	30*	ND		

		(µg/d)	(µg/d)			
Copper	Component of enzymes in iron metabolism			Organ meats, seafood, nuts, seeds, wheat bran cereals, whole grain products, cocoa products	Gastrointestinal distress, liver damage	Individuals with Wilson's disease, Indian childhood cirrhosis, and idiopathic copper toxicosis may be at increased risk of adverse effects from excess copper intake.
	Lactation					
	≤18 y	44*	ND			
	19–30 y	45*	ND			
	31–50 y	45*	ND			
	Infants					
	0–6 mo	200*	ND			
	7–12 mo	220*	ND			
	Children					
	1–3 y	340	1000			
	4–8 y	440	3000			
	Males					
	9–13 y	700	5000			
	14–18 y	890	8000			
	19–30 y	900	10,000			
	31–50 y	900	10,000			
	51–70 y	900	10,000			
	>70 y	900	10,000			
	Females					
	9–13 y	700	5000			
	14–18 y	890	8000			
	19–30 y	900	10,000			

Table continued on following page

Table 3-2	DIETARY REFERENCE INTAKES: ELEMENTS *(Continued)*						
Nutrient	Function	Life Stage Group	RDA/AI*	UL	Selected Food Sources	Adverse Effects of Excessive Consumption	Special Considerations
		31–50 y	**900**	10,000			
		51–70 y	**900**	10,000			
		>70 y	**900**	10,000			
		Pregnancy					
		≤18 y	**1000**	8000			
		19–30 y	**1000**	10,000			
		31–50 y	**1000**	10,000			
		Lactation					
		≤18 y	**1300**	8000			
		19–30 y	**1300**	10,000			
		31–50 y	**1300**	10,000			
			(mg/d)	*(mg/d)*			
Fluoride	Inhibits the initiation and progression of dental caries and stimulates	Infants			Fluoridated water, teas, marine fish, fluoridated dental products	Enamel and skeletal fluorosis	None
		0–6 mo	0.01*	0.7			
		7–12 mo	0.5*	0.9			
		Children					
		1–3 y	0.7*	1.3			
		4–8 y	1*	2.2			

new bone formation.

Males		
9–13 y	2*	10
14–18 y	3*	10
19–30 y	4*	10
31–50 y	4*	10
51–70 y	4*	10
>70 y	4*	10
Females		
9–13 y	2*	10
14–18 y	3*	10
19–30 y	3*	10
31–50 y	3*	10
51–70 y	3*	10
>70 y	3*	10
Pregnancy		
≤18 y	3*	10
19–30 y	3*	10
31–50 y	3*	10
Lactation		
≤18 y	3*	10
19–30 y	3*	10
31–50 y	3*	10

Table continued on following page

Table 3-2	DIETARY REFERENCE INTAKES: ELEMENTS *(Continued)*						
Nutrient	Function	Life Stage Group	RDA/AI*	UL	Selected Food Sources	Adverse Effects of Excessive Consumption	Special Considerations
			(*µg/d*)	(*µg/d*)			
Iodine	Component of the thyroid hormones; prevents goiter and cretinism.	Infants			Marine origin, processed foods, iodized salt	Elevated thyroid stimulating hormone (TSH) concentration	Individuals with autoimmune thyroid disease, previous iodine deficiency, or nodular goiter are distinctly susceptible to the adverse effect of excess iodine intake. Therefore, individuals with these conditions may not be protected by the UL for iodine intake for the general population.
		0–6 mo	110*	ND			
		7–12 mo	130*	ND			
		Children					
		1–3 y	**90**	200			
		4–8 y	**90**	300			
		Males					
		9–13 y	**120**	600			
		14–18 y	**150**	900			
		19–30 y	**150**	1100			
		31–50 y	**150**	1100			
		51–70 y	**150**	1100			
		>70 y	**150**	1100			
		Females					
		9–13 y	**120**	600			
		14–18 y	**150**	900			
		19–30 y	**150**	1100			

	31–50 y	150	1100
	51–70 y	150	1100
	>70 y	150	1100
	Pregnancy		
	≤18 y	220	900
	19–30 y	220	1100
	31–50 y	220	1100
	Lactation		
	≤18 y	290	900
	19–30 y	290	1100
	31–50 y	290	1100

		(mg/d)	(mg/d)
Iron	Infants		
Component of hemoglobin and numerous enzymes; prevents microcytic hypochromic anemia.	0–6 mo	0.27*	40
	7–12 mo	11	40
	Children		
	1–3 y	7	40
	4–8 y	10	40
	Males		
	9–13 y	8	40
	14–18 y	11	45
	19–30 y	8	45

Sources: Fruits, vegetables, fortified bread and grain products such as cereal (non-heme iron sources), meat and poultry (heme iron sources)

Toxicity: Gastrointestinal distress

Notes: Non-heme iron absorption is lower for those consuming vegetarian diets than for those eating non-vegetarian diets. Therefore, it has been suggested that the iron requirement for

Table continued on following page

Table 3-2	DIETARY REFERENCE INTAKES: ELEMENTS *(Continued)*						
Nutrient	Function	Life Stage Group	RDA/AI*	UL	Selected Food Sources	Adverse Effects of Excessive Consumption	Special Considerations
		31–50 y	8	45			those consuming a vegetarian diet is approximately two-fold greater than for those consuming a nonvegetarian diet.
		51–70 y	8	45			
		>70 y	8	45			
		Females					
		9–13 y	8	40			
		14–18 y	15	45			
		19–30 y	18	45			Recommended intake assumes 75% of iron is from heme iron sources.
		31–50 y	18	45			
		51–70 y	8	45			
		>70 y	8	45			
		Pregnancy					
		≤18 y	27	45			
		19–30 y	27	45			
		31–50 y	27	45			
		Lactation					
		≤18 y	10	45			
		19–30 y	9	45			
		31–50 y	9	45			

Table continued on following page

Magnesium	Cofactor for enzyme systems		(mg/d)	(mg/d)	Green leafy vegetables, unpolished grains, nuts, meat, starches, milk	There is no evidence of adverse effects from the consumption of naturally occurring magnesium in foods.	None
		Infants					
		0–6 mo	30*	ND			
		7–12 mo	75*	ND			
		Children					
		1–3 y	80	65			
		4–8 y	130	110			
		Males				Adverse effects from magnesium-containing supplements may include osmotic diarrhea.	
		9–13 y	240	350			
		14–18 y	410	350			
		19–30 y	400	350			
		31–50 y	420	350			
		51–70 y	420	350			
		>70 y	420	350			
		Females				The UL for magnesium represents intake from a pharmacologic agent only and does not include intake from food and water.	
		9–13 y	240	350			
		14–18 y	360	350			
		19–30 y	310	350			
		31–50 y	320	350			
		51–70 y	320	350			
		>70 y	320	350			

Table 3-2	DIETARY REFERENCE INTAKES: ELEMENTS (Continued)						
Nutrient	Function	Life Stage Group	RDA/AI*	UL	Selected Food Sources	Adverse Effects of Excessive Consumption	Special Considerations
		Pregnancy					
		≤18 y	**400**	350			
		19–30 y	**350**	350			
		31–50 y	**360**	350			
		Lactation					
		≤18 y	**360**	350			
		19–30 y	**310**	350			
		31–50 y	**320**	350			
			(mg/d)	(mg/d)			
Manganese	Involved in the formation of bone, as well as in enzymes involved in amino acid, cholesterol, and carbohydrate metabolism.	Infants			Nuts, legumes, tea, whole grains	Elevated blood concentration and neurotoxicity	Because manganese in drinking water and supplements may be more bioavailable than manganese from food, caution should be taken when using manganese supplements
		0–6 mo	0.0003*	ND			
		7–12 mo	0.6*	ND			
		Children					
		1–3 y	1.2*	2			
		4–8 y	1.5*	3			
		Males					
		9–13 y	1.9*	6			
		14–18 y	2.2*	9			

				Food Sources	Adverse Effects
	19–30 y	2.3*	11		especially among those persons already consuming large amounts of manganese from diets high in plant products.
	31–50 y	2.3*	11		
	51–70 y	2.3*	11		
	>70 y	2.3*	11		
	Females				In addition, individuals with liver disease may be distinctly susceptible to the adverse effects of excess manganese intake.
	9–13 y	1.6*	6		
	14–18 y	1.6*	9		
	19–30 y	1.8*	11		
	31–50 y	1.8*	11		
	51–70 y	1.8*	11		
	>70 y	1.8*	11		
	Pregnancy				
	≤18 y	2.0*	9		
	19–30 y	2.0	11		
	31–50 y	2.0	11		
	Lactation				
	≤18 y	2.6*	9		
	19–30 y	2.6*	11		
	31–50 y	2.6*	11		
		(μg/d)	(μg/d)		
Molybdenum	Infants			Legumes, grain products, nuts	Reproductive effects as observed in animal studies.
Cofactor for enzymes involved in catabolism	0–6 mo	2*	ND		Individuals who are deficient in dietary copper or have some
	7–12 mo	3*	ND		

Table continued on following page

Table 3–2	DIETARY REFERENCE INTAKES: ELEMENTS *(Continued)*						
Nutrient	Function	Life Stage Group	RDA/AI*	UL	Selected Food Sources	Adverse Effects of Excessive Consumption	Special Considerations
	of sulphur amino acids, purines, and pyridines	Children					dysfunction in copper metabolism that makes them copper-deficient could be at increased risk of molybdenum toxicity.
		1–3 y	**17**	300			
		4–8 y	**22**	600			
		Males					
		9–13 y	**34**	1100			
		14–18 y	**43**	1700			
		19–30 y	**45**	2000			
		31–50 y	**45**	2000			
		51–70 y	**45**	2000			
		>70 y	**45**	2000			
		Females					
		9–13 y	**34**	1100			
		14–18 y	**43**	1700			
		19–30 y	**45**	2000			
		31–50 y	**45**	2000			
		51–70 y	**45**	2000			
		>70 y	**45**	2000			

	Life Stage Group		(mg/d)	Selected Food Sources	Adverse Effects
	Pregnancy				
	≤18 y	50	1700		
	19–30 y	50	2000		
	31–50 y	50	2000		
	Lactation				
	≤18 y	50	1700		
	19–30 y	50	2000		
	31–50 y	50	2000		
Nickel					
No clear biological function in humans has been identified. May serve as a cofactor of metallo-enzymes and facilitate iron absorption or metabolisms in microorganisms.	**Infants**			Nuts, legumes, cereals, sweeteners, chocolate milk powder, chocolate candy	Decreased body weight gain. Note: As observed in animal studies. Individuals with preexisting nickel hypersensitivity (from previous dermal exposure) and kidney dysfunction are distinctly susceptible to the adverse effects of excess nickel intake.
	0–6 mo	ND	ND		
	7–12 mo	ND	ND		
	Children				
	1–3 y	ND	0.2		
	4–8 y	ND	0.3		
	Males				
	9–13 y	ND	0.6		
	14–18 y	ND	1.0		
	19–30 y	ND	1.0		
	31–50 y	ND	1.0		
	51–70 y	ND	1.0		
	>70 y	ND	1.0		

Table continued on following page

Table 3-2	DIETARY REFERENCE INTAKES: ELEMENTS *(Continued)*						
Nutrient	Function	Life Stage Group	RDA/AI*	UL	Selected Food Sources	Adverse Effects of Excessive Consumption	Special Considerations
		Females					
		9–13 y	ND	0.6			
		14–18 y	ND	1.0			
		19–30 y	ND	1.0			
		31–50 y	ND	1.0			
		51–70 y	ND	1.0			
		>70 y	ND	1.0			
		Pregnancy					
		≤18 y	ND	1.0			
		19–30 y	ND	1.0			
		31–50 y	ND	1.0			
		Lactation					
		≤18 y	ND	1.0			
		19–30 y	ND	1.0			
		31–50 y	ND	1.0			
			(mg/d)	*(mg/d)*			
Phosphorus	Maintenance of pH, storage and transfer	Infants			Milk, yogurt, ice cream, cheese, peas,	Metastatic calcification, skeletal porosity,	Athletes and others with high energy expenditure
		0–6 mo	100*	ND			
		7–12 mo	275*	ND			

of energy and nucleotide synthesis			meat, eggs, some cereals and breads	interference with calcium absorption	frequently consume amounts from food greater than the UL without apparent effect.
Children					
1–3 y	**460**	3000			
4–8 y	**500**	3000			
Males					
9–13 y	**1250**	4000			
14–18 y	**1250**	4000			
19–30 y	**700**	4000			
31–50 y	**700**	4000			
51–70 y	**700**	4000			
>70 y	**700**	3000			
Females					
9–13 y	**1250**	4000			
14–18 y	**1250**	4000			
19–30 y	**700**	4000			
31–50 y	**700**	4000			
51–70 y	**700**	4000			
>70 y	**700**	3000			
Pregnancy					
≤18 y	**1250**	3500			
19–30 y	**700**	3500			
31–50 y	**700**	3500			

Table continued on following page

Table 3–2	DIETARY REFERENCE INTAKES: ELEMENTS *(Continued)*					
Nutrient	Function	Life Stage Group	RDA/AI*	UL	Selected Food Sources	Adverse Effects of Excessive Consumption	Special Considerations
		Lactation					
		≤18 y	**1250**	4000			
		19–30 y	**700**	4000			
		31–50 y	**700**	4000			
			(mg/d)	*(mg/d)*			
Selenium	Defense against oxidative stress and regulation of thyroid hormone action, and the reduction and oxidation status of vitamin C and other molecules	Infants			Organ meats, seafood, plants (depending on soil selenium content)	Hair and nail brittleness and loss	None
		0–6 mo	15*	45			
		7–12 mo	20*	60			
		Children					
		1–3 y	**20**	90			
		4–8 y	**30**	150			
		Males					
		9–13 y	**40**	280			
		14–18 y	**55**	400			
		19–30 y	**55**	400			
		31–50 y	**55**	400			
		51–70 y	**55**	400			
		>70 y	**55**	400			

Silicon	No biological function in humans has been identified.		
	Involved in bone		

Females			
9–13 y	**40**	280	
14–18 y	**55**	400	
19–30 y	**55**	400	
31–50 y	**55**	400	
51–70 y	**55**	400	
>70 y	**55**	400	

Pregnancy		
≤18 y	**60**	400
19–30 y	**60**	400
31–50 y	**60**	400

Lactation		
≤18 y	**70**	400
19–30 y	**70**	400
31–50 y	**70**	400

Infants		
0–6 mo	ND	ND
7–12 mo	ND	ND

Children		
1–3 y	ND	ND
4–8 y	ND	ND

Plant-based foods

There is no evidence that silicon that occurs naturally in food and water produces adverse health effects.

None

Table continued on following page

Table 3-2	DIETARY REFERENCE INTAKES: ELEMENTS (Continued)						
Nutrient	Function	Life Stage Group	RDA/AI*	UL	Selected Food Sources	Adverse Effects of Excessive Consumption	Special Considerations
	function in animal studies.	Males					
		9–13 y	ND	ND			
		14–18 y	ND	ND			
		19–30 y	ND	ND			
		31–50 y	ND	ND			
		51–70 y	ND	ND			
		>70 y	ND	ND			
		Females					
		9–13 y	ND	ND			
		14–18 y	ND	ND			
		19–30 y	ND	ND			
		31–50 y	ND	ND			
		51–70 y	ND	ND			
		>70 y	ND	ND			
		Pregnancy					
		≤18 y	ND	ND			
		19–30 y	ND	ND			
		31–50 y	ND	ND			

		Life Stage Group			(mg/d)	Selected Food Sources	Adverse Effects of Excessive Consumption	Special Considerations
Vanadium	No biological function in humans has been identified.	Lactation				Mushrooms, shellfish, black pepper, parsley, dill seed	Renal lesions as observed in animal studies	None
		≤18 y	ND	ND	ND			
		19–30 y	ND	ND	ND			
		31–50 y	ND	ND	ND			
		Infants						
		0–6 mo	ND	ND	ND			
		7–12 mo	ND	ND	ND			
		Children						
		1–3 y	ND	ND	ND			
		4–8 y	ND	ND	ND			
		Males						
		9–13 y	ND	ND	ND			
		14–18 y	ND	ND	ND			
		19–30 y	ND	ND	ND			
		31–50 y	ND	ND	1.8			
		51–70 y	ND	ND	1.8			
		>70 y	ND	ND	1.8			
		Females						
		9–13 y	ND	ND	ND			
		14–18 y	ND	ND	ND			
		19–30 y	ND	ND	1.8			

Table continued on following page

Table 3–2	DIETARY REFERENCE INTAKES: ELEMENTS *(Continued)*						
Nutrient	Function	Life Stage Group	RDA/AI*	UL	Selected Food Sources	Adverse Effects of Excessive Consumption	Special Considerations
		31–50 y	ND	1.8			
		51–70 y	ND	1.8			
		>70 y	ND	1.8			
		Pregnancy					
		≤18 y	ND	ND			
		19–30 y	ND	ND			
		31–50 y	ND	ND			
		Lactation					
		≤18 y	ND	ND			
		19–30 y	ND	ND			
		31–50 y	ND	ND			
			(mg/d)	*(mg/d)*			
Zinc	Component of multiple enzymes and proteins;	Infants			Fortified cereals, red meats, certain seafood	Reduced copper status	Zinc absorption is lower for those consuming vegetarian diets
		0–6 mo	2*	4			
		7–12 mo	3	5			

than for those eating nonvegetarian diets. Therefore, it has been suggested that the zinc requirement for those consuming a vegetarian diet is approximately twofold greater than for those consuming a nonvegetarian diet.

involved in the regulation of gene expression.

Children		
1–3 y	3	7
4–8 y	5	12
Males		
9–13 y	8	23
14–18 y	11	34
19–30 y	11	40
31–50 y	11	40
51–70 y	11	40
>70 y	11	40
Females		
9–13 y	8	23
14–18 y	9	34
19–30 y	8	40
31–50 y	8	40
51–70 y	8	40
>70 y	8	40
Pregnancy		
≤18 y	13	34
19–30 y	12	40
31–50 y	12	40

Table continued on following page

Table 3-2	DIETARY REFERENCE INTAKES: ELEMENTS *(Continued)*						
Nutrient	Function	Life Stage Group	RDA/AI*	UL	Selected Food Sources	Adverse Effects of Excessive Consumption	Special Considerations
		Lactation					
		≤18 y	**13**	34			
		19–30 y	**12**	40			
		31–50 y	**12**	40			

*Recommended Dietary Allowances (RDAs) are in **bold type**. Adequate Intake (AIs) are denoted with an asterisk (*). RDAs and AIs may both be used as goals for individual intake. RDAs are set to meet the needs of almost all (97% to 98%) individuals in a group. For healthy breastfed infants, the AI is the mean intake. The AI for other life stage and gender groups is believed to cover the needs of all individuals in the group, but lack of data prevent being able to specify with confidence the percentage of individuals covered by this intake.

UL. The maximum level of daily nutrient intake that is likely to pose no risk of adverse effects. Unless otherwise specified, the UL represents total intake from food, water, and supplements. Due to lack of suitable data, ULs could not be established for vitamin K, thiamine, riboflavin, vitamin B$_{12}$, pantothenic acid, biotin or carotenoids. In the absence of ULs, extra caution may be warranted in consuming levels above recommended intakes.

ND. Not determinable due to lack of data of adverse effects in this age group and concern with regard to lack of ability to handle excess amounts. Source of intake should be from food only to prevent high levels of intake.

Sources: Refs. 1–4. These reports may be accessed via www.nap.edu. Copyright 2001 by The National Academies. All rights reserved. Published with permission.

Table 3-3 DIETARY REFERENCE INTAKES: MACRONUTRIENTS

Nutrient	Function	Life Stage Group	RDA/AI* (g/d)	AMDR	Selected Food Sources	Adverse Effects of Excessive Consumption
Carbohydrate—Total digestible	RDA based on its role as the primary energy source for the brain; AMDR based on its role as a source of kilocalories to maintain body weight.	Infants			Starch and sugar are the major types of carbohydrates. Grains and vegetables (corn, pasta, rice, potatoes, breads) are sources of starch. Natural sugars are found in fruits and juices. Sources of added sugars are soft drinks, candy, fruit drinks, and desserts.	While no defined intake level at which potential adverse effects of total digestible carbohydrate was identified, the upper end of the AMDR was based on decreasing risk of chronic disease and providing adequate intake of other nutrients. It is suggested that the maximal intake of added sugars be limited to providing no more than 25 percent of energy
		0–6 mo	60*	ND		
		7–12 mo	95*	ND		
		Children				
		1–3 y	130	45–65		
		4–8 y	130	45–65		
		Males				
		9–13 y	130	45–65		
		14–18 y	130	45–65		
		19–30 y	130	45–65		
		31–50 y	130	45–65		
		51–70 y	130	45–65		
		>70 y	130	45–65		
		Females				
		9–13 y	130	45–65		
		14–18 y	130	45–65		
		19–30 y	130	45–65		
		31–50 y	130	45–65		

Table continued on following page

Table 3–3	DIETARY REFERENCE INTAKES: MACRONUTRIENTS *(Continued)*					
Nutrient	Function	Life Stage Group	RDA/AI* (g/d)	AMDR	Selected Food Sources	Adverse Effects of Excessive Consumption
		51–70 y	**130**	45–65		
		>70 y	**130**	45–65		
		Pregnancy				
		≤18 y	**175**	45–65		
		19–30 y	**175**	45–65		
		31–50 y	**175**	45–65		
		Lactation				
		≤18 y	**210**	45–65		
		19–30 y	**210**	45–65		
		31–50 y	**210**	45–65		
Total fiber	Improves laxation, reduces risk of coronary heart disease, assists in maintaining normal blood glucose levels.	Infants			Includes dietary fiber naturally present in grains (such as found in oats, wheat, or unmilled rice) and functional fiber synthesized or isolated from plants or animals and shown to be	Dietary fiber can have variable compositions and therefore it is difficult to link a specific source of fiber with a particular adverse effect, especially when phylate is also present in the natural fiber source. It is concluded that as part of an overall
		0–6 mo	ND			
		7–12 mo	ND			
		Children				
		1–3 y	19*			
		4–8 y	25*			
		Males				
		9–13 y	31*			

	14–18 y	38*	of benefit to health.
	19–30 y	38*	
	31–50 y	38*	
	51–70 y	30*	
	>70 y	30*	
	Females		
	9–13 y	26*	
	14–18 y	26*	
	19–30 y	25*	
	31–50 y	25*	
	51–70 y	21*	
	>70 y	21*	
	Pregnancy		
	≤18 y	28*	
	19–30 y	28*	
	31–50 y	28*	
	Lactation		
	≤18 y	29*	
	19–30 y	29*	
	31–50 y	29*	
	Infants		
	0–6 mo	31*	
	7–12 mo	30*	

healthy diet, a high intake of dietary fiber will not produce deleterious effects in healthy individuals. While occasional adverse gastrointestinal symptoms are observed when consuming some isolated or synthetic fibers, serious chronic adverse effects have not been observed. Due to the bulky nature of fibers, excess consumption is likely to be self-limiting. Therefore, a UL was not set for individual functional fibers.

Total fat

Energy source: when found in foods, is a source of *n*-6 and *n*-3

Butter, margarine, vegetable oils, whole milk, visible fat on

While no defined intake level at which potential adverse effects of total fat was

Table continued on following page

Table 3-3 DIETARY REFERENCE INTAKES: MACRONUTRIENTS (Continued)

Nutrient	Function	Life Stage Group	RDA/AI* (g/d)	AMDR	Selected Food Sources	Adverse Effects of Excessive Consumption
	polyunsaturated fatty acids. Its presence in the diet increases absorption of fat soluble vitamins and precursors such as vitamin A and pro-vitamin A carotenoids.	Children			meat and poultry products, invisible fat in fish, shellfish, some plant products such as seeds and nuts, bakery products	identified, the upper end of AMDR is based on decreasing risk of chronic disease and providing adequate intake of other nutrients. The lower end of the AMDR is based on concerns related to the increase in plasma triacylglycerol concentrations and decreased HDL cholesterol concentrations seen with very low fat (and thus high carbohydrate) diets.
		1–3 y		30–40		
		4–8 y		25–35		
		Males				
		9–13 y		25–35		
		14–18 y		25–35		
		19–30 y		20–35		
		31–50 y		20–35		
		51–70 y		20–35		
		>70 y		20–35		
		Females				
		9–13 y		25–35		
		14–18 y		25–35		
		19–30 y		20–35		
		31–50 y		20–35		
		51–70 y		20–35		
		>70 y		20–35		
		Pregnancy				
		≤18 y		20–35		

		AI	AMDR
	19–30 y		20–35
	31–50 y		20–35
	Lactation		
	≤18 y		20–35
	19–30 y		20–35
	31–50 y		20–35
n-6 Polyunsaturated fatty acids (linolenic acid)	Infants		
Essential component of structural membrane lipids, involved with cell signaling, and precursor of eicosanoids. Required for normal skin function.	0–6 mo	4.4*	ND
	7–12 mo	4.6*	ND
	Children		
	1–3 y	7*	5–10
	4–8 y	10*	5–10
	Males		
	9–13 y	12	5–10
	14–18 y	16*	5–10
	19–30 y	17*	5–10
	31–50 y	17*	5–10
	51–70 y	14*	5–10
	>70 y	14*	5–10
	Females		
	9–13 y	10*	5–10
	14–18 y	11*	5–10

Sources: Nuts, seeds, and vegetable oils such as soybean, safflower, and corn oil.

While no defined intake level at which potential adverse effects of n-6 polyunsaturated fatty acids was identified, the upper end of the AMDR is based on the lack of evidence that demonstrates long-term safety along with human in vitro studies that show increased free-radical formation and lipid peroxidation with higher amounts of n-6 fatty acids. Lipid peroxidation is thought to be a component in the development of

Table continued on following page

Table 3-3	DIETARY REFERENCE INTAKES: MACRONUTRIENTS *(Continued)*				
Nutrient	Function	Life Stage Group	RDA/AI* (g/d)	AMDR	Selected Food Sources	Adverse Effects of Excessive Consumption
		19–30 y	12*	5–10		atherosclerotic plaques.
		31–50 y	12*	5–10		
		51–70 y	12*	5–10		
		>70 y	11*	5–10		
		Pregnancy				
		≤18 y	13*	5–10		
		19–30 y	13*	5–10		
		31–50 y	13*	5–10		
		Lactation				
		≤18 y	13*	5–10		
		19–30 y	13*	5–10		
		31–50 y	13*	5–10		
n-3 Polyunsaturated fatty acids (α-linolenic acid)	Involved with neurological development and growth. Precursor of eicosanoids.	**Infants**			Vegetable oils such as soybean, canola, and flax seed oil, fatty fish oils, fatty fish, with smaller amounts in meats and eggs.	While no defined intake level at which potential adverse effects of *n*-3 polyunsaturated fatty acids was identified, the upper end of AMDR is based on maintaining
		0–6 mo	0.5*	ND		
		7–12 mo	0.5*	ND		
		Children				
		1–3 y	0.7*	0.6–1.2		
		4–8 y	0.9*	0.6–1.2		

the appropriate balance with n-6 fatty acids and on the lack of evidence that demonstrates long-term safety, along with human in vitro studies that show increased free-radical formation and lipid peroxidation with higher amounts of polyunsaturated fatty acids. Lipid peroxidation is thought to be a component in the development of atherosclerotic plaques.

Males		
9–13 y	1.2*	0.6–1.2
14–18 y	1.6*	0.6–1.2
19–30 y	1.6*	0.6–1.2
31–50 y	1.6*	0.5–1.2
51–70 y	1.6*	0.6–1.2
>70 y	1.6*	0.6–1.2
Females		
9–13 y	1.0*	0.6–1.2
14–18 y	1.1*	0.6–1.2
19–30 y	1.1*	0.6–1.2
31–50 y	1.1*	0.6–1.2
51–70 y	1.1*	0.6–1.2
>70 y	1.1*	0.6–1.2
Pregnancy		
≤18 y	1.4*	0.6–1.2
19–30 y	1.4*	0.6–1.2
31–50 y	1.4*	0.6–1.2
Lactation		
≤18 y	1.3*	0.6–1.2
19–30 y	1.3*	0.6–1.2
31–50 y	1.3*	0.6–1.2

Table continued on following page

Table 3–3 **DIETARY REFERENCE INTAKES: MACRONUTRIENTS** *(Continued)*

Nutrient	Function	Life Stage Group	RDA/AI* (g/d)	AMDR	Selected Food Sources	Adverse Effects of Excessive Consumption
Saturated and *trans* fatty acids, and cholesterol	No required role for these nutrients other than as energy sources was identified; the body can synthesize its needs for saturated fatty acids and cholesterol from other sources.	Infants 0–6 mo 7–12 mo	ND ND		Saturated fatty acids are present in animal fats (meat fats and butter fat), and coconut and palm kernel oils. Sources of cholesterol include liver, eggs and foods that contain eggs such as cheesecake and custard pies. Sources of *trans* fatty acids include stick margarines and foods containing hydrogenated or partially	There is an incremental increase in plasma total and low-density lipoprotein concentrations with increased intake of saturated or *trans* fatty acids or with cholesterol at even very low levels in the diet. Therefore, the intakes of each should be minimized while consuming a nutritionally adequate diet.
		Children 1–3 y 4–8 y				
		Males 9–13 y 14–18 y 19–30 y 31–50 y 51–70 y >70 y				
		Females 9–13 y 14–18 y 19–30 y 31–50 y				

Nutrient and function	Life stage group		AMDR	Sources	Comments
	50–70 y			hydrogenated vegetable shortenings.	
	>70 y				
	Pregnancy				
	≤18 y				
	19–30 y				
	31–50 y				
	Lactation				
	≤18 y				
	19–30 y				
	31–50 y				
Protein and amino acids†	Infants			Proteins from animal sources, such as meat, poultry, fish, eggs, milk, cheese, and yogurt, provide all nine indispensable amino acids in adequate amounts, and for this reason are	While no defined intake level at which potential adverse effects of protein was identified, the upper end of AMDR was based on complementing the carbohydrate and fat for the various age groups. The lower end of the AMDR is set at approximately the RDA.
Serves as the major structural components of all cells in the body, and functions as enzymes, in membranes, as transport carriers, and as some hormones. During digestion	0–6 mo	9.1*	ND		
	7–12 mo	13.5	ND		
	Children				
	1–3 y	13	5–20		
	4–8 y	19	10–30		
	Males				
	9–13 y	34	10–30		
	14–18 y	52	10–30		
	19–30 y	56	10–35		

Table continued on following page

Table 3-3	DIETARY REFERENCE INTAKES: MACRONUTRIENTS *(Continued)*				
Nutrient	Function	Life Stage Group	RDA/AI* (g/d)	AMDR	Selected Food Sources	Adverse Effects of Excessive Consumption
	and absorption, dietary proteins are broken down to amino acids, which become the building blocks of these structural and functional compounds. Nine of the amino acids must be provided in the diet; these are termed indispensable amino acids. The body can	31–50 y	56	10–35	considered "complete proteins." Proteins from plants, legumes, grains, nuts, seeds and vegetables tend to be deficient in one or more of the indispensable amino acids and are called "incomplete proteins." Vegan diets adequate in total protein content can be "complete" by	
		51–70 y	56	10–35		
		>70 y	56	10–35		
		Females				
		9–13 y	34	10–30		
		14–18 y	46	10–30		
		19–30 y	46	10–35		
		31–50 y	46	10–35		
		51–70 y	46	10–35		
		>70 y	46	10–35		
		Pregnancy				
		≤18 y	71	10–35		
		19–30 y	71	10–35		
		31–50 y	71	10–35		
		Lactation				
		≤18 y	71	10–35		

make the other amino acids needed to synthesize specific structures from other amino acids.	19–30 y 31–50 y	**71** **71**	**10–35** **10–35**	combining sources of incomplete proteins, which lack different indispensable amino acids.

*Recommended Dietary Allowances (RDAs) are in **bold type.** Adequate Intakes (AIs) are denoted by an asterisk. RDAs and AIs may both be used as goals for individual intake. RDAs are set to meet the needs of almost all (97% to 98%) individuals in a group. For healthy breastfed infants, the AI is the mean intake. The AI for other life stage and gender groups is believed to cover the needs of all individuals in the group, but lack of data prevents being able to specify with confidence the percentage of individuals covered by this intake.

AMDR, Acceptable Macronutrient Distribution Range is the range of intake for a particular energy source that is associated with reduced risk of chronic disease while providing intakes of essential nutrients. If an individual consumes in excess of the AMDR, there is a potential of increasing the risk of chronic diseases and insufficient intakes of essential nutrients.

ND, Not determinable due to lack of data of adverse effects in this age group and concern with regard to lack of ability to handle excess amounts. Source of intake should be from food only to prevent high levels of intake.

†RDA/AI for protein and amino acids is based on 1.5 g/kg/day for infants, 1.1 g/kg/day for 1–3 y, 0.95 g/kg/day for 4–13 y, 0.85 g/kg/day for 14–18 y, 0.8 g/kg/day for adults, and 1.1 g/kg/day for pregnant (using prepregnancy weight) and lactating women.

Sources: Ref. 5. This report may be accessed via www.nap.edu. Published with permission.

Table 3–4	DIETARY REFERENCE INTAKES: INDISPENSABLE AMINO ACIDS*			
Nutrient	Function	IOM/FNB 2002 Scoring Pattern	Mg/g Protein	Adverse Effects of Excessive Consumption
Histidine	The building blocks of all proteins in the body and some hormones. These nine amino acids must be provided through diet and thus are termed indispensable amino acids. The body can make the other amino acids needed to synthesize specific structures from other amino acids and carbohydrate precursors.	Histidine	18	Since there is no evidence that amino acids found in usual or even high intakes of protein from food present any risk, attention was focused on intakes of the L-form of these and other amino acids found in dietary protein and amino acid supplements. Even from well-studied amino acids, adequate dose-response data from human or animal studies on which to base a UL were not available. While no defined intake level at which potential adverse effects of protein was identified for any amino acid, this does not mean that there is no potential for adverse effects resulting from high intakes of amino acids from dietary supplements. Since data on the adverse effects of high levels of amino acid intakes from dietary supplements are limited, caution may be warranted.
Isoleucine		Isoleucine	25	
Lysine		Lysine	55	
Leucine		Leucine	51	
Methionine and Cysteine		Methionine and Cysteine	25	
Phenylalanine and Tyrosine		Phenylalanine and Tyrosine	47	
Threonine		Threonine	27	
Tryptophan		Tryptophan	7	
Valine		Valine	32	

*Based on the amino acid requirements derived for preschool children (1–3 y): (EAR for amino acid ÷ EAR for protein); for 1–3 y group where EAR for protein = 0.88 g/kg/d.

IOM/FNB, Institute of Medicine Food and Nutrition Board.

Source: Ref. 5. This report may be accessed via www.nap.edu. Published with permission.

Table 3-5	DIETARY REFERENCE INTAKES: VITAMINS					
Nutrient	Function	Life Stage Group	RDA/AI*	UL	Selected Food Sources	Adverse Effects of Excessive Consumption	Special Considerations
Biotin	Coenzyme in synthesis of fat, glycogen. and amino acids		(µg/d)		Liver and smaller amounts in fruits and meats	No adverse effects of biotin in humans or animals were found. This does not mean that there is no potential for adverse effects resulting from high intakes. Because data on the adverse effects of biotin are limited, caution	None
		Infants					
		0–6 mo	5*	ND			
		7–12 mo	6*	ND			
		Children					
		1–3 y	8*	ND			
		4–8 y	12*	ND			
		Males					
		9–13 y	20*	ND			
		14–18 y	25*	ND			
		19–30 y	30*	ND			
		31–50 y	30*	ND			
		51–70 y	30*	ND			
		>70 y	30*	ND			
		Females					
		9–13 y	20*	ND			

Table continued on following page

Table 3-5	DIETARY REFERENCE INTAKES: VITAMINS *(Continued)*						
Nutrient	Function	Life Stage Group	RDA/AI*	UL	Selected Food Sources	Adverse Effects of Excessive Consumption	Special Considerations
		14–18 y	25*	ND		may be warranted.	
		19–30 y	30*	ND			
		31–50 y	30*	ND			
		51–70 y	30*	ND			
		>70 y	30*	ND			
		Pregnancy					
		≤18 y	30*	ND			
		19–30 y	30*	ND			
		31–50 y	30*	ND			
		Lactation					
		≤18 y	35*	ND			
		19–30 y	35*	ND			
		31–50 y	35*	ND			
			(mg/d)	*(mg/d)*			
Choline	Precursor for acetylcholine, phospholipids, and betaine	Infants 0–6 mo	125*	ND	Milk, liver, eggs, peanuts	Fishy body odor, sweating, salivation, hypotension,	Individuals with trimethylaminuria, renal disease, liver
		7–12 mo	150*	ND			

			hepato-toxicity	disease.
Children				depression, and
1–3 y	200*	1000		Parkinson's
4–8 y	250*	1000		disease may be
				at risk of
Males				adverse effects
9–13 y	375*	2000		with choline
14–18 y	550*	3000		intakes at the UL.
19–30 y	550*	3500		
31–50 y	550*	3500		Although AIs have
51–70 y	550*	3500		been set for
>70 y	550*	3500		choline, there
				are few data to
Females				assess whether
9–13 y	375*	2000		a dietary supply
14–18 y	400*	3000		of choline is
19–30 y	425*	3500		needed at all
31–50 y	425*	3500		stages of the
51–70 y	425*	3500		life cycle, and it
>70 y	425*	3500		may be that the
				choline
Pregnancy				requirement
≤18 y	450*	3000		can be met by
19–30 y	450*	3500		endogenous
31–50 y	450*	3500		

Table continued on following page

| Table 3–5 | DIETARY REFERENCE INTAKES: VITAMINS (Continued) |

Nutrient	Function	Life Stage Group	RDA/AI*	UL	Selected Food Sources	Adverse Effects of Excessive Consumption	Special Considerations
		Lactation					synthesis at some of these stages.
		≤18 y	550*	3000			
		19–30 y	550*	3500			
		31–50 y	550*	3500			
			(μg/d)	(μg/d)			
Folate	Coenzyme in the metabolism of nucleic and amino acids; prevents megaloblastic anemia.	Infants			Enriched cereal grains, dark leafy vegetables, enriched and whole-grain breads and bread products, fortified ready-to-eat cereals	Masks neurological complication in people with vitamin B_{12} deficiency.	In view of evidence linking folate intake with neural tube defects in the fetus, it is recommended that all women capable of becoming pregnant consume 400 μg from supplements or fortified foods
(Also known as folic acid, folacin, and pteroylpoly-glutamates. Note: Given as dietary folate equivalents (DFE). 1 DFE = 1 μg food folate = 0.6 μg of folate from fortified food or as a supplement consumed with		0–6 mo	65*	ND			
		7–12 mo	80*	ND			
		Children				No adverse effects associated with folate from food or supplements have been reported.	
		1–3 y	150	300			
		4–8 y	200	400			
		Males					
		9–13 y	300	600			
		14–18 y	400	800			
		19–30 y	400	1000			
		31–50 y	400	1000			
		51–70 y	400	1000			
		>70 y	400	1000			

food = 0.5 μg of a supplement taken on an empty stomach.)

Female			This does not mean that there is no potential for adverse effects resulting from high intakes. Because data on the adverse effects of folate are limited, caution may be warranted.	in addition to intake of food folate from a varied diet.
9-13 y	300	600		It is assumed that women will continue consuming 400 μg from supplements or fortified food until their pregnancy is confirmed and they enter prenatal care, which ordinarily occurs after the end of the periconceptional period—the critical time for formation of the neural tube.
14-18 y	400	800		
19-30 y	400	1000		
31-50 y	400	1000		
51-70 y	400	1000		
>70 y	400	1000		
Pregnancy				
≤18 y	600	800		
19-30 y	600	1000		
31-50 y	600	1000		
Lactation			The UL for folate applies to synthetic forms obtained from supplements and/or fortified foods.	
≤18 y	500	800		
19-30 y	500	1000		
31-50 y	500	1000		

Table continued on following page

Table 3-5 DIETARY REFERENCE INTAKES: VITAMINS *(Continued)*

Nutrient	Function	Life Stage Group	RDA/AI* (mg/d)	UL (mg/d)	Selected Food Sources	Adverse Effects of Excessive Consumption	Special Considerations
Niacin	Coenzyme or cosubstrate in many biological reduction and oxidation reactions, thus required for energy metabolism	Infants			Meat, fish poultry, enriched and whole-grain breads and bread products, fortified ready-to-eat cereals	There is no evidence of adverse effects from the consumption of naturally occurring niacin in foods.	Extra niacin may be required by persons treated with hemodialysis or peritoneal dialysis, or those with malabsorption syndrome.
(Includes nicotinic acid, nicotinic amide, nicotinic acid (pyridine-3-carboxylic acid), and derivatives that exhibit the biological activity of nicotinamide.		0–6 mo	2*	ND			
		7–12 mo	4*	ND			
		Children					
		1–3 y	6	10			
		4–8 y	8	15			
Note: Given as niacin equivalents (NE).		Males				Adverse effects from niacin-containing supplements may include flushing and gastrointestinal distress.	
		9–13 y	12	20			
		14–18 y	16	30			
1 mg of niacin = 60 mg of		19–30 y	16	35			
tryptophan;		31–50 y	16	35			
0–6 months = preformed niacin [not NEJ.)		51–70 y	16	35			
		>70 y	16	35			
		Females					
		9–13 y	12	20			
		14–18 y	14	30			
		19–30 y	14	35			

Nutrient	Function	Life Stage Group	(mg/d)	(mg/d)	Food Sources	Adverse Effects
		31–50 y	14	35		The UL for niacin applies to synthetic forms obtained from supplements, fortified foods, or a combination of the two.
		51–70 y	14	35		
		>70 y	14	35		
		Pregnancy				
		≤18 y	18	30		
		19–30 y	18	35		
		31–50 y	18	35		
		Lactation				
		≤18 y	17	30		
		19–30 y	17	35		
		31–50 y	17	35		
Pantothenic acid	Coenzyme in fatty acid metabolism				Chicken, beef, potatoes, oats, cereals, tomato products, liver, kidney, yeast, egg yolk, broccoli, whole grains	None
		Infants				No adverse effects associated with pantothenic acid from food or supplements have been reported. This does not mean that there is no potential for adverse
		0–6 mo	1.7*	ND		
		7–12 mo	1.8*	ND		
		Children				
		1–3 y	2*	ND		
		4–8 y	3*	ND		
		Males				
		9–13 y	4*	ND		
		14–18 y	5*	ND		
		19–30 y	5*	ND		

Table continued on following page

Table 3-5	DIETARY REFERENCE INTAKES: VITAMINS *(Continued)*					
Nutrient	Function	Life Stage Group	RDA/AI*	UL	Selected Food Sources	Adverse Effects of Excessive Consumption	Special Considerations
		31–50 y	5*	ND		effects resulting from high intakes. Because data on the adverse effects of pantothenic acid are limited, caution may be warranted.	
		51–70 y	5*	ND			
		>70 y	5*	ND			
		Females					
		9–13 y	4*	ND			
		14–18 y	5*	ND			
		19–30 y	5*	ND			
		31–50 y	5*	ND			
		51–70 y	5*	ND			
		>70 y	5*	ND			
		Pregnancy					
		≤18 y	6*	ND			
		19–30 y	6*	ND			
		31–50 y	6*	ND			
		Lactation					
		≤18 y	7*	ND			
		19–30 y	7*	ND			
		31–50 y	7*	ND			

Riboflavin (Also known as Vitamin B$_2$.)	Coenzyme in numerous redox reactions		(mg/d)	(mg/d)	Organ meats, milk, bread products, fortified cereals	No adverse effects associated with riboflavin consumption from food or supplements have been reported. This does not mean that there is no potential for adverse effects resulting from high intakes. Because data on the adverse effects of riboflavin are limited, caution may be warranted.	None
		Infants					
		0–6 mo	0.3*	ND			
		7–12 mo	0.4*	ND			
		Children					
		1–3 y	0.5	ND			
		4–8 y	0.6	ND			
		Males					
		9–13 y	0.9	ND			
		14–18 y	1.3	ND			
		19–30 y	1.3	ND			
		31–50 y	1.3	ND			
		51–70 y	1.3	ND			
		>70 y	1.3	ND			
		Females					
		9–13 y	0.9	ND			
		14–18 y	1.0	ND			
		19–30 y	1.1	ND			
		31–50 y	1.1	ND			
		51–70 y	1.1	ND			
		>70 y	1.1	ND			

Table continued on following page

Table 3–5	DIETARY REFERENCE INTAKES: VITAMINS *(Continued)*						
Nutrient	Function	Life Stage Group	RDA/AI*	UL	Selected Food Sources	Adverse Effects of Excessive Consumption	Special Considerations
		Pregnancy					
		≤18 y	**1.4**	ND			
		19–30 y	**1.4**	ND			
		31–50 y	**1.4**	ND			
		Lactation					
		≤18 y	**1.6**	ND			
		19–30 y	**1.6**	ND			
		31–50 y	**1.6**	ND			
			(mg/d)				
Thiamin	Coenzyme in the metabolism of carbohydrates and branched-chain amino acids	Infants			Enriched, fortified, or whole-grain products; bread and bread products, mixed foods whose main ingredient is	No adverse effects associated with thiamin from food or supplements have been reported. This does not mean that	Persons who may have increased needs for thiamin include those being treated with hemodialysis or peritoneal dialysis, or individuals with
(Also known as Vitamin B_1 and Aneurin)		0–6 mo	0.2*	ND			
		7–12 mo	0.3*	ND			
		Children					
		1–3 y	**0.5**	ND			
		4–8 y	**0.6**	ND			
		Males					
		9–13 y	**0.9**	ND			

14–18 y	1.2	ND
19–30 y	1.2	ND
31–50 y	1.2	ND
51–70 y	1.2	ND
>70 y	1.2	ND
Females		
9–13 y	0.9	ND
14–18 y	1.0	ND
19–30 y	1.1	ND
31–50 y	1.1	ND
51–70 y	1.1	ND
>70 y	1.1	ND
Pregnancy		
≤18 y	1.4	ND
19–30 y	1.4	ND
31–50 y	1.4	ND
Lactation		
≤18 y	1.4	ND
19–30 y	1.4	ND
31–50 y	1.4	ND

grain, and ready-to-eat cereals

there is no potential for adverse effects resulting from high intakes. Because data on the adverse effects of thiamin are limited, caution may be warranted.

malabsorption syndrome.

Table continued on following page

| Table 3-5 | DIETARY REFERENCE INTAKES: VITAMINS *(Continued)* | | | | | | | |

Nutrient	Function	Life Stage Group	RDA/AI*	UL	Selected Food Sources	Adverse Effects of Excessive Consumption	Special Considerations
			(μg/d)	(μg/d)			
Vitamin A	Required for normal vision, gene expression, reproduction, embryonic development and immune function	Infants			Liver, dairy products, fish, darkly colored fruits and leafy vegetables	Teratological effects, liver toxicity	Individuals with high alcohol intake, pre-existing liver disease, hypertlipidemia or severe protein malnutrition may be distinctly susceptible to the adverse effects of excess preformed vitamin A intake.
(Includes provitamin A carotenoids that are dietary precursors of retinol. Note: Given as retinol activity equivalents (RAEs). 1 RAE = 1 μg retinol, 12 μg β-carotene, 24 μg α-carotene, or 24 μg β-cryptoxanthin. To calculate RAEs from REs of provitamin A carotenoids in foods, divide the		0–6 mo	400*	600			
		7–12 mo	500*	600		Note: From preformed vitamin A only.	
		Children					
		1–3 y	300	600			
		4–8 y	400	900			
		Males					β-carotene supplements are advised only to serve as a provitamin A
		9–13 y	600	1700			
		14–18 y	900	2800			
		19–30 y	900	3000			
		31–50 y	900	3000			
		51–70 y	900	3000			
		>70 y	900	3000			
		Females					
		9–13 y	600	1700			
		14–18 y	700	2800			
		19–30 y	700	3000			

		(mg/d)	(mg/d)		
REs by 2. For preformed vitamin A in foods or supplements and for provitamin A carotenoids in supplements, 1 RE = 1 RAE)	31–50 y	**700**	3000		source for individuals at risk of vitamin A deficiency.
	51–70 y	**700**	3000		
	>70 y	**700**	3000		
	Pregnancy				
	≤18 y	**750**	2800		
	19–30 y	**770**	3000		
	31–50 y	**770**	3000		
	Lactation				
	≤18 y	**1200**	2800		
	19–30 y	**1300**	3000		
	31–50 y	**1300**	3000		None
Vitamin B$_6$		(mg/d)	(mg/d)		
Coenzyme in the metabolism of amino acids, glycogen, and sphingoid bases.	Infants			Fortified cereals, organ meats, fortified soy-based meat substitutes	No adverse effects associated with vitamin B$_6$ from food have been reported. This does not mean that there is no potential for adverse effects resulting from high intakes.
	0–6 mo	0.1*	ND		
	7–12 mo	0.3*	ND		
(Vitamin B$_6$ comprises a group of six related compounds: pyridoxal, pyridoxine, pyridoxamine, and 5'-phosphates [PLP, PNP, PMP].)	Children				
	1–3 y	**0.5**	30		
	4–8 y	**0.6**	40		
	Males				
	9–13 y	**1.0**	60		
	14–18 y	**1.3**	80		
	19–30 y	**1.3**	100		

Table continued on following page

Table 3-5	DIETARY REFERENCE INTAKES: VITAMINS *(Continued)*						
Nutrient	Function	Life Stage Group	RDA/AI*	UL	Selected Food Sources	Adverse Effects of Excessive Consumption	Special Considerations
		31–50 y	1.3	100		Because data on the adverse effects of vitamin B$_6$ are limited, caution may be warranted.	
		>70 y	1.7	100			
		Females					
		9–13 y	1.0	60			
		14–18 y	1.2	80			
		19–30 y	1.3	100		Sensory neuropathy has occurred from high intakes of supplemental forms.	
		31–50 y	1.3	100			
		51–70 y	1.3	100			
		>70 y	1.5	100			
		Pregnancy					
		≤18 y	1.9	80			
		19–30 y	1.9	100			
		31–50 y	1.9	100			
		Lactation					
		≤18 y	2.0	80			
		19–30 y	2.0	100			
		31–50 y	2.0	100			

Vitamin B₁₂	Coenzyme in nucleic acid metabolism; prevents megaloblastic anemia	Life stage	(μg/d)		Fortified cereals, meat, fish, poultry	No adverse effects have been associated with the consumption of the amounts of vitamin B₁₂ normally found in foods or supplements. This does not mean that there is no potential for adverse effects resulting from high intakes. Because data on the adverse effects of vitamin B₁₂ are limited, caution may be warranted.	Because 10% to 30% of older people may malabsorb food-bound vitamin B₁₂, it is advisable for those older than 50 to meet their RDA mainly by consuming foods fortified with vitamin B₁₂ or a supplement containing vitamin B₁₂.
(Also known as Cobalamin)		Infants					
		0–6 mo	0.4*	ND			
		7–12 mo	0.5*	ND			
		Children					
		1–3 y	0.9	ND			
		4–8 y	1.2	ND			
		Males					
		9–13 y	1.8	ND			
		14–18 y	2.4	ND			
		19–30 y	2.4	ND			
		31–50 y	2.4	ND			
		51–70 y	2.4	ND			
		>70 y	2.4	ND			
		Females					
		9–13 y	1.8	ND			
		14–18 y	2.4	ND			
		19–30 y	2.4	ND			
		31–50 y	2.4	ND			
		51–70 y	2.4	ND			
		>70 y	2.4	ND			

Table continued on following page

Table 3–5	DIETARY REFERENCE INTAKES: VITAMINS *(Continued)*						
Nutrient	Function	Life Stage Group	RDA/AI*	UL	Selected Food Sources	Adverse Effects of Excessive Consumption	Special Considerations
		Pregnancy					
		≤18 y	**2.6**	ND			
		19–30 y	**2.6**	ND			
		31–50 y	**2.6**	ND			
		Lactation					
		≤18 y	**2.8**	ND			
		19–30 y	**2.8**	ND			
		31–50 y	**2.8**	ND			
			(mg/d)	*(mg/d)*			
Vitamin C	Cofactor for reactions requiring reduced copper or iron metalloenzyme and as a protective antioxidant	Infants			Citrus fruits, tomatoes, tomato juice, potatoes, Brussels sprouts, cauliflower, broccoli, strawberries, cabbage, spinach	Gastrointestinal disturbances, kidney stones, excess iron absorption	Individuals who smoke require an additional 35 mg/d of vitamin C over that needed by nonsmokers.
(Also known as Ascorbic acid and Dehydro-ascorbic acid [DHA])		0–6 mo	40*	ND			
		7–12 mo	50*	ND			Nonsmokers regularly exposed to tobacco smoke
		Children					
		1–3 y	**15**	400			
		4–8 y	**25**	650			
		Males					
		9–13 y	**45**	1200			
		14–18 y	**75**	1800			

are encouraged to ensure they meet the RDA for vitamin C.

19–30 y	**90**	2000
31–50 y	**90**	2000
51–70 y	**90**	2000
>70 y	**90**	2000
Females		
9–13 y	**45**	1200
14–18 y	**65**	1800
19–30 y	**75**	2000
31–50 y	**75**	2000
51–70 y	**75**	2000
>70 y	**75**	2000
Pregnancy		
≤18 y	**80**	1800
19–30 y	**85**	2000
31–50 y	**85**	2000
Lactation		
≤18 y	**115**	1800
19–30 y	**120**	2000
31–50 y	**120**	2000
	($\mu g/d$)	($\mu g/d$)
Infants		
0–6 mo	5*	25
7–12 mo	5*	25

Vitamin D

(Also known as Calciferol.)

Maintain serum calcium and

Fish liver oils, flesh of fatty fish,

Elevated plasma 25 (OH) D concentration

Patients on glucocorticoid therapy may

Table continued on following page

Table 3-5 DIETARY REFERENCE INTAKES: VITAMINS *(Continued)*

Nutrient	Function	Life Stage Group	RDA/AI*	UL	Selected Food Sources	Adverse Effects of Excessive Consumption	Special Considerations
Note: 1 µg calciferol = 40 IU vitamin D. The DRI values are based on the absence of adequate exposure to sunlight.)	phosphorus concentrations.	Children			liver and fat from seals and polar bears, eggs from hens that have been fed vitamin D, fortified milk products, fortified cereals	causing hypercalcemia	require additional vitamin D.
		1–3 y	5*	50			
		4–8 y	5*	50			
		Males					
		9–13 y	5*	50			
		14–18 y	5*	50			
		19–30 y	5*	50			
		31–50 y	5*	50			
		51–70 y	10*	50			
		>70 y	15*	50			
		Females					
		9–13 y	5*	50			
		14–18 y	5*	50			
		19–30 y	5*	50			
		31–50 y	5*	50			
		51–70 y	10*	50			
		>70 y	15*	50			

		(mg/d)	(mg/d)		
Vitamin E	A metabolic function has not yet been identified. Vitamin E's major function appears to be as a non-specific chain-breaking antioxidant.			Vegetable oils, unprocessed cereal grains, nuts, fruits, vegetables, meats	There is no evidence of adverse effects from the consumption of vitamin E naturally occurring in foods.
(Also known as α-tocopherol. Note: α-Tocopherol includes RRR-α-tocopherol, the only form of α-tocopherol that occurs naturally in foods, and the 2R-stereoisomeric forms of α-tocopherol (RRR-, RSR-, RRS-,					
Pregnancy					
≤18 y		5*	50		
19–30 y		5*	50		
31–50 y		5*	50		
Lactation					
≤18 y		5*	50		
19–30 y		5*	50		
31–50 y		5*	50		
Infants					Adverse effects from vitamin E-containing supplements
0–6 mo		4*	ND		
7–12 mo		5*	ND		
Children					
1–3 y		**6**	200		
4–8 y		**7**	300		
Males					
9–13 y		**11**	600		
14–18 y		**15**	800		Patients on anticoagulant therapy should be monitored when taking vitamin E supplements.
19–30 y		**15**	1000		
31–50 y		**15**	1000		
51–70 y		**15**	1000		
>70 y		**15**	1000		

Table continued on following page

Table 3-5	DIETARY REFERENCE INTAKES: VITAMINS *(Continued)*					
Nutrient	Function	Life Stage Group	RDA/AI*	UL	Selected Food Sources	Special Considerations
and *RSS-α-*tocopherol) that occur in fortified foods and supplements. It does not include the 2S-stereoisomeric forms of α-tocopherol (*SRR-, SSR-, SRS-,* and *SSS-*α-tocopherol), also found in fortified foods and supplements.)		Females				
		9–13 y	**11**	600		may include hemorrhagic toxicity.
		14–18 y	**15**	800		
		19–30 y	**15**	1000		The UL for vitamin E applies to any form of α-tocopherol obtained from supplements, fortified foods, or a combination of the two.
		31–50 y	**15**	1000		
		51–70 y	**15**	1000		
		>70 y	**15**	1000		
		Pregnancy				
		≤18 y	**15**	800		
		19–30 y	**15**	1000		
		31–50 y	**15**	1000		
		Lactation				
		≤18 y	**19**	800		
		19–30 y	**19**	1000		
		31–50 y	**19**	1000		

Vitamin K	Coenzyme during the synthesis of many proteins involved in blood clotting and bone metabolism		(μg/d)	Green vegetables (collards, spinach, salad greens, broccoli), Brussels sprouts, cabbage, plant oils, margarine	No adverse effects associated with vitamin K consumption from food or supplements have been reported in humans or animals. This does not mean that there is no potential for adverse effects resulting from high intakes. Because data on the adverse effects of vitamin K are limited, caution may be warranted.	Patients on anticoagulant therapy should monitor vitamin K intake.
	Infants					
	0–6 mo	2.0*	ND			
	7–12 mo	2.5*	ND			
	Children					
	1–3 y	30*	ND			
	4–8 y	55*	ND			
	Males					
	9–13 y	60*	ND			
	14–18 y	75*	ND			
	19–30 y	120*	ND			
	31–50 y	120*	ND			
	51–70 y	120*	ND			
	>70 y	120*	ND			
	Females					
	9–13 y	60*	ND			
	14–18 y	75*	ND			
	19–30 y	90*	ND			
	31–50 y	90*	ND			
	51–70 y	90*	ND			
	>70 y	90*	ND			

Table continued on following page

Table 3-5	DIETARY REFERENCE INTAKES: VITAMINS *(Continued)*						
Nutrient	Function	Life Stage Group	RDA/AI*	UL	Selected Food Sources	Adverse Effects of Excessive Consumption	Special Considerations
		Pregnancy					
		≤18 y	75*	ND			
		19–30 y	90*	ND			
		31–50 y	90*	ND			
		Lactation					
		≤18 y	75*	ND			
		19–30 y	90*	ND			
		31–50 y	90*	ND			

*Recommended Dietary Allowances (RDAs) are in **bold type**. Adequate Intakes (AIs) are denoted with an asterisk. RDAs and AIs may both be used as goals for individual intakes. RDAs are set to meet the needs of almost all (97% to 98 %) individuals in a group. For healthy breastfed infants, the AI is the mean intake. The AI for other life stage and gender groups is believed to cover the needs of all individuals in the group, but lack of cata prevent being able to specify with confidence the percentage of individuals covered by this intake.

UL, The maximum level of daily nutrient intake that is likely to pose no risk of adverse effects. Unless otherwise specified, the UL represents total intake from food, water, and supplements. Due to lack of suitable data, Uls could not be established for vitamin K, thiamine, riboflavin, vitamin B_{12}, pantothenic acid, biotin, or carotenoids. In the absence of Uls, extra caution may be warranted in consuming levels above recommended intakes.

ND, Not determinable due to lack of data of adverse effects in this age group and concern with regard to lack of ability to handle excess amounts. Source of intakes should be from food only to prevent high levels of intake.

Sources: Refs. 1–4. These reports may be accessed via www.nap.edu. Copyright 2001 by The National Academies. All rights reserved. Published with permission.

requirements, vitamins act not only as cofactors but also as pharmacologic agents; in some cases, these two actions are very different. Therefore, it cannot be assumed that at high doses the effects of a supplement are simply those of lower doses amplified.

Because some of the fat-soluble vitamins are stored in the body, excess intake can result in accumulation of toxic quantities. For example, vitamin A taken by an adult in daily doses greater than 50,000 IU for several months can precipitate headaches from increased intracranial pressure (pseudotumor cerebri), liver abnormalities, bone and joint pain, hypercalcemia, and scaling of the skin.

Because most water-soluble vitamins, when present in excess amounts, are excreted in the urine, it has often been said that water-soluble vitamins are less likely to cause toxicity. Although this is true for the most part, water-soluble vitamins can be toxic. Prolonged intake of large doses of vitamin B_6 (pyridoxine) can cause peripheral neuropathy with numbness and paresthesias, especially in the lower extremities. Because these symptoms have been caused by doses as low as 200 mg/day for several months and do not always completely resolve after discontinuation, such use of pyridoxine should be discouraged. The adult UL for pyridoxine is 100 mg/day.

More subtle potential toxicities of high-dose vitamins have emerged only when large populations were carefully monitored. A meta-analysis of large randomized trials of vitamin E supplementation found increased all-cause mortality with doses greater than 400 IU per day.[7] In women with diabetes, daily consumption of 300 mg or more of vitamin C from supplements was associated with increased cardiovascular mortality.[8] The fact that these risks were not observed with multivitamin-dose supplements or with high vitamin intakes from foods indicates that health care practitioners should demand substantial risk-benefit evidence before recommending that healthy people take high-dose micronutrient supplements.

Text continued on p. 136.

Table 3-6	NUTRIENTS: FUNCTIONS, STORES, DEFICIENCIES, ASSESSMENT, TREATMENT, AND TOXICITIES

Proteins/Amino Acids

Functions
Constituents of structural proteins (e.g., muscle), enzymes, antibodies, hormones, neurotransmitters, nucleic acids. Transport other substances in the blood; perform many other vital functions. Diet must provide some (essential); body can synthesize others (nonessential). Provide 4 kcal/g.

Stores, Longevity with Minimal Intake
All lean tissues, months (depends on total energy intake)

Conditions Predisposing to Deficiency
Acute, critical illness (see Chapters 9 and 23); monotonous low-protein diet

Clinical Signs, Symptoms, Syndromes of Deficiency
Hypoproteinemia, edema, easy hair pluckability, skin changes, poor wound healing, lymphopenia, impaired immune function, and many others; many signs due to functional metabolic impairment caused by illness, and not dietary deficiency (see Chapter 9)

Treatment of Deficiency
1.5–4.0 g/kg/day orally, enterally, or parenterally

Lab Tests (normal values)
Serum albumin (3.5–5.5 g/dL)
Serum total iron binding capacity (TIBC) (240–450 µg/dL)
Serum transferrin (200–400mg/dL)

Toxicity/Side Effects
Azotemia can occur at high doses, especially in patients with impaired renal function.

Carbohydrates

Functions
Source of energy (provides 4 kcal/g, 3.4 kcal/g for IV dextrose); stored as glycogen mainly in liver and muscle; main source of dietary fiber

Stores, Longevity with Minimal Intake
Liver and muscle (glycogen), hours (see Chapter 9)

Conditions Predisposing to Deficiency
Diets restricted in total carbohydrate (ketosis) or limited to refined and/or simple carbohydrates (inadequate fiber)

Clinical Signs, Symptoms, Syndromes of Deficiency
Ketosis; constipation from inadequate fiber

Treatment of Deficiency
Adequate amount to prevent ketosis (usually 60 g/day for adults)

	NUTRIENTS: FUNCTIONS, STORES, DEFICIENCIES,
Table 3-6	ASSESSMENT, TREATMENT, AND
	TOXICITIES *(Continued)*

Carbohydrates *(Continued)*

Toxicity/Side Effects
Obesity (calories), dental caries (simple sugars), flatulence and
bulky stools (fiber)

Fats

Functions
Source of energy (provides 9 kcal/g); precursors or constituents of cell
membranes and steroid hormones; essential fatty acids (EFA)
are precursors of prostaglandins, thromboxanes, prostacyclins, and
leukotrienes

Stores, Longevity with Minimal Intake
Adipose tissue, months (depends on total energy intake)

Conditions Predisposing to Deficiency
Anorexia from various causes (energy); prolonged fat-free
parenteral nutrition (EFA, rare)

Clinical Signs, Symptoms, Syndromes of Deficiency
Weight loss if total energy intake is inadequate (see Chapter 9);
EFA deficiency—dry, scaling skin and poor wound healing

Treatment of Deficiency
EFA—250–500 mL lipid intravenously at least 2–3 times/week.
EFA deficiency prevention in TPN patients by daily application of
15–30 mL vegetable oil to the skin (but not a reliable treatment).

Lab Tests (normal values)
EFA (reference laboratory)
Lipoproteins (see Chapter 20)

Toxicity/Side Effects
Obesity; high saturated-fat diets associated with increased risk of
coronary artery disease (see Chapter 20)

Vitamin A (Fat-soluble)

Functions
Ocular rod and cone formation, embryonic development and bone
growth, sperm formation; necessary for growth and
differentiation of epithelial tissues; antioxidant (mainly
β-carotene)

Stores, Longevity with Minimal Intake
Liver (not exclusively), >1year

Table continued on following page

Table 3–6	**NUTRIENTS: FUNCTIONS, STORES, DEFICIENCIES, ASSESSMENT, TREATMENT, AND TOXICITIES** *(Continued)*

Vitamin A (Fat-soluble) *(Continued)*

Conditions Predisposing to Deficiency
Chronic fat malabsorption, insufficient intake (children), inadequate diet (common in developing countries), smoking (β-carotene)

Clinical Signs, Symptoms, Syndromes of Deficiency
Follicular hyperkeratosis, scaling skin, night blindness, male sterility, growth retardation, xerophthalmia, keratomalacia, Bitot's spots, blindness; increased risk for or morbidity from infection, e.g., measles

Treatment of Deficiency
5,000–30,000 IU/day orally; single 100,000 IU injection intramuscularly (IM), possibly repeated after 1–4 weeks

Lab Tests (normal values)
Plasma retinol (25–70 µg/dL)
Plasma total carotene (60–200 µg/dL); can also be fractionated into α- and β-carotene, lutein, zeaxanthin.

Indications for Therapeutic Doses/Megadoses
Measles, Darier's disease

Toxicity/Side Effects
Higher vitamin A intakes associated with decreased bone mineral density and increased hip fracture risk: >50,000 IU/day—dry and itching skin, desquamation, erythematous dermatitis, hair loss, headaches and papilledema from increased intracranial pressure, bone and joint pain, liver injury, hypercalcemia, anorexia, fatigue; >10,000 IU/day during pregnancy—increased the risk of birth defects. High-dose β-carotene supplements increase lung cancer incidence and all-cause mortality in smokers.

Thiamin (Vitamin B$_1$ [Water-soluble])

Functions
Coenzyme in decarboxylation of α-keto acids and in transketolation in the hexosemonophosphate shunt

Stores, Longevity with Minimal Intake
None appreciable, weeks

Conditions Predisposing to Deficiency
Alcohol abuse; inadequate diet, especially with superimposed glucose load (e.g., IV fluids); gastric bypass surgery

Clinical Signs, Symptoms, Syndromes of Deficiency
Precipitated by carbohydrate loading (e.g., IV glucose)
Wet beriberi—cardiomegaly, tachycardia, high-output congestive heart failure

Table 3-6	**NUTRIENTS: FUNCTIONS, STORES, DEFICIENCIES, ASSESSMENT, TREATMENT, AND TOXICITIES** *(Continued)*

Thiamin (Vitamin B$_1$ [Water-soluble]) *(Continued)*

Dry beriberi—peripheral polyneuropathy with paresthesias, hypesthesia, anesthesia
Alcoholic polyneuropathy—myelopathy, cerebellar signs, anorexia, hypothermia
Wernicke-Korsakoff syndrome—confabulation, disorientation, ophthalmoplegia, cerebellar ataxia

Treatment of Deficiency
At least 10–15 mg/day, up to 100 mg/day p.o., IM, or IV (parenteral route is preferable in alcoholics due to decreased absorption)

Lab Tests (normal values)
Whole-blood thiamin (preferred) (1.6–4.0 μg/dL)
Plasma thiamin (0.2–2.0 μg/dL)
Erythrocyte transketolase activity coefficient (deficiency indicated by high level) (1.00–1.23)
Urinary thiamin (≥100 μg/24hr)

Indications for Therapeutic Doses/Megadoses
Transketolase defect (Wernicke-Korsakoff), branched-chain keto acid dehydrogenase and/or decarboxylase deficiency (maple syrup urine disease), pyruvate dehydrogenase deficiency (subacute necrotizing encephalopathy), pyruvate kinase deficiency, thiamine-responsive megaloblastic anemia (in diabetes mellitus)

Toxicity/Side Effects
None documented up to 200 times RDA

Riboflavin (Vitamin B$_2$ [Water-soluble])

Functions
Coenzyme (FAD, FMN) of active prosthetic group of flavoproteins involved with tissue oxidation and respiration

Stores, Longevity with Minimal Intake
None appreciable, weeks

Conditions Predisposing to Deficiency
Inadequate diet (uncommon); alcohol abuse

Clinical Signs, Symptoms, Syndromes of Deficiency
Soreness and burning of lips, mouth, tongue; angular stomatitis; swelling, pain, and magenta coloration of tongue; tearing, burning, and itching of eyes; desquamation and seborrhea (especially nasolabial folds and scrotum)

Treatment of Deficiency
10–15 mg/day p.o. for 1 week

Table continued on following page

| Table 3-6 | **NUTRIENTS: FUNCTIONS, STORES, DEFICIENCIES, ASSESSMENT, TREATMENT, AND TOXICITIES** *(Continued)* |

Riboflavin (Vitamin B$_2$ [Water-soluble]) *(Continued)*

Lab Tests (normal values)
Erythrocyte glutathione reductase (EGR) activity coefficient
(deficiency indicated by high level) (1.00–1.67)
Urine riboflavin (children: >270 µg/g creatinine;
adults ≥80 µg/g creatinine)

Indications for Therapeutic Doses/Megadoses
Carnitine synthetase deficiency with lipid myopathy; acyl-coenzyme A
dehydrogenase deficiency; ethyl-adipic aciduria

Toxicity/Side Effects
None documented at doses well above RDA

Niacin (Vitamin B$_3$ [Water-soluble])

Functions
Component of coenzymes NAD and NADP involved in glycolysis and
tissue respiration

Stores, Longevity with Minimal Intake
None appreciable, weeks

Conditions Predisposing to Deficiency
Inadequate dietary niacin and tryptophan (uncommon), alcohol abuse

Clinical Signs, Symptoms, Syndromes of Deficiency
Pellagra—diarrhea, dermatitis (hyperpigmented scaling in sun-exposed
areas), dementia; tongue can be scarlet, raw, depapillated, painful,
and fissured
Hartnup disease—aminoaciduria, pellagra-like rash, cerebellar ataxia

Treatment of Deficiency
50–500 mg/day p.o. or IV

Lab Tests (normal values)
No reliable clinical assay of niacin status available

Indications for Therapeutic Doses/Megadoses
Hartnup disease (nicotinamide or nicotinic acid), elevated LDL and/or
VLDL cholesterol (nicotinic acid)

Toxicity/Side Effects
Doses >100 mg—flushing (manageable with gradual increase in dose
or use of sustained-release form); possible nausea, vomiting,
diarrhea, liver injury

Pyridoxine (Vitamin B$_6$ [Water-soluble])

Functions
Cofactor in numerous reactions, mostly associated with amino acid
metabolism

	NUTRIENTS: FUNCTIONS, STORES, DEFICIENCIES,
Table 3-6	**ASSESSMENT, TREATMENT, AND**
	TOXICITIES *(Continued)*

Pyridoxine (Vitamin B₆ [Water-soluble]) *(Continued)*

Stores, Longevity with Minimal Intake
None appreciable; weeks (inversely related to protein intake)

Conditions Predisposing to Deficiency
Inadequate diet, especially with high protein intake (clinically
uncommon); drugs that interact

Clinical Signs, Symptoms, Syndromes of Deficiency
Polyneuropathy, oxalate stone formation, seborrheic dermatitis,
microcytic anemia, glossitis, cheilosis, muscular twitching,
convulsions

Treatment of Deficiency
At least 2 mg/day, up to 50 mg/day

Lab Tests (normal values)
Plasma total pyridoxine (5–30 ng/mL)
Erythrocyte aspartate aminotransferase (AST or GOT) activity coefficient
(deficiency indicated by high level) (1.15–1.89)

Indications for Therapeutic Doses/Megadoses
Infantile convulsive disorders, cystathioninuria, homocystinuria,
kynureninase deficiency, ornithine γ-amino transferase deficiency,
sideroblastic anemia, oxaluria

Toxicity/Side Effects
Ataxia and sensory neuropathy with doses as low as 200 mg/day for
several months

Folic Acid (Folacin, Folate [Water-soluble])

Functions
1-carbon (formyl) group transfer; biosynthesis of purine bases, histidine,
choline, and serine; methylation of biological molecules, e.g., DNA

Stores, Longevity with Minimal Intake
Liver, months

Conditions Predisposing to Deficiency
Inadequate diet, intestinal malabsorption, pregnancy, smoking,
antifolate medications

Clinical Signs, Symptoms, Syndromes of Deficiency
Macrocytic anemia, leukopenia, thrombocytopenia, glossitis, stomatitis,
diarrhea, malabsorption (see Chapter 26)
Neural tube defects in babies born to genetically susceptible mothers
with less than optimal diets

Treatment of Deficiency
1 mg/day p.o. or IV

Table continued on following page

| Table 3–6 | **NUTRIENTS: FUNCTIONS, STORES, DEFICIENCIES, ASSESSMENT, TREATMENT, AND TOXICITIES** *(Continued)* |

Folic Acid (Folacin, Folate [Water-soluble]) *(Continued)*

Lab Tests (normal values)
Plasma folate (0–3.3 ng/mL: deficient, 3.4–5.3 ng/mL: indeterminate, 5.4–40.0 ng/mL: normal)
RBC folate (280–903 ng/mL)

Indications for Therapeutic Doses/Megadoses
400 μg/day supplementation recommended for women with child-bearing potential. Megadoses indicated for formiminotransferase deficiency, folate reductase deficiency, hyperhomocysteinemia, homocystinuria; to reverse effects of antifolates such as methotrexate

Toxicity/Side Effects
Can mask vitamin B_{12} deficiency (methyl-folate trap)

Vitamin B_{12} (Water-soluble)

Functions
Isomerization of methylmalonyl CoA to succinyl CoA; interacts with folic acid in methionine synthetase, homocysteine/methionine conversion, methylation reactions, and synthesis of proteins, purines, and pyrimidines

Stores, Longevity with Minimal Intake
Liver, several years

Conditions Predisposing to Deficiency
Pernicious anemia, gastric bypass surgery, resection or disease (e.g., Crohn's) of terminal ileum or stomach, pancreatic insufficiency, intestinal bacterial overgrowth; strict vegetarianism; advanced age

Clinical Signs, Symptoms, Syndromes of Deficiency
Macrocytic anemia (mainly pernicious anemia), leukopenia, thrombocytopenia, stomatitis, glossitis (see Chapter 26), includes peripheral and central neuropathy with decreased vibratory and position senses, paresthesia, unsteady gait, delusions, even psychosis

Treatment of Deficiency
100 μg IM per day for several days or 1000 μg IM once. Maintenance: 100 μg IM or 500 μg nasal gel monthly, or 1000 μg p.o. daily

Lab Tests (normal values)
Plasma B_{12} (200–900 pg/mL)
Serum methylmalonic acid (B_{12} deficiency indicated by elevated level) (0.00–0.40 μmol/L)
Schilling test (see Chapter 26)

Vitamin B$_{12}$ (Water-soluble) *(Continued)*

Indications for Therapeutic Doses/Megadoses
Rare congenital B$_{12}$ metabolism defect (e.g., B$_{12}$-responsive methylmalonic acidemia), homocystinuria

Toxicity/Side Effects
None documented

Biotin (Water-soluble)

Functions
Cofactor for carboxylase enzymes involved in fatty acid, carbohydrate, protein, and cholesterol metabolism

Stores, Longevity with Minimal Intake
Unknown, influenced by intestinal flora synthesis and avidin intake

Conditions Predisposing to Deficiency
Substantial, prolonged consumption of avidin (raw egg whites)

Clinical Signs, Symptoms, Syndromes of Deficiency
Biotin deficiency—hair loss, dermatitis, diarrhea, atrophic lingual papillae, graying of mucous membranes, hypercholesterolemia, electrocardiographic abnormalities
Holoenzyme synthetase deficiency—erythematous rash, persistent vomiting, impaired immune function
Biotinidase deficiency—delayed neuromotor development, nystagmus, hypotonia, impaired immune function, ketosis, accumulation of lactate in tissues

Treatment of Deficiency
300 µg/day for several days

Lab Tests (normal values)
Whole blood biotin (200–500 pg/mL)
Urinary biotin (6–100 µg/24hrs)

Indications for Therapeutic Doses/Megadoses
Holoenzyme synthetase deficiency, biotinidase deficiency, propionic acidemia, β-methylcrotonyl glycinuria

Toxicity/Side Effects
None documented

Vitamin C (Ascorbic Acid [Water-soluble])

Functions
Affects growth of developing cartilage and bone (fibroblasts, osteoblasts, and odontoblasts), hydroxylation of proline and lysine, formation of neurotransmitters (dopamine to norepinephrine, tryptophan to 5-hydroxytryptophan), enhances GI iron absorption and inhibits copper absorption; antioxidant

Table continued on following page

| Table 3–6 | NUTRIENTS: FUNCTIONS, STORES, DEFICIENCIES, ASSESSMENT, TREATMENT, AND TOXICITIES *(Continued)* |

Vitamin C (Ascorbic Acid [Water-soluble]) *(Continued)*

Stores, Longevity with Minimal Intake
None, about 6 weeks

Conditions Predisposing to Deficiency
Inadequate diet with or without physiologic stress from illness; smoking

Clinical Signs, Symptoms, Syndromes of Deficiency
Scurvy—follicular hyperkeratosis, corkscrew hairs, perifollicular
  petechiae, ecchymoses, bleeding of gums (in patients with teeth)
  and multiple other sites, dry skin, dry mouth, scorbutic arthritis,
  impaired wound healing

Treatment of Deficiency
Up to 1–2 g/day

Lab Tests (normal values)
Plasma vitamin C (0.4–2.0 mg/dL); scurvy indicated when level <0.2

Indications for Therapeutic Doses/Megadoses
Chédiak-Higashi disease; 1–2 g/day to enhance compromised wound
  healing

Toxicity/Side Effects
Occasional diarrhea; increased uric acid excretion; possible interference
  with tests for urine glucose (false positive with copper reagents,
  false negative with glucose-oxidase method) and stool occult blood
  (false negative); possible impairment of anticoagulant therapy;
  possible increased cardiovascular mortality with supplements
  ≥300 mg per day in women with diabetes.

Pantothenic Acid (Water-soluble)

Functions
Integral component of coenzyme A, involved in fatty acid and
  cholesterol synthesis, and lipid, carbohydrate, and amino acid
  metabolism

Stores, Longevity with Minimal Intake
Unknown, weeks

Conditions Predisposing to Deficiency
Rare genetic defect in pantothenate-kinase 2 enzyme

Clinical Signs, Symptoms, Syndromes of Deficiency
None well documented

Treatment of Deficiency
Uncertain because of unclear existence of deficiency

Lab Tests (normal values)
Whole blood pantothenic acid (100 to 300 µg/dL)

Table 3-6	**NUTRIENTS: FUNCTIONS, STORES, DEFICIENCIES, ASSESSMENT, TREATMENT, AND TOXICITIES** *(Continued)*

Pantothenic Acid (Water-soluble) *(Continued)*

Indications for Therapeutic Doses/Megadoses
None

Toxicity/Side Effects
Occasional diarrhea with 10–20 g/day

Vitamin D (Fat-soluble)

Functions
Facilitates calcium and phosphorus absorption and utilization, maintenance of skeletal integrity

Stores, Longevity with Minimal Intake
Liver and skin, months to years (depends on sun exposure)

Conditions Predisposing to Deficiency
Chronic fat malabsorption, gastric bypass surgery, renal insufficiency; breast feeding without supplemental vitamin D; inadequate sun exposure, advanced age

Clinical Signs, Symptoms, Syndromes of Deficiency
Rickets (children)—bony deformities due to enlargement of epiphyseal growth plates, stunted growth
Osteomalacia (adults)—bone pain and tenderness, pathologic fractures, proximal muscle weekness, hypocalcemia, hypophosphatemia (see Chapter 28)

Treatment of Deficiency
Rickets—1,000 IU/day
Osteomalacia—50,000 IU/day vitamin D_3 or 50 µg/day calcifediol

Lab Tests (normal values, higher in summer, lower in winter)
Serum 25-OH vitamin D (20–57 ng/mL (as reported by clinical laboratories; a lower limit of 32 ng/mL may be more appropriate to prevent secondary hyperparathyroidism and bone loss)
Serum 1,25-$(OH)_2$ vitamin D (15–75 pg/mL)

Indications for Therapeutic Doses/Megadoses
Osteoporosis, vitamin D dependency, familial hypophosphatemia

Toxicity/Side Effects
Serum 25-OH vitamin D level >400 ng/mL associated with weakness, fatigue, headache, nausea, vomiting, hypercalcemia, and impaired renal function; can cause growth arrest in children

Vitamin E (Fat-soluble)

Functions
Antioxidant, free radical scavenger (primarily in membranes)

Table continued on following page

Table 3–6	**NUTRIENTS: FUNCTIONS, STORES, DEFICIENCIES, ASSESSMENT, TREATMENT, AND TOXICITIES** (Continued)

Vitamin E (Fat-soluble) (Continued)

Stores, Longevity with Minimal Intake
Liver, cell membranes, all lipid-rich tissues; years

Conditions Predisposing to Deficiency
Severe long-term fat malabsorption, prematurity, genetic defects
    (Friedreich's ataxia, a-beta-lipoproteinemia)

Clinical Signs, Symptoms, Syndromes of Deficiency
Hemolytic anemia, retinopathy, and bronchopulmonary dysplasia in
    premature newborns
Neuropathy and myopathy with creatinuria in adults with severe,
    longstanding malabsorption

Treatment of Deficiency
0.2–2 g/day (200–2000 IU) p.o.

Lab Tests (normal values)
Serum tocopherol (0.6–1.4 mg/dL, lower in patients with low blood
    lipids, higher in patients with hyperlipidemia)

Indications for Therapeutic Doses/Megadoses
Premature birth, chronic cholestasis, pancreatic insufficiency,
    uncontrolled celiac disease
Inborn errors such as glucose-6-phosphate dehydrogenase deficiency,
    glutathione peroxidase deficiency, glutathione synthetase deficiency,
    thalassemia major, and sickle cell anemia
Intermittent claudication (peripheral atherosclerosis)

Toxicity/Side Effects
Generally thought to be harmless, but supplementary doses
    ≥400 IU/day may increase risk of bleeding and
    all-cause mortality

Vitamin K (Fat-soluble)

Functions
Carboxylation of glutamic acid residues in formation of clotting
    factors II, VII, IX, and X, and bone proteins

Stores, Longevity with Minimal Intake
Liver, cell membranes; weeks (despite synthesis by intestinal flora,
    shortened by antibiotic use)

Conditions Predisposing to Deficiency
Hemolytic disease of the newborn; anticoagulant therapy;
    fat malabsorption; inadequate diet plus antibiotic use (uncommon
    except in hospitalized patients)

Clinical Signs, Symptoms, Syndromes of Deficiency
Increased prothrombin time, ecchymoses, bleeding

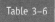

Vitamin K (Fat-soluble) *(Continued)*

Treatment of Deficiency
5–10 mg IV or IM to restore prothrombin time to normal
Newborn infants: routine single dose of 0.5–1.0 mg IM at birth

Lab Tests (normal values)
Prothrombin time (12.0–15.5 seconds; International Normalized
  Ratio (INR) used in patients on warfarin anticoagulation therapy)

Indications for Therapeutic Doses/Megadoses
Parenchymal liver disease with hypoprothrombinemia

Toxicity/Side Effects
None documented

Calcium

Functions
Forms structure of bones and teeth; integral to neurotransmission,
  muscle contraction, and blood clotting

Stores, Longevity with Minimal Intake
Bones, years

Conditions Predisposing to Deficiency
Inadequate diet, malabsorption, vitamin D deficiency, magnesium
  deficiency; gastric bypass surgery

Clinical Signs, Symptoms, Syndromes of Deficiency
Hypoparathyroidism: paresthesias, neuromuscular excitability, muscle
  cramps, tetany, and convulsions
Osteoporosis and osteomalacia: bone fractures, bone pain, height loss
  (see Chapter 28)

Treatment of Deficiency
Osteoporosis, osteomalacia, and hypoparathyroidism: supplementation
  with calcium (see Table 3–2) and vitamin D (see above)

Lab Tests (normal values)
Serum calcium (8.5–10.5 mg/dL)
Urine calcium (30–250 mg/24 hr)

Indications for Therapeutic Doses/Megadoses
None

Toxicity/Side Effects
Constipation, rarely kidney stones

Chloride

Functions
Principal extracellular anion, plays a key role in fluid and
  electrolyte balance; acidifies gastric juice

Table continued on following page

Table 3-6	**NUTRIENTS: FUNCTIONS, STORES, DEFICIENCIES, ASSESSMENT, TREATMENT, AND TOXICITIES** *(Continued)*

Chloride *(Continued)*

Stores, Longevity with Minimal Intake
None, days (depletion very unusual without sodium depletion)

Conditions Predisposing to Deficiency
Chloride-free parenteral fluids, sodium depletion (e.g., heavy sweating), gastric suction or prolonged vomiting

Clinical Signs, Symptoms, Syndromes of Deficiency
Volume depletion

Treatment of Deficiency
About 60 mEq/day NaCl p.o. or IV

Lab Tests (normal values)
Serum chloride (95–108 mEq/L)

Indications for Therapeutic Doses/Megadoses
None

Toxicity/Side Effects
Possible elevated blood pressure

Chromium

Functions
Cofactor for insulin in glucose metabolism

Stores, Longevity with Minimal Intake
Unknown

Conditions Predisposing to Deficiency
Chromium-free parenteral nutrition (rare)

Clinical Signs, Symptoms, Syndromes of Deficiency
Glucose intolerance, peripheral neuropathy, weight loss

Treatment of Deficiency
200 µg/day chromium chloride or 10 g/day Brewer's yeast

Lab Tests
Serum and urine chromium used clinically only to detect toxic levels

Indications for Therapeutic Doses/Megadoses
Toxicity/Side Effects
Only documented after industrial exposure; none documented at 50–200 µg/day

Copper

Functions
Influences iron absorption and mobilization; a component of a number of metalloenzymes, e.g., ceruloplasmin, lysyloxidase, cytochrome C, superoxide dismutase

Table 3–6	**NUTRIENTS: FUNCTIONS, STORES, DEFICIENCIES, ASSESSMENT, TREATMENT, AND TOXICITIES** (Continued)

Copper (Continued)

Stores, Longevity with Minimal Intake
Unknown

Conditions Predisposing to Deficiency
Upper gastrointestinal resection or bypass; copper-free parenteral
nutrition

Clinical Signs, Symptoms, Syndromes of Deficiency
Menkes' Disease (genetic)—mental deterioration, hypothermia, defective
keratinization of hair, metaphyseal lesions, degeneration of aortic
elastin, depigmentation of hair
Microcytic anemia indistinguishable from iron deficiency anemia;
neutropenia (see Chapter 26)

Treatment of Deficiency
Copper sulfate 2–4 mg/day p.o or 2.5 mg/day IV

Lab Tests (normal values)
Serum copper (70–190 µg/dL [adults])
Serum ceruloplasmin (20–60 mg/dL)
Urine copper (3–50 µg/24 hrs)

Indications for Therapeutic Doses/Megadoses
None

Toxicity/Side Effects
Doses >15 mg can cause nausea, vomiting, headache, diarrhea, and
abdominal cramps
Wilson Disease (genetic)—possible chronic copper toxicity (hepatic
cirrhosis, accumulation in kidney and brain)

Fluoride (Fluorine)

Functions
Protects against dental caries

Stores, Longevity with Minimal Intake
Unknown

Clinical Signs, Symptoms,
Syndromes of Deficiency
Dental caries (true requirement in humans is debatable)

Treatment of Deficiency
1–2 mg/day sodium fluoride for persons living in nonfluoridated
areas

Indication for Therapeutic Doses/Megadoses
Toxicity/Side Effects
Dental and skeletal fluorosis (mottling)

Table continued on following page

Table 3-6	**NUTRIENTS: FUNCTIONS, STORES, DEFICIENCIES, ASSESSMENT, TREATMENT, AND TOXICITIES** *(Continued)*

Iodine

Functions
Component of thyroid hormones

Stores, Longevity with Minimal Intake
Thyroid gland, unknown

Conditions Predisposing to Deficiency
Inadequate diet (common in developing countries)

Clinical Signs, Symptoms, Syndromes of Deficiency
Goiter, hypothyroidism

Treatment of Deficiency
2 g/day iodized salt

Lab Tests (normal values)
Serum thyroxine (T_4) (5–14 µg/dL)
Serum total triiodothyronine (T_3) (80–200 ng/dL)
Seum TSH (0.3–5 mU/L)

Indications for Therapeutic Doses/Megadoses
None

Toxicity/Side Effects
>2 mg/day may induce goiter

Iron

Functions
Oxygen transport (hemoglobin and myoglobin), electron transport (cytochromes)

Stores, Longevity with Minimal Intake
Bone marrow, liver, spleen (ferritin, hemosiderin); months

Conditions Predisposing to Deficiency
Blood loss (commonly menstrual or gastrointestinal); inadequate diet (common in infancy and adolescence); gastrectomy, gastric bypass surgery; pregnancy

Clinical Signs, Symptoms, Syndromes of Deficiency
Microcytic anemia, pallor, fatigue, glossitis, tachycardia (see Chapter 26)

Treatment of Deficiency
325 mg ferrous sulfate p.o. t.i.d., preferably with vitamin C, for 2–6 months to rebuild iron stores; ~1,000 mg IV × 1 when GI absorption is impaired

Lab Tests (normal values)
Serum iron (30–170 µg/dL)
Total iron binding capacity (240–450 µg/dL)

Table 3-6	**NUTRIENTS: FUNCTIONS, STORES, DEFICIENCIES, ASSESSMENT, TREATMENT, AND TOXICITIES** *(Continued)*

Iron *(Continued)*

Indications for Therapeutic Doses/Megadoses
Chronic Blood Loss, Malabsorption
Toxicity/Side Effects
Hemochromatosis and/or hemosiderosis (iron overload)

Magnesium

Functions
Associated with more than 300 enzyme systems, especially
  in metabolism of ATP; therefore, participates in glucose
  utilization, synthesis of proteins, fats, and nucleic acids,
  muscle contraction, membrane transport systems, and
  neurotransmission

Stores, Longevity with Minimal Intake
Bones, muscles, soft tissues; about 3 weeks

Conditions Predisposing to Deficiency
Malabsorption, alcohol abuse, protein-energy malnutrition

Clinical Signs, Symptoms, Syndromes of Deficiency
Hypocalcemia, hypokalemia, paresthesias, neuromuscular
  excitability, muscle spasms, progressing to tetany, seizures,
  and coma

Treatment of Deficiency
250–500 mg magnesium oxide p.o. b.i.d. to q.i.d.; or 1–2 g/day
  IV or IM

Lab Tests (normal values)
Serum magnesium (1.8–2.4 mg/dL)
Urinary magnesium (12–200 mg/24 hrs)

Indications for Therapeutic Doses/Megadoses
Constipation

Toxicity/Side Effects
Diarrhea; accumulation in patients with impaired renal function
  can cause decreased neurotransmission and cardiorespiratory
  dysfunction

Manganese

Functions
Cofactor in many enzymes; involved in glycosyl transferases,
  gluconeogenesis, lipid metabolism, and mucopolysaccharide
  metabolism

Stores, Longevity with Minimal Intake
Unknown

Table continued on following page

Table 3-6	**NUTRIENTS: FUNCTIONS, STORES, DEFICIENCIES, ASSESSMENT, TREATMENT, AND TOXICITIES** *(Continued)*

Manganese *(Continued)*

Clinical Signs, Symptoms, Syndromes of Deficiency
None well documented

Treatment of Deficiency—Lab Tests (normal values)
Serum manganese (0–8 µg/L)

Indications for Therapeutic Doses/Megadoses
None

Toxicity/Side Effects
Manganese oxide inhaled by miners can cause neuropsychiatric
    problems

Molybdenum

Functions
Cofactor in oxidase enzymes

Stores, Longevity with Minimal Intake
Unknown

Conditions Predisposing to Deficiency
Prolonged molybdenum-free parenteral nutrition (rare)

Clinical Signs, Symptoms, Syndromes of Deficiency
Tachycardia, tachypnea, stupor, and coma reported in one long-term
    parenterally fed patient

Treatment of Deficiency
300 µg/day IV

Lab Tests (normal values)
Serum molybdenum (2.9–12 nmol/L)

Indications for Therapeutic Doses/Megadoses
None

Toxicity/Side Effects
No clear syndrome documented

Phosphorus

Functions
Constituent of nucleic acids and cell membranes; essential in
    glycolysis and (as ATP) in all energy-requiring reactions; involved in
    modulation of tissue calcium concentrations and maintenance
    of acid/base equilibrium

Stores, Longevity with Minimal Intake
Bones, years (serum levels can drop within hours in starved patients
    given glucose loads)

Table 3–6	**NUTRIENTS: FUNCTIONS, STORES, DEFICIENCIES, ASSESSMENT, TREATMENT, AND TOXICITIES** (Continued)

Phosphorus (Continued)

Conditions Predisposing to Deficiency
Glucose load (e.g., parenteral nutrition) in starved cachectic patients (see Chapter 11); vitamin D deficiency, hyperparathyroidism, chronic acidosis; alcohol abuse, phosphate-binding antacids

Clinical Signs, Symptoms, Syndromes of Deficiency
Depletion caused by renal tubular disease or parenteral nutrition without adequate phosphorus supplementation can cause muscle weakness with cardiorespiratory failure, glucose intolerance, diminished red blood cell, leukocyte, and platelet function (see Chapter 11)

Children also show growth retardation, skeletal deformities, and bone pain

Treatment of Deficiency
Serum phosphorus 1.0–2.5 mg/dL: 1 mmol/kg IV or p.o. over 24 hrs

Serum phosphorus <1.0 mg/dL: 1.5 mmol/kg IV over 24 hrs

Lab Tests (normal values)
Serum phosphorus (adults: 2.5–4.5 mg/dl; children [varies by age]: 4.0–7.0 mg/dL)

Urinary phosphorus (400–1300 mg/24 hrs)

Indications for Therapeutic Doses/Megadoses
Toxicity/Side Effects
Diarrhea resulting from oral phosphorus supplementation; secondary hyperparathyroidism and calcification of soft tissues from poor excretion in renal disease

Potassium

Functions
Principal intracellular cation; nerve impulse transmission; skeletal and autonomic muscle contraction; blood pressure maintenance

Stores, Longevity with Minimal Intake
None; days

Conditions Predisposing to Deficiency
Gastrointestinal fluid losses (e.g., gastric suctioning, vomiting, diarrhea), renal reabsorptive defects, diuretics, laxatives, potassium-free parenteral fluids

Clinical Signs, Symptoms, Syndromes of Deficiency
Muscle weakness, tetany, cardiac arrhythmias, hypotension, respiratory failure, ileus

Table continued on following page

Table 3-6	**NUTRIENTS: FUNCTIONS, STORES, DEFICIENCIES, ASSESSMENT, TREATMENT, AND TOXICITIES** *(Continued)*

Potassium *(Continued)*

Treatment of Deficiency
20–60 mEq KCL p.o. or (gradually) IV

Lab Tests (normal values)
Serum potassium (3.3–5.0 mEq/L)

Indications for Therapeutic Doses/Megadoses
None

Toxicity/Side Effects
Cardiac arrhythmias and arrest

Selenium

Functions
Scavenges free radicals and protects against lipid peroxidation, as a component of glutathione peroxidase and in association with vitamin E

Stores, Longevity with Minimal Intake
None appreciable; years

Conditions Predisposing to Deficiency
Consumption of foods from areas with low soil selenium content; prolonged low-selenium parenteral nutrition (rare)

Clinical Signs, Symptoms, Syndromes of Deficiency
Cardiomyopathy (Keshan Disease) and increased cancer rates (both mainly reported in China), nail changes

Treatment of Deficiency
200–400 µg/day

Lab Tests (normal values)
Serum or whole blood selenium (23–190 µg/L)

Indications for Therapeutic Doses/Megadoses
None

Toxicity/Side Effects
Hair loss, brittle fingernails, fatigue, irritability

Sodium

Functions
Principal extracellular cation; primary regulator of fluid and electrolyte balance; blood pressure maintenance

Stores, Longevity with Minimal Intake
None, days

Table 3-6	**NUTRIENTS: FUNCTIONS, STORES, DEFICIENCIES, ASSESSMENT, TREATMENT, AND TOXICITIES** *(Continued)*

Sodium *(Continued)*

Conditions Predisposing to Deficiency
Sodium-free parenteral fluids; heavy sweating; gastrointestinal fluid losses (e.g., gastric suctioning, vomiting, diarrhea); diuresis from drugs or other causes; inappropriate antidiuretic hormone secretion (SIADH); psychogenic polydypsia

Clinical Signs, Symptoms, Syndromes of Deficiency
Volume depletion

Treatment of Deficiency
NaCl, ≥60 mEq/day, p.o. or IV

Lab Test (normal values)
Serum sodium (135–145 mEq/L)

Indications for Therapeutic Doses/Megadoses
None

Toxicity/Side Effect
Edema, hypertension

Zinc

Functions
Cofactor for over 70 enzymes involved in growth, sexual maturation, fertility and reproduction, night vision, taste acuity, and immune function

Stores, Longevity with Minimal Intake
Bone, muscle (available pool is small), months (influenced by dietary protein, phosphorus, and iron)

Conditions Predisposing to Deficiency
Malabsorption or chronic losses or drainage of upper intestinal fluid or exudative material; critical illness (e.g., trauma, burns, surgery), sickle-cell disease, nephrotic syndrome, dialysis

Clinical Signs, Symptoms, Syndromes of Deficiency
Growth retardation, hypogonadism, impaired taste and smell, poor wound healing, lethargy, poor appetite; dry, scaling, hyperpigmented skin; cellular immune deficiency, acrodermatitis enteropathica (hereditary)

Treatment of Deficiency
60 mg elemental zinc (e.g., zinc sulfate 220 mg) p.o. q.d. to t.i.d. or 5–10 mg/day element zinc IV

Lab Tests (normal values)
Serum zinc (65–290 µg/dL)
Urinary zinc (150–1200 µg/24 hrs)

Table continued on following page

Table 3-6	**NUTRIENTS: FUNCTIONS, STORES, DEFICIENCIES, ASSESSMENT, TREATMENT, AND TOXICITIES** (Continued)

Zinc (Continued)

Indications for Therapeutic Doses/Megadoses

Therapeutic doses (same levels as for deficiency) for possible enhancement of compromised wound healing in patients with increased requirements resulting from severe physiologic stress or with increased zinc losses

Toxicity/Side Effects

Possible interference with iron or copper metabolism (sideroblastic anemia); possible impairment of immune function

---

For additional information on functions, food sources, and potential adverse effects of excessive consumption, see the DRI tables (Tables 3–1 through 3–5). For detailed nutrient content data, see the USDA Nutrient Data Laboratory website, http://www.nal.usda.gov/fnic/foodcomp/.

Conditions predisposing to deficiency are generally those encountered in the United States. Many of these conditions can result in deficiency even when intake of the nutrient is consistent with the RDA. Specific (e.g., inherited) syndromes in which the nutrient deficiency is a central feature are considered under the heading *Clinical signs, symptoms, syndromes of deficiency*.

Normal values vary among laboratories and age groups, and should be considered approximate. Many of those listed were obtained at http://www.aruplab.com. Activity coefficients, which are derived from a laboratory method to assess thiamin, riboflavin, and pyridoxine status, involve measuring the plasma or erythrocyte activity of an enzyme that requires the respective vitamin as a cofactor. The equation used to calculate activity coefficient follows:

Enzyme activity with the vitamin added to the assay tube

Enzyme activity without additional vitamin

When a vitamin deficiency is present, the enzyme activity increases with addition of the vitamin to the assay tube, making the ratio greater than 1; therefore, high activity coefficients indicate deficiency.

The term *megadoses* is used to indicate established or widely accepted uses of nutrients at levels beyond those required to maintain nutritional sufficiency (RDA) or to correct deficiency. Generally, a megadose is greater than 10 times the RDA.

The known toxicities of other vitamins and minerals are listed in Table 3–6; clinical findings in some vitamin toxicities are also shown in Table 10–2.

REFERENCES

1. Food and Nutrition Board, Institute of Medicine: Dietary Reference Intakes for Calcium, Phosphorus, Magnesium, Vitamin D, and Fluoride. Washington, DC, Institute of Medicine, National Academy Press, 1997; http://www.nap.edu/books/0309063507/html/index.html.

2. Food and Nutrition Board, Institute of Medicine: Dietary Reference Intakes for Thiamin, Riboflavin, Niacin, Vitamin B6, Folate, Vitamin B12, Pantothenic Acid, Biotin, and Choline. Washington, DC, Institute of Medicine, National Academy Press, 1998; http://www.nap.edu/books/0309065542/html/index.html.

3. Food and Nutrition Board, Institute of Medicine: Dietary Reference Intakes for Vitamin C, Vitamin E, Selenium, and Carotenoids. Washington, DC, Institute of Medicine, National Academy Press, 2000; http://www.nap.edu/books/0309069351/html/index.html.

4. Food and Nutrition Board, Institute of Medicine: Dietary Reference Intakes for Vitamin A, Vitamin K, Arsenic, Boron, Chromium, Copper, Iodine, Iron, Manganese, Molybdenum, Nickel, Silicon, Vanadium, and Zinc. Washington, DC, Institute of Medicine, National Academy Press, 2000; http://www.nap.edu/books/0309072794/html/index.html.

5. Food and Nutrition Board, Institute of Medicine: Dietary Reference Intakes for Energy, Carbohydrate, Fiber, Fat, Fatty Acids, Cholesterol, Protein, and Amino Acids (Macronutrients). Washington, DC, Institute of Medicine, National Academy Press, 2002; http://www.nap.edu/books/0309085373/html/index.html.

6. Food and Nutrition Board, Institute of Medicine: Dietary Reference Intakes for Water, Potassium, Sodium, Chloride, and Sulfate. Washington, DC, Institute of Medicine, National Academy Press, 2004; http://www.nap.cdu/books/0309091691/html/index.html.

7. Miller ER, Pastor-Barriuso R, Dalal D, et al: Meta-analysis: High-dosage vitamin E supplementation may increase all-cause mortality. Ann Intern Med 142:37–46, 2005.

8. Lee D-H, Folsom AR, Harnack L, et al: Does supplemental vitamin C increase cardiovascular disease risk in women with diabetes? Am J Clin Nutr 80:1194–1200, 2005.

SUGGESTED READINGS

Fairfield KM, Fletcher RH: Vitamins for chronic disease prevention in adults: Scientific review. JAMA 287:3116–3126, 2002.

Fletcher RH, Fairfield KM: Vitamins for chronic disease prevention in adults: Clinical applications. JAMA 287:3127–3129, 2002.

Heimburger DC, McLaren DS, Shils ME: Clinical manifestations of micronutrient deficiencies and toxicities: A resume. In Shils ME, Shike M, Ross AC, et al (eds): Modern Nutrition in Health and Disease, 10th ed. Baltimore, Lippincott Williams & Wilkins, 2005.

4

Pregnancy and Lactation

JANET D. TISDALE, MPH, RD

Pregnancy and lactation are critical times when maternal nutrition is important in influencing the health of both mother and infant. Women of childbearing age need to maintain good nutritional status before, during, and after pregnancy. Pregnancy causes major metabolic and physiologic changes that influence the nutritional needs of a woman during pregnancy.

Normal Changes in Pregnancy

Many changes occur during pregnancy that maintain the mother's health while allowing for the development of the fetus (Table 4–1). These changes affect the mother's

Table 4-1	NORMAL CHANGES AND DISCOMFORTS IN PREGNANCY		
Change	**Basis for Change**	**Trimester**	**Relief Measures**
GI System Taste Nausea and vomiting Digestion	Progesterone $\in\downarrow$GI motility HCG/Estrogen Nausea and vomiting	All	Small meals $\uparrow$Carbohydrate $\uparrow$Fiber $\uparrow$Water
Cardiovascular and Pulmonary Systems Dyspnea $\Uparrow$Cardiac Output Edema	Progesterone $\uparrow$O$_2$ $\downarrow$CO$_2$ Vasodilatation Hypotension	1st and 2nd 3rd	Avoid sudden changes Good posture Small meals Adequate fluids
Urinary System Frequent Urination	$\uparrow$Renal filtration	All	Drink fluids early in the day

nutritional status by increasing her energy and nutrient needs. An increase in reproductive hormone levels significantly alters maternal metabolism. Increased levels of human chorionic gonadatropin, human placental lactogen, progesterone, estrogen, prolactin, and cortisol support fetal growth and development. In addition, the plasma volume increases out of proportion to the expansion of red blood cells, causing hemodilution and a drop in the hematocrit. As a result of the increased circulating plasma volume, there is an increase in cardiac output and basal metabolic rate.

Physiologic changes also affect the gastrointestinal, pulmonary, renal, and endocrine systems. Changes in the gastrointestinal tract produce symptoms that can have a major impact on the mother's nutritional status. Heartburn results from the enlarging uterus pushing against the stomach and intestines. Progesterone decreases the integrity of the lower esophageal sphincter, allowing reflux of food and acid. Constipation results from progesterone slowing the peristaltic action of smooth muscles in the bowel along with the displacement of internal organs by the enlarging uterus. Morning sickness or nausea and vomiting is also a common problem during pregnancy.

Maternal and Fetal Weight Gain

Birth weight is the best indicator of a newborn's health. Low prepregnant weight and inadequate weight gain during pregnancy are the most significant contributors to intrauterine growth retardation and low birth weight. Prepregnancy body mass index (BMI) is used to establish a target for total weight gain in pregnancy (Table 4–2). Special consideration should be given to women with low (BMI <19.8) and high (BMI >29) prepregnant weights. Excessive weight gain, especially in women with a BMI >29, should be discouraged to prevent poor maternal and fetal outcomes including postpartum weight retention. Aside from the weight of the developing baby, additional fat is laid down between maternal organs. Expanded uterus and breast tissue add to the weight gain of the

Table 4-2	RECOMMENDED WEIGHT GAIN IN PREGNANCY	
Prepregnancy BMI	**Pounds**	**Kilograms**
Low (BMI <19.8)	28–40	12.5–18
Normal (BMI 19.8–26)	25–35	11.5–16
High (BMI 26–29)	15–25	7–11.5
Obese (BMI >29)	>15	>7
Twins	34–45	15.9–20.4
Triplets/Multiples	>50	>22.7

BMI, Body mass index.
Source: Position of the American Dietetic Association: Nutrition and lifestyle for a healthy pregnancy outcome. J Am Diet Assoc 102: 1479–1490, 2002.

mother, as does a dramatic increase in fluid and blood volume. Table 4-3 details the components of maternal weight gain.

Maternal characteristics associated with low gestational weight gain include age at time of conception (younger than 18 or older than 35); low socioeconomic status; history of previous pregnancy complications (spontaneous abortion, birth weight of less than 2750 grams, or delivery before 37 weeks of gestation); maternal height less than 62 inches; hypertension; use of alcohol, tobacco, or drugs; and restrictive eating habits

Table 4-3	NORMAL COMPONENTS OF MATERNAL WEIGHT GAIN DURING PREGNANCY
Organ, Tissue, or Fluid	**Weight (g)**
Uterus	970
Breasts	450
Blood	1250
Water	1680
Fat	3350
Maternal Components	*= 7700*
Fetus	3400
Placenta	650
Amniotic fluid	800
Non-Maternal Components	*= 4850*
Total (All Components)	*= 12550*

or excessive exercise. Maintaining activity and exercise at lower intensity levels (such as walking or swimming) is encouraged during pregnancy. However, pregnant women who continue to exercise should maintain an adequate intake of calories, nutrients, and fluids to support weight gain.

Specific Nutrient Needs during Pregnancy and Lactation

Pregnancy

A pregnant woman's energy needs do not increase during the first trimester of pregnancy. During the second and third trimesters, the energy demands of pregnancy increase by approximately 300–400 kcal per day. This should be matched by a balanced increase in calorie intake from proteins, fats, and carbohydrates. The major fuel source for the mother is fat, whereas carbohydrates or glucose are the major fuel source for the fetus. The Dietary Reference Intake (DRI) for protein during pregnancy is an additional 25 g over the non-pregnant state, or 1.2 g/kg body weight. In addition to being a major fuel source for the mother, dietary fat is also key for supporting fetal growth and brain development. Specifically, docosahexaenoic acid (DHA) and arachidonic acid (AA)—two long chain polyunsaturated fats (PUFA)—are critical during the third trimester of pregnancy and the first months of life. DHA, an omega-3 fatty acid, is found primarily in fish (tuna, salmon, sardines, etc.). However, the U.S. Food and Drug Administration (FDA) warns against pregnant women eating large predatory fish (shark, swordfish, king mackerel, or tilefish) due to high levels of mercury in these fish. To reduce exposure to the harmful effects of mercury, it is recommended that pregnant women eat up to 12 ounces (two average meals) a week of shrimp, canned light tuna, salmon, pollock, and catfish or up to 6 ounces of albacore ("white") tuna.

Adequate fetal growth requires more than just a supply of energy and protein. It is important to consider the role of vitamins and minerals in growth and development of new cells. Specific nutrients to consider are folic acid, calcium, iron, and zinc. The DRI for folic acid during pregnancy is 600 µg. The U.S. Public Health Service has recommended that all women of childbearing age capable of becoming pregnant should consume 400 µg of folic acid daily to reduce the incidence of neural tube defects such as spina bifida and myelomeningocele. The American College of Obstetricians and Gynecologists recommends that women who are planning a pregnancy and have previously had a child with a neural tube defect take 4 mg of folic acid daily beginning 1 month prior to conception and continuing through the first 3 months of pregnancy. As of January 1998, the FDA requires all enriched cereal grains to be fortified with folic acid (140 µg of folic acid per 100 g of grain).

The Adequate Intake (AI) for calcium during pregnancy is between 1000 and 1300 mg, depending on the woman's age. Because of increased efficiency of calcium absorption, calcium requirements during pregnancy are similar to that of nonpregnant women. Supplementation is necessary for those who do not drink milk or eat dairy products. Vitamin D intake should be 5 µg per day (200 IU) to facilitate absorption of calcium. Vitamin D deficiency during pregnancy can lead to poor tooth enamel development and hypocalcemia in the fetus. Excesses should also be avoided, because infantile hypercalcemia syndrome may result.

The DRI for iron during pregnancy is 27 mg, compared to 18 mg for nonpregnant women. Unfortunately, many women start pregnancy with poor or depleted iron stores. Because the target iron intake is often not achieved from diet alone, supplementation with 30 mg ferrous iron per day is recommended for all pregnant women, especially during the second and third trimesters. The DRI for zinc, needed for the synthesis of DNA and RNA, is 11 to 13 mg per day. To achieve this, supplementation is recommended by the Institute of Medicine (IOM); adequate amounts are found in most multivitamin/multimineral supplements intended for pregnant women. Large doses of iron can interfere with zinc absorption.

Lactation

During lactation, the energy needs of the infant must be met by the mother. This is accomplished in part by mobilizing the extra maternal fat stores deposited during pregnancy, but even so, the mother must consume additional calories above the nonpregnant state requirements. The DRI for energy during lactation is approximately 400 kcal per day above the nonpregnant state. Lactation results in a small net energy deficit as a result of milk production and mobilization of fat stores. Therefore, lactating women typically lose 1 to 2 pounds per month, and the loss of the extra body fat is usually complete by the time the infant is 6 months old. Women who do not breastfeed are more likely to have difficulty losing weight after delivery.

Lactating women need about the same amount of protein per day as pregnant women, roughly 71 g or 1.2 g/kg. Other important nutrients in the lactating woman's diet include calcium, vitamin D, magnesium, zinc, folate, and vitamin B_6. Adequate fluids, rest, and family support are also essential for successful lactation.

Milk production in healthy well-nourished women is directly regulated by frequency and duration of infant suckling—the greater the nipple stimulation, the greater the milk volume. Milk composition is quite constant even if dietary intake of nutrients is below the DRIs. However, it appears that during lactation a balance between total energy intake and total energy expenditure is a requirement for normal milk production and infant growth.

Implementation of Nutrition Guidelines

Women should eat enough food to gain weight at the recommended rate. Fruits, vegetables, grains, meats, and dairy products should be included in meals and snacks daily. As noted earlier, adequate dairy and overall energy intakes are particularly important. Women should be encouraged to eat or drink at least 3 servings of dairy products daily. Four to five servings per day are recommended for women younger than 18 years. For better absorption of iron, meals should include meat, poultry or fish, and a vitamin C source such as orange juice or other citrus fruit.

The U.S. Department of Agriculture/Department of Health and Human Services (USDA/DHHS) Food Guide Pyramid recommends a range of servings for each major food group. For most pregnant women, the following revisions to the pyramid are appropriate: 6 to 9 servings from the starch group, 2 to 3 servings of fruits, 3 to 5 servings of vegetables, 2 to 3 servings from the meat group, and at least 3 servings of dairy products per day. The same dietary advice applies to lactating women. A well-balanced, varied diet should be encouraged with special attention given to adequate intake of energy, calcium, zinc, and fluids.

Prenatal Vitamins

A well-planned diet can meet many of the nutrient needs of pregnant and lactating women. However, vitamin and mineral supplementation may be appropriate for the nutrients described earlier (folic acid, calcium, vitamin D, iron, and zinc). Pregnant and lactating women should be careful not to exceed the tolerable upper limits for any vitamin or mineral.

Specific groups of women with increased risk for inadequate nutrient intake particularly benefit from vitamin and mineral supplementation. These include women who have low incomes, inadequate food supply or inadequate dietary choices, strict food restrictions including vegan dietary practices, substance abuse problems, pica (see section later in this chapter), chronic illnesses or medical conditions including iron deficiency anemia, and those who are carrying more than one fetus. Supplementation should begin by the 12th week of gestation with the exception of folic acid, which preferably should begin before pregnancy. Patients should be cautioned that excessive doses of some vitamins can be harmful to the fetus. A general prenatal vitamin, which includes the nutrients listed in Box 4–1, is usually recommended.

BOX 4-1   Prenatal Supplement Guidelines for
Women at Risk for Deficiency*

Iron	30–60 mg
Zinc	15 mg
Copper	2 mg
Calcium	250 mg
Vitamin D	400 IU
Vitamin C	50 mg
Folic acid	400 µg
Vitamin B_6	2 mg
Vitamin B_{12}	2 µg

*Recommended by Institute of Medicine.

Additional iron may be required for women with anemia (except for sickle cell anemia). A supplement of 60 to 120 mg of iron should be taken if the hemoglobin level falls below 11 g/dL during the first or third trimester or below 10.5 g/dL during the second trimester.

Other Recommendations

Sodium

Salt should not be restricted during pregnancy unless it is necessary because of a medical problem. Pregnant women should be advised to salt food to taste because the need for salt increases somewhat during pregnancy.

Caffeine

Evidence about the effects of caffeine on pregnancy is equivocal. Although one study suggested that moderate to heavy users of caffeine were more likely to have spontaneous abortions in the late first trimester and second trimester, there is no convincing evidence that caffeine affects embryonic development. It is best to advise pregnant women to limit coffee and other caffeinated beverages to 2 to 3 servings per day.

Alcohol, Tobacco, and Drugs

Tobacco, alcohol, and illicit drugs are best avoided entirely during pregnancy because of the potential for impaired fetal growth, fetal alcohol syndrome, and inadequate maternal food intake while using them. Cigarette smoking and alcohol use also increase requirements for some nutrients.

Artificial Sweeteners

The FDA has approved several non-nutritive sweeteners for general use. It is best to moderate their use during pregnancy. The most commonly used artificial sweeteners are sucralose (Splenda), aspartame (Equal) and saccharin (Sweet'N Low). Sucralose is the most recent high intensity sweetener approved as safe for human consumption. Aspartame is considered safe for individuals who do not have phenylketonuria (PKU). Saccharin crosses the placenta and may remain in fetal tissue due to slow fetal clearance. Use of saccharin in pregnancy is cautioned.

Medicinal Herb Use

Little is known about the pharmacokinetic action of herbs used during pregnancy or lactation. Pregnant women should consider herbal treatments as suspect until their safety in pregnancy is well established. Medicinal herbs should be viewed as drugs having both pharmacologic and toxicologic potential. Table 4–4 shows herbal and botanical supplements that may not be safe for use during pregnancy and lactation.

High Risk Considerations

Pica

Pica is characterized by the ingestion of non-nutritive materials such as dirt, clay, laundry starch, cornstarch, ice, chalk, burnt matches, baking soda, hair, stone, gravel, charcoal, cigarette ashes, mothballs, coffee grounds, and even tire inner tubes. Groups with a higher prevalence

Table 4–4	HERBAL AND BOTANICAL SUPPLEMENTS THAT MAY NOT BE SAFE FOR USE DURING PREGNANCY		
Agnus castus	Aloes	Angelica	Apricot kernal
Asafoetida	Aristolchia	Avens	Blue flag
Bogbean	Boldo	Boneset	Borage
Broom	Buchu	Buckthorn	Burdock
Calamus	Calendula	Cascara	German chamomile
Roman chamomile	Chaparral	Black cohosh	Blue cohosh
Cola	Coltsfoot	Comfrey	Cottonroot
Cornsilk	Crotalaria	Damiana	Devil's claw
Dong quai	Dogbane	Ephedra	Eucalyptus
Eupatorium	Euphorbia	Fenugreek	Feverfew
Foxglove	Frangula	Fucus	Gentian
Germander	Ginseng	Goldenseal	Ground ivy
Grounsel	Guarana	Hawthorne	Heliotropium
Hops	Horehound	Horsetail	Horseradish
Hydorcotyle	Jamaica dogwood	Juniper	Liferoot
Licorice	Lobelia	Mandrake	Mate
Male fern	Meadowsweet	Melliot	Mistletoe
Motherwort	Myrrh	Nettle	Osha
Passionflower	Pennyroyal	Petasites	Plantain
Pleurisy root	Podophyllium	Pokeroot	Poplar
Prickly ash	Pulsatilla	Queen's delight	Raqwort
Raspberry	Red clover	Rhubarb	Rue
Sassafras	Scullcap	Senna	Shephard's purse
Skunk cabbage	Stephania	Squill	St. John's wort
Tansy	Tonka bean	Uva-Ursi	Vervain
Wild carrot	Willow	Wormwood	Yarrow
Yellow dock	Yohimbe		

Source: Position of the American Dietetic Association: Nutrition and lifestyle for a healthy pregnancy outcome. J Am Diet Assoc 102:1479–1490, 2002.

of pica (up to 20%) include those living in rural areas, persons with a childhood or family history of pica, and African Americans. Some reasons given for pica behavior include the relief of nausea or nervous tension, having a pleasant sensation when chewing, an inherent craving for the substance, and encouragement by family members. Possible risks from the practice include hematological and gastrointestinal disorders and interference with nutrient ingestion and absorption. Pica has also been associated with reduced maternal serum ferritin and hemoglobin levels.

Health professionals counseling patients who practice pica should remain non-judgmental while strongly encouraging discontinuation of the practice. The substance being ingested and the reason for ingestion should be determined, and the dangers explained in a way that is culturally appropriate.

Gestational Diabetes Mellitus

Gestational diabetes mellitus (GDM) appears during pregnancy in women with no prior history of diabetes. GDM is associated with increased incidence of prematurity, macrosomia, and perinatal mortality. Pregnant women should be screened to detect GDM between 24 and 28 weeks of gestation, using a 1-hour, 50-g non-fasting oral glucose challenge. If the plasma glucose level is >140 mg/dL (>7.8 mM) after 1 hour, a 3-hour, 100-g oral glucose tolerance test (GTT) should be performed. Different sets of 3-hour oral GTT diagnostic criteria for GDM have been promulgated by the National Diabetes Data Group and by Carpenter and Coustan (Table 4–5). Outcome data are currently insufficient to support one set of criteria over the other. In patients with GDM, the goal is to provide all required nutrients, prevent hyperglycemia and ketosis, and insure appropriate weight gain.

Table 4-5	TWO DIAGNOSTIC CRITERIA FOR GESTATIONAL DIABETES MELLITUS			
	Plasma or Serum Glucose Level, Carpenter/ Coustan Criteria*		Plasma Level, National Diabetes Data Group Criteria*	
Status	mg/dL	mmol/L	mg/dL	mmol/L
Fasting	95	5.3	105	5.8
1 hour	180	10.0	190	10.6
2 hour	155	8.6	165	9.2
3 hours	140	7.8	145	8.0

*Gestational diabetes is diagnosed if two or more of the levels are met or exceeded.
Source: American College of Obstetricians and Gynecologists: Gestational diabetes, ACOG practice bulletin 30. Obstet Gynecol 98:525–538, 2001.

The meal plan is individualized for the patient; blood glucose self-monitoring may be required.

As the incidence of diabetes increases in the general population, more women will enter pregnancy with pre-existing diabetes. Patients with diabetes are at increased risk for pregnancy complications and should be counseled before becoming pregnant. Those requiring insulin may need to monitor their blood glucose levels 4 to 8 times daily both before and during pregnancy, with adjustment of insulin as necessary. The hemoglobin A_1C concentration, which reflects blood glucose levels over the past 4 to 6 weeks, should be maintained no higher than 5.5% to 6.5%. This is accomplished if blood glucose levels average between 110 and 150 mg/dL. Urine ketones should be checked whenever the blood glucose exceeds 200 mg/dL (11 mM). The diet should be individualized according to the patient's prepregnancy intake, and adjusted to achieve the recommended weight gain.

Preeclampsia, or Pregnancy-Induced Hypertension

Preeclampsia is characterized by hypertension, proteinuria, and edema developing after the 20th week of pregnancy. It occurs most often in primiparas younger than 20 and older than 35 years of age. Eclampsia ("toxemia") includes grand mal seizures or coma, and is often fatal. When all signs of preeclampsia are present, the baby must be delivered immediately. Patients with pregnancy-induced hypertension (PIH) should be counseled on a diet that is liberal in protein, energy, and fluids. Sodium restriction is not necessary.

HIV and AIDS

Transmission of the human immunodeficiency virus (HIV) from mother to fetus is a major concern during pregnancy. Administration of combination antiretroviral therapy during the second and third trimesters of pregnancy, labor, and early postpartum period has dramatically reduced rates of transmission. Pregnancy does not appear to have an adverse effect on the natural progression of HIV. In the United States and other developed countries, breastfeeding is discouraged because of the risk of viral transmission. As with any high-risk condition in pregnancy, low maternal weight gain can compromise fetal weight and pregnancy outcome. Along with HIV medications and a prenatal vitamin, adequate caloric and protein intake needs to be assured for appropriate weight gain. Nausea and vomiting from HIV medications can compromise adequate intake. Calorie supplements can help meet additional needs during pregnancy (see Table 13–1).

Nutrition Counseling

Health providers should coordinate efforts to educate women in childbearing years about the importance of good nutritional status before, during, and after pregnancy. Good prenatal care includes dietary assessment and nutrition education. A registered dietitian can be a valuable resource in assessing current dietary intake, identifying problems that may affect nutrient intake or absorption, and educating the patient. Taking a good dietary history will indicate whether the mother is omitting a major food group from her diet. Nondietary factors that may influence a woman's nutritional requirements and intake, such as inadequate housing, poor access to food, and substance abuse, should be identified and appropriate referrals made. The woman's attitude toward weight gain and concern about body size should also be assessed.

After the initial nutrition assessment, the pregnant woman should be counseled on a diet that addresses her individual needs and takes into consideration her cultural food preferences and practices. As mentioned previously, the Food Guide Pyramid and the U.S. *Dietary Guidelines* can be used as a good basis for nutrition education. Regular exercise during pregnancy and lactation should also be encouraged.

Strategies for managing common symptoms in pregnancy are listed in Boxes 4–2, 4–3, and 4–4.

BOX 4-2   **Recommendations for Nausea and Vomiting**

Eat crackers, melba toast, or dry cereal before getting out
of bed in the morning.
Eat small, frequent meals.
Try to take adequate fluids even if solid foods are not tolerated.
Avoid drinking coffee and tea.
Avoid or limit intake of fatty and spicy foods.

BOX 4-3   **Recommendations for Heartburn**

Eat small low-fat meals, slowly.
Drink fluids mainly between meals.
Avoid spices.
Avoid lying down for 1 to 2 hours after eating or drinking.
Wear loose-fitting clothing.

BOX 4-4   **Recommendations for Constipation**

Drink 2 to 3 quarts of fluids daily.
Eat high-fiber foods, including cereals, whole grains, legumes, and
fresh fruits and vegetables.
Be physically active.
Avoid taking laxatives.

Food and Nutrition Resources

The Food Stamp Program is available for U.S. citizens from
low income households. Eligibility is determined after
formal application to local public assistance or social
service agencies. The Special Supplemental Nutrition
Program for Women, Infants, and Children (WIC) is
available in each county throughout the United States.
Eligibility requirements are based on income level and
nutritional risk (e.g., anemia). Women who are pregnant,
postpartum (up to 6 months), and breastfeeding (up to
1 year) are eligible. The benefits include individualized
food packages and nutrition education. Upon completion
of certification, food vouchers are provided, in most cases

on the day of application. Health professionals who refer a client to the WIC program should provide the patient's hemoglobin or hematocrit, medical risks, and height and weight. Local WIC agencies can provide standard referral forms.

SUGGESTED READINGS

American College of Obstetricians and Gynecologists: Gestational diabetes, ACOG Practice Bulletin 30. Obstet Gynecol 98:525–538, 2001.

Position of the American Dietetic Association: Breaking the barriers to breastfeeding. J Am Diet Assoc 101:1213–1220, 2001.

Position of the American Diabetic Association: Nutrition and lifestyle for a healthy pregnancy outcome. J Am Diet Assoc 102:1279–1490, 2002.

Meek JY (ed): New Mother's Guide to Breastfeeding. Elk Grove, Ill, American Academy of Pediatrics, 2002.

WEB SITES

La Leche League, http://www.lalecheleague.org

March of Dimes, http://www.modimes.org

National Women's Health Information Center, http://www.4woman.gov

5

Infancy

FRANK A. FRANKLIN, JR., MD •
REINALDO FIGUEROA, MD

The First Year of Life

The first year of life is characterized by rapid growth and changes in body composition. Adequate nutrition is required to promote optimal growth and development, avoid illness, and allow infants to interact with and explore their environments. Infant nutritional requirements are different from those of adults. For example, protein, fat, and energy (which are important for growth) and iron, zinc, and calcium are required in greater proportions for infants.

Body Composition

Knowledge of the infant's body composition at various stages is of considerable importance. Characterizing changes in body composition is a way to understand the process of growth and changes in function that affect the nutritional needs of a growing infant. The body is composed of fat and fat-free body mass (FFBM), which includes water, protein, carbohydrates, and minerals. The percent of body weight that is fat increases throughout infancy from approximately 14% at birth to 23% by 1 year of age (Table 5–1). The accompanying decrease in the percentage of FFBM is principally the result of a decrease in water content. The contribution of protein, minerals, and carbohydrates remains relatively constant throughout infancy.

Body composition can be viewed in terms of its functional units, such as organs (brain, heart, liver, kidney),

Table 5-1	BODY COMPOSITION OF REFERENCE INFANTS (AGE 0–1 YEAR; 50TH PERCENTILE)[1,2]						
		Fat		Fat-free Body Mass			
Age (months)	Weight (kg)	(Kg)	(%)	Kg	(%)	Length (cm)	Head Circumference (cm)
Boys							
Birth	3.5	0.5	14	3.1	86	50.5	34.8
3	6.4	1.5	23	4.9	77	61.1	40.6
6	8	2	25	6	75	67.8	43.8
9	9.2	2.2	24	7	76	72.3	45.8
12	10.2	2.3	23	7.9	77	76.1	47
Girls							
Birth	3.3	0.5	15	2.8	85	49.9	34.3
3	5.7	1.4	24	4.4	76	59.5	39.5
6	7.3	1.9	26	5.3	74	65.9	42.4
9	8.3	2.1	25	6.2	75	70.4	44.3
12	9.2	2.2	24	7	76	74.3	45.6

muscle mass, energy reserves (fat mass), extracellular fluid, and supporting structures (connective tissue, bone). The major organs and muscle mass account for most of the body protein; the fat mass is primarily used for energy when energy intake is inadequate; and bone contains a reserve of calcium, phosphorus, and other minerals.

Growth

Growth increments in weight, length, and head circumference are extremely rapid before birth and during the first year of life (see Table 5-1 and growth charts in Chapter 6). A normal 1-month-old infant grows approximately 1 cm per week and gains 20 to 30 g per day, a rate that gradually decreases to 0.5 cm per week in length and 10 g per day in weight by 12 months of age. An average newborn weighs 3.5 kg; weight generally doubles by 4 months and triples by 12 months of age. The energy cost of growth is the cost of depositing fat and protein. Because fat deposition requires 10.8 kcal/g and protein deposition requires 13.4 kcal/g, depositing fat is more energy efficient than building muscle.

During early postnatal development, all organs appear to grow by cell division (hyperplasia) followed by a pattern of increasing cell size (hypertrophy). At birth, 15% of an infant's body weight is organ mass, 25% is muscle mass, 14% is fat, and 15% is bone and connective tissue. Throughout infancy these organ systems continue to grow and mature at a rapid rate. Cell number, measured by increments of DNA, continues to increase rapidly in the brain, heart, kidney, liver, and spleen. The brain doubles in size by 1 year of age. Energy or nutrient deficiencies during this period of rapid cell replication may limit the number of cells formed and possibly cause permanent deficits in the developing brain and nervous system.

Organ Maturation

The number and magnitude of obstacles newborns face in maintaining nutrient balance are inversely related to gestational age. The gastrointestinal tract of the preterm and sometimes the term infant may not be ready to perform the vital functions of nutrient intake, processing, assimilation, metabolism, and distribution to other organs. The term infant has mature coordination of sucking and swallowing but poor coordination of esophageal motility, decreased lower esophageal sphincter pressure (which enhances the risk of gastroesophageal reflux), limited gastric volume and delayed gastric emptying, and variable maturity of several enzymatic and hormonal systems.

The kidneys fine-tune water and electrolyte excretion in relation to intake to maintain a body-fluid composition that supports optimal functioning. The term infant has the full number of nephrons but a low glomerular filtration rate in the first 48 hours, a higher fractional excretion of sodium than in adults, relative difficulty excreting a high-acid load, and normal diluting but limited concentrating capabilities. These limitations adversely affect the ability of the newborn to handle renal solute loads derived from the catabolism of excess protein to urea.

Breastfeeding

Exclusive breastfeeding is adequate for the first 4 to 6 months of age for almost all infants. One of the U.S. government's *Healthy People 2010* goals is to increase to at least 75% the proportion of mothers who breastfeed their babies in the early postpartum period, to at least 50% the proportion who breastfeed up to 6 months, and to at least 25% the proportion who breastfeed up to 1 year. In 1998 these proportions were 64%, 29%, and 16%, respectively.[1] Recommended strategies to promote breastfeeding include education programs, postpartum support and peer counseling, hospital rooming-in of mother with infant, encouraging early maternal contact and frequent, on-demand breastfeeding, elimination of commercial discharge packages for new mothers, and discouraging the early use of artificial nipples and pacifiers. Differences in energy requirements between breastfed and formula-fed infants result from lower energy excretion in breastfed infants and higher energy cost of tissue synthesis (greater fat deposition) in formula-fed infants. Some of the advantages and disadvantages of breast milk are presented in Table 5–2.

Table 5-2	ADVANTAGES AND DISADVANTAGES OF BREAST MILK
Advantages (Antibacterial and Antiviral Properties)	**Comments**
Humoral Factors	
IgA	Confers passive mucosal protection of gastrointestinal tract against penetration of intestinal organisms and antigens
Bifidus factor	Supports growth of *Lactobacillus bifidus,* a microorganism that converts lactose to acetic and lactic acids; low resulting pH—inhibits growth of *E.coli* and protects against *Staphylococus aureus, Shigella,* and protozoal infections
Lysozymes	Bacteriolytic enzymes that act against *Enterobacteriaceae* and gram-positive bacteria
Lactoferrin	Iron-binding whey protein; bacteriostatic effect on *S. aureus* and *E. coli* by limiting iron available for their growth
Interferon	Antiviral protein
Cellular Factors	
Macrophages	Phagocytize bacteria and viruses in the gut; synthesize complement lysozyme, and lactoferrin
Lymphocytes	T-cells: may transfer delayed hypersensitivity from mother to infant; B-cells: synthesize Ig
Advantages (Nutritional Properties)	**Comments**
Protein Quality	
60:40 whey/casein ratio	Forms small, soft, easily digestible curd in stomach; essential amino acids (cysteine) provided in higher concentration by whey
Nucleotides	Nonprotein nitrogen postulated to play a role in anabolism and growth
Hypoallergenic	Reduces potential for allergenic reactions

Table continued on following page

Table 5–2	ADVANTAGES AND DISADVANTAGES OF BREAST MILK *(Continued)*

Advantages (Nutritional Properties) *(Continued)*	Comments
Lipid Quality	
High oleic acid content	Improves digestibility and absorbability of lipid by increasing lipotytic enzymes ability to act stereospecifically
Lipolytic activity	Improves fat absorption
Cholesterol	Possibly facilitates formation of nerve tissue and synthesis of bile salts; necessary for optimal development of cholesterol regulatory mechanism
Mineral/Electrolyte Content	
Ca^{++}/P ratio = 2:1	Improves absorption of calcium in gut
Low renal solute load (one-third of cow milk)	More suited to immature capacity for renal solute excretion
Iron	High bioavailability (40%–50% absorption) compared to commercial formulas (<10% absorption)
Other	
Infant-maternal bonding	Potential long-term advantage
Possible decreased risk for obesity	High lipid and protein content at the end of breast milk feedings may signal satiety and inhibit overconsumption; may postpone introduction of solids

Disadvantages	Comments
Possible nutrient inadequacies	May develop vitamin D and iron deficiencies with prolonged breast feeding if supplements or a variety of solid foods are not initiated
Inborn errors of metabolism	Inappropriate nutrient composition
Maternal drugs (antithyroid, antimetabolite, anticoagulant)	May be hazardous to the nursing infant
Environmental contaminants (herbicides, pesticides, insecticides, radioisotopes)	Have unknown effects on exposed children; no practical way to monitor contamination of human milk
Human immunodeficiency virus	Possible transmission to infant

Nutritional Advantages of Breast Milk

Human milk is tailored precisely for the growth and development needs of the human infant. The protein content of breast milk is lower than that of other species (1 % versus 3 % in cow milk) whose young double their birth weight and wean quickly in days or weeks. The profile of amino acids in human milk is ideal not only for absorption but for utilization, especially by the brain. The composition of human milk relative to infant needs for essential amino acids is shown in Table 5-3. The main protein in cow milk, casein, forms a somewhat indigestible curd and has high levels of phenylalanine, tyrosine, and methionine for which the infant has little digestive enzyme resources. Cow milk contains little lactalbumin and cysteine, which the infant can digest readily. Human milk contains taurine, an important nutrient for brain and nerve growth, whereas cow milk contains none, so taurine must be added to most infant formulas.

The fat profile of human milk is predominantly saturated and monounsaturated fats (only about 15 % polyunsaturated fats) with a stable amount of cholesterol,

Table 5-3	ESSENTIAL AMINO ACID COMPOSITION OF BREAST MILK AND A CASEIN-BASED FORMULA RELATIVE TO INFANT REQUIREMENTS		
	Intake (150 mL/kg/day)		
Essential Amino Acid	**Breast Milk**	**Casein-based Formula**	**Requirement (mg/kg/day)**
Histidine	37	45	28
Isoleucine	90	112	70
Leucine	155	210	161
Lysine	105	155	103
Methionine and cystine	68	82	58
Phenylalanine and tyrosine	135	190	125
Threonine	75	100	87
Tryptophan	30	30	17
Valine	100	120	93
Taurine	7.5	7	—

Table 5–4	FAT COMPOSITION OF BREAST MILK RELATIVE TO A WHEY-BASED FORMULA	
	Breast Milk	**Whey-based Formula**
Total (g/dL)	3.5–4.5	3.8
Triglycerides (%)	98–99	99
Cholesterol (mg/dL)	10–15	—
Phospholipids (mq/dL)	15–20	30
Fatty Acids (%)		
Oleic (18:1)	35	16
Palmitic (16:0)	22	10
Linoleic (18:2, n-6)	15	32
Myristic (14:0)	6	9
Lauric (12:0)	4	22
Linolenic (18:3, omega-3)	1	1
Medium-chain triglycerides	10	8

regardless of the mother's cholesterol intake (Table 5–4). Cholesterol is an important constituent of brain and nerve tissue as well as a precursor of steroid hormones and bile acids. Most formulas contain no cholesterol and contain fats of varying quality as compared with cow-milk fat. Animal and human studies suggest a strong relationship between intake of the long-chain omega-3 polyunsaturated fatty acid docosahexaenoic acid (DHA; 22:6, n-3) and visual acuity and cognitive function. DHA is present in human milk but absent from cow milk; some commercial formulas are now fortified with DHA from single cell oils (0.2 % of the fatty acids).

Human milk is rich in vitamins A, C, and E. The B-vitamin content depends on maternal intake and meets calculated standards. Because the primary source of vitamin B_6 and the only source of vitamin B_{12} are animal products, vegetarian mothers (especially strict vegans) may produce milk that is deficient in these vitamins unless they supplement their diets. It is recommended that all infants, including those who are exclusively breastfed and those with formula intakes less than 500 ml, should have a minimum intake of 200 IU of vitamin D daily beginning in the first 2 months. The vitamin D content of human milk (25 IU/L) is lower than that of cow milk, so supplementation is advisable in breastfed infants if sun exposure is restricted. All newborns should receive a 0.5- to 1-mg injection or a 2-mg oral dose of vitamin K immediately after birth, regardless of whether breastfeeding or bottle-feeding will be used.

Variations in Composition

The composition of milk varies during each feeding and as the child matures. When a feeding is initiated, the mother's milk "lets down" and the first milk, or foremilk, is released from the ducts as the lacteal cells respond to the surge of prolactin. The first milk is lower in fat and slightly higher in cells, protein, and lactose. The hind-milk is high in fat because the fat globules take more time to form and pass across the cell membrane. Human milk goes through three phases: colostrum, transitional milk, and mature milk. Produced at delivery and during the first few days postpartum, colostrum is high in protein, especially immunoglobulins such as secretory IgA that provide the infant with initial protection against infection. Colostrum is also high in carotene, giving it a yellow color. Colostrum provides enzymes that stimulate gut maturation, facilitate digestion (especially of fats by lipase), and stimulate the gut to pass meconium. There is a gradual change from colostrum to transitional milk and then mature milk over the first 7 to 10 days postpartum. The profile of mature milk persists until about 6 months postpartum when there is a slight decrease in protein content. The immune properties are measurable throughout lactation. During weaning, the milk increases in protein, sodium, and chloride as the supply diminishes. Mothers who are not fully lactating or are experiencing lactation failure have milk that is higher in sodium and chloride than mature milk.

Other Components of Human Milk

Living cells are present in concentrations of $4000/mm^3$ in colostrum and $1500/mm^3$ in mature milk. They include macrophages that phagocytize bacteria and viruses in the gut and lymphocytes from the mother's Peyer patches that also provide immunologic protection in the infant's intestines. The normal flora of the newborn gut include lactobacilli, whose growth is stimulated by the bifidus factor and slightly acidic pH of human milk. The growth of *Escherichia coli* is suppressed by lactoferrin in human milk, which binds the iron that *E. coli* need for survival, whereas growth of *E. coli* is enhanced by iron provided in the diet. Secretory IgA in human milk impedes translocation of organisms across the intestinal wall and mucous membranes from the mouth onward and reduces respiratory disease, diarrhea, and sepsis. Other humoral factors (whose precise roles have not all been identified) found in human milk include nucleotides, resistance factor, lysozyme, interferon, complement, and vitamin B_{12}-binding protein. All these properties are unique to human milk, and attempts to fortify infant formulas with some of them (e.g., nucleotides) have not been shown to prevent disease.

Fully breastfed infants experience a lower incidence of and morbidity from bacterial, especially respiratory, illnesses. Both retrospective and prospective epidemiologic studies also suggest that infants who are fully breastfed for at least 4 to 6 months may have relative protection against type 1 diabetes, cancers (such as lymphoma), celiac disease, Crohn's disease, and obesity. The incidence of significant allergic disease (eczema, asthma, and allergic rhinitis) is significantly reduced in the first 2 years of life by breastfeeding, at least in part because of decreased intestinal permeability.

Contraindications to Breastfeeding

Maternal infections in general do not contraindicate breastfeeding, and in most cases they even provide additional protection for the infant via the milk. At one time hepatitis B represented a contraindication to breastfeeding. However, now that all infants born to mothers with hepatitis B are given hepatitis B immune globulin in the first 12 hours of life and then a vaccine before hospital discharge, breastfeeding is safe even if the virus passes into the milk.

The disease that is currently causing significant concern is acquired immunodeficiency syndrome (AIDS). Not all infants born to HIV-1-positive mothers are infected with the virus at birth, but those who are infected cannot be identified immediately because they have passive maternal antibodies. In the United States where the survival of healthy bottle-fed babies is assured, mothers with HIV-1 disease should not breastfeed. By contrast, breastfeeding is encouraged in developing countries where there is less than an 18% additional risk of an infant acquiring AIDS by breastfeeding from an HIV-1-positive mother but a potentially higher risk of death in the infant who is not breastfed. Information should be presented to the mother so that she can make an informed decision about the type of infant feeding.

Maternal Medications and Substances of Abuse

Although medications pass into milk in varying amounts depending on the pharmacologic properties of the compound, most medications are safe for breastfeeding mothers to take. Medications that are necessary and the most effective and safest alternatives that deliver the lowest amounts to the infant should be selected. Timing medication doses as far away as possible from feedings minimizes the levels received by the infant. Over-the-counter drugs such as aspirin, acetaminophen, and ibuprofen are usually acceptable in moderate doses for temporary use. Although most antibiotics pass into milk to some degree, those that can be given directly to infants are safe for lactating mothers to take. Anti-anxiety drugs, antidepressants, and neuroleptic drugs have unknown effects but may be of concern for long-term neurodevelopmental effects. Extensive lists of drugs transferred through the placenta or breast milk, and therefore contraindicated during pregnancy and lactation, are available.[2] In most cases acceptable substitutes can be found for contraindicated drugs.

Although drugs of abuse represent a risk to nursing infants, in the case of marijuana the risk-to-benefit ratio favors breastfeeding over bottle-feeding. The mother who is bottle-feeding and smokes marijuana in the presence of her infant creates risk in addition to losing the benefits of breastfeeding. Cigarette smoking has been associated with decreased breastfeeding duration, but breastfed infants of smoking mothers have fewer respiratory infections than bottle-fed infants whose mothers smoke. Mothers should be cautioned never to smoke in the presence of the infant and not to smoke within 30 minutes before a feeding to avoid suppressing the let-down reflex and to decrease the possibility of nicotine appearing in the milk. Pregnancy and lactation should be used as opportunities to help mothers to stop smoking.

Mothers who have received a radioactive pharmaceutical as a single dose for clinical diagnosis should temporarily stop breastfeeding. The breasts should be pumped to maintain lactation, but the milk should be discarded. When radioactive drugs are used in multiple doses for treatment, breastfeeding must be completely discontinued, because no amount of radioactive material is safe for an infant.

Common Misunderstandings

Breastfeeding success is enhanced by early initiation. Ideally, the baby should be offered the breast immediately after birth. No test water is necessary when the Apgar scores are good and secretions modest. Subsequent feedings should be "on demand" but never more than 4 to 5 hours apart in the first week. This is important not only for nourishing and hydrating the infant but also for stimulating the breast to produce milk. Breastfeeding is an infant-driven process. Ending feedings with water, glucose water, and especially formula is a recipe for lactation failure. Carefully controlled studies have demonstrated clearly that infants who are given water, glucose water, or formula instead of human milk exclusively in the first week lose weight, regain it more slowly, and have higher bilirubin levels and fewer stools.

The average infant nurses every 2 hours for 10 to 12 feedings a day during the first few weeks. The stomach's emptying time with human milk is no more than 90 minutes, whereas with formula it is more than 3 hours and up to 6 hours with homogenized milk. Weight gain should be consistent, at least 1 oz per day after 10 to 14 days when the milk supply is well established. Initial weight loss should not exceed 10% of birth weight and usually averages about 8% when the mother is primiparous. An additional means of monitoring adequate breast milk intake is to count the number of the infant's urinary voidings, which should total at least six per day and include some soaking. Stools are an important indication of adequate food in the gut. In the first few weeks, infants produce stool every day, often with every feeding. Signs such as failure to gain weight or infrequent stools and voidings should be evaluated.

Sore nipples are associated more with the position of the infant during breastfeeding, problems in "latching on," and release of suction than with the length of feedings. When mothers complain of sore nipples, observe the infant while breastfeeding, taking particular note of positioning; the baby's abdomen should face the mother's abdomen, and the infant should directly face the breast.

Infant Formulas

When breastfeeding is not feasible, commercially prepared infant formulas are an acceptable alternative. The manufacturers of routine infant formulas attempt to approximate the composition of breast milk. They are stable mixtures of emulsified fats, proteins, carbohydrates, minerals, and vitamins and come in ready-to-feed, concentrated liquid, or powdered preparations. Standard infant formulas have an energy density of 20 kcal/oz and an osmolarity of 300 mOsm/L. The American Academy of Pediatrics suggests a caloric distribution of 30% to 55% fat (2.7% of the calories as linoleic acid), 7% to 16% protein, and the remaining 35% to 65% of energy from carbohydrate. Details of the compositions of infant formulas are available on the manufacturers' websites listed at the end of this chapter. The modular feeding products listed in Table 5–5 were developed to help physicians treat infants and children with medical problems. Most of these products are not complete diets, so care must be used to avoid producing nutrient deficiencies.

Solid Food

The introduction of solid food (complementary foods) should be based on the individual infant's growth, activity, gastrointestinal maturity, and neuromuscular development. Infants do not have the oral motor skills to consume solid food or eat from a spoon until 4 to 6 months of age when the oral extrusion reflex is extinguished. A recommended schedule for introducing solid food is shown in Box 5–1. The potential disadvantages of introducing solid food in advance of the schedule are shown in Box 5–2.

Table 5-5	COMMERCIAL MODULAR FEEDING COMPONENTS		
Product	**Manufacturer**	**Composition**	**Energy Content**
Moducal	Novartis	Maltodextrin	3.8 kcal/g
Polycose liquid	Ross Laboratories	Glucose polymer	2 kcal/mL
Polycose powder	Ross Laboratories	Glucose polymer	3.8 kcal/g
Corn oil	—	—	9 kcal/mL
Microlipid	Novartis	Emulsified long-chain triglycerides	4.5 kcal/mL
Medium-chain triglyceride oil	Novartis	Fractionated coconut oil	7.7 kcal/mL
Casec	Novartis	Calcium caseinate, egg-white solids	3.7 kcal/g

BOX 5–1   Age Schedule for Introducing Solid Food

Age 1 to 6 months
Breast milk or formula only

Age 6 to 7 months
Iron-fortified cereal
Fruit (strained or mashed); cup introduced

Age 7 to 8 months
Vegetables (strained or mashed)

Age 8 to 9 months
Finger food (e.g., crackers, bananas) and chopped (junior)
  baby food

Age 9 months
Meat and citrus juice

Age 10 to 11 months
Bite-size cooked food

Age 12 months
All table food

BOX 5–2   Potential Disadvantages of Introducing
Solid Food Before 6 Months of Age

Poor oral-motor coordination
Insufficient energy and nutrient replacement for breast milk or
  infant formula
Increased risk of food allergies
Increased renal solute load and hyperosmolarity
Disturbance of appetite regulation possibly encouraging
  overfeeding
Increased likelihood of infant desiring sugar and salt later
  in life

When adding solid food to an infant's diet, one new, single-ingredient food should be introduced every 3 to 5 days. This allows the parent to watch for allergic reactions and gives the infant time to become accustomed to new tastes. Other suggested guidelines for introducing solids are shown in Box 5–3. The sequence of introducing food is not critical, although iron-fortified, dry baby cereal is usually added first. Rice cereal is commonly the first food added because rice is the least allergenic. Eggs and wheat should be avoided during the first 6 to 9 months of age to minimize the possibility of an allergic reaction. Combination foods such as strained cereal with fruit, vegetables with meat, high-meat dinners, and other infant or toddler foods may be introduced after single-ingredient foods are well tolerated. Introducing foods of increasing texture (lumpy foods), variety, color, and taste over the period of 6 to 10 months decreases the chance of food refusal related to texture and need for chewing. Finger foods can be introduced by 8 months. Unsweetened fruit juice should be introduced when the infant can drink from a cup. Juice should be given in a cup and not a bottle, as the latter may predispose

---

BOX 5–3   Guidelines for Introducing Solid Food

Begin with single-ingredient foods; add one at a time.
Introduce a small amount of each new food beginning with 1 to 2 tsp, and gradually increase the amount to 3 to 4 tsp per feeding.
Wait 3 to 5 days before adding another new food; discontinue the last food if an adverse reaction occurs.
Ultimately, offer a wide variety of food. For older infants, include meat, milk, fruit, vegetable, bread, and cereal for nutritional adequacy and diversity.
Avoid mixing solids with fluids so that the infant can learn textures and flavors and develop facial muscles, (Exception: For infants with reflux, add rice cereal to thicken meals.)
Never put a baby to bed with a bottle or allow a baby to suck a bottle continuously during the day to maximize the risk of dental caries and adverse tooth eruption.
Provide solids with textures that are compatible with the infant's ability to chew and swallow.

the infant to nursing-bottle caries. The protein content of breast milk decreases gradually as lactation duration increases, so high-protein baby food intake should be encouraged and have a significant content of highly bioavailable iron. Sugar and salt should not be added during the preparation of homemade baby food, and frozen or canned foods containing sugar and salt should be avoided. At 12 months, children can eat the same foods as consumed by the rest of the family (see Box 5-3).

Between 6 and 12 months of age, infants show increasing interest in self-feeding and develop the ability to grasp and pick up food. Finger foods should be offered once the ability to chew is acquired. These should be carefully selected to allow for easy manipulation in the mouth and minimize the potential for choking and aspiration (Box 5-4). Establishing a healthy feeding relationship involves recognition of the role of the parent to provide appropriate foods and for the child to decide whether and how much to eat; a balance between the child's need for assistance with feeding and parental encouragement of self-feeding; parental responsiveness to cues from the child about hunger and satiety; and slow, patient feeding while encouraging but not forcing

---

BOX 5-4   Finger Foods for Infants

Preferred

Bread: bread, toast, unsalted crackers
Fruit: items that are fresh or canned (unsweetened), soft, and
    without seeds or peels (bananas, apples, peaches, apricots)
Meat, poultry, fish: items that are tender and in small cooked
    pieces or strips without bones (meatballs, meat sticks,
    hamburger, meat loaf, chicken nuggets, turkey, fish sticks)
Vegetables: items that are tender and in cooked whole pieces
    or chunks (carrots, green beans, squash, potato)

Avoid

Popcorn, nuts, seeds, unmashed peas, raw carrots, raisins,
    potato chips, hard candies, corn kernels (because of
    potential for choking and aspiration)

intake and minimizing distractions. Repeated exposure to new foods enhances their acceptance and overcomes the child's innate fears of new and different tastes (neophobia).

Nutritional Requirements of Infants

The characteristics of the Dietary Reference Intakes (DRIs) and Recommended Dietary Allowances (RDAs) are discussed in Chapter 3, and age-specific recommendations for individual nutrients are listed in Tables 3–1 through 3–5. The RDAs for infants up to 6 months of age are based primarily on the amounts of nutrients provided by breast milk. Those for infants from 6 months to 1 year of age assume consumption of infant formula and increasing amounts of solid food.

Energy

The energy balance of infants may be described simply as

Gross energy intake = Energy expended + Energy excreted (losses) + Energy stored (growth)

The components of energy expenditure are basal metabolic rate (energy needed to maintain body temperature; support the minimal work of the brain, heart, and respiratory muscles; and supply the minimal energy requirements of tissues at rest), the thermic effect of feeding (energy used for digestion, transport, and conversion of absorbed nutrients into their respective storage forms), and physical activity. Changes in the partitions of energy requirements during the first 6 months of life are shown in Figure 5–1. Energy requirements per kilogram of body weight gradually decline throughout infancy as a result of decreases in basal metabolic rate per kilogram due to decreasing relative contribution of the most metabolically active organs (brain, heart, lungs, liver, and kidneys) to body weight and growth rate. The proportion of energy intake used for growth decreases from about 27% at birth to about 5% by 1 year of age.

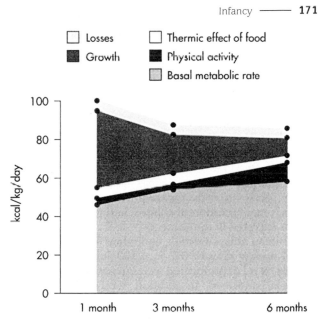

Figure 5–1. Changes in energy requirements in the first 6 months of life.

Water

Water is necessary for the infant to replace losses from the skin and lungs (evaporative loss), feces, and urine; a small amount is also needed for growth. Under most conditions water intake exceeds the requirements for evaporative losses, renal excretion of solutes, and growth, and any excess is excreted in the urine.

Human milk, cow milk, and infant formulas of conventional energy density (67 kcal/100 mL) provide approximately 89 mL of preformed water in each 100 mL of milk or formula consumed. In addition, food yields water when oxidized; the combustion of 1 g of protein, fat, and carbohydrate yields 0.41 mL, 1.07 mL, and 0.55 mL of water, respectively. In milks and formulas, preformed water and oxidation water amount to approximately 95% of the volume consumed.

Carbohydrates

Carbohydrates should comprise 35% to 65% of the total energy intake of the term infant and are usually consumed in the form of disaccharides or glucose polymers. Glucose is the principal nutrient the neonatal brain utilizes, and inadequate carbohydrate intake can lead to hypoglycemia, ketosis, and excessive protein catabolism. Most milk-based formulas contain lactose, a disaccharide of glucose and galactose, as the principal carbohydrate in amounts similar to that of human milk (6 to 7 g/100 mL). Several soy formulas and special formulas contain sucrose, maltose, fructose, dextrins, and glucose polymers as their carbohydrate sources. Because they are lactose free, they are useful in managing disorders such as galactosemia and primary lactase deficiency and recovering from secondary lactose intolerance.

Fat

Dietary fat serves as a concentrated source of energy, carries fat-soluble vitamins, and provides essential fatty acids (EFAs). EFAs are precursors for the synthesis of prostaglandins and serve other essential functions. The American Academy of Pediatrics recommends that 30% to 55% of total energy intake be from fat and 2.7% from linoleic acid. Table 5–4 compares the fat composition of breast milk with that of a whey-based formula.

Breast milk is unique in containing maternal lipases that aid in the digestion of fat. Fat digestion begins in the stomach with the additional action of lingual lipase, an enzyme secreted from lingual serous glands, and gastric lipase secreted from glands in the gastric mucosa. Further digestion takes place in the small intestine through the action of pancreatic and intestinal lipases.

The fat content of infant formulas is derived from a variety of long-chain vegetable triglycerides such as soy, corn, safflower, and coconut oil and from medium-chain triglycerides (MCTs). Linoleic acid is found only in the long-chain vegetable oils in various concentrations. Breast milk contains 8% to 10% of total calories as linoleic acid, and most infant formulas have at least 10%. Some special formulas contain MCTs (fatty acids from 8 to 12 carbons in length) compared with long-chain triglycerides (fatty acids more than 14 carbons long). MCTs are partially soluble in water and not dependent on bile acids for solubilization, so they can be absorbed by patients with malabsorption or hepatobiliary disease. Because of their solubility, MCTs can appose the mucosal surface and be hydrolyzed by mucosal lipases. This obviates the need for pancreatic lipase, which is deficient in patients with pancreatic insufficiency. A large percentage of absorbed MCTs are transported directly into the portal circulation, bypassing the lymphatic channels necessary to transport long-chain triglycerides packaged in chylomicrons. For this reason, MCT oil is useful in managing diseases such as intestinal lymphangiectasia, chylous ascites, and chylothorax. The disadvantages of MCTs are that they are not very palatable, have a cathartic effect when given in large amounts, are expensive, and do not contain EFAs.

Protein

Protein provides nitrogen and amino acids for the synthesis of body tissues, enzymes, hormones, and antibodies that regulate and perform physiologic and metabolic functions. Excess dietary proteins are metabolized for energy, producing urea that increases the renal solute load, water requirements, and the risk for dehydration when excess water losses occur, such as during diarrhea. The American Academy of Pediatrics recommends that 7% to 16% of total energy be from protein, or 1.6 to 2.2 g/kg/day. Healthy term infants may grow well with a protein intake (from breast milk) slightly below 1.6 g/kg/day.

The protein in most commercial infant formulas typically comes from cow milk, which has a whey/casein ratio of 20:80. Several recently developed infant formulas contain whey/casein ratios of 60:40, which is closer to the 65:35 or 70:30 ratio and amino acid composition of breast milk. The curd formed from whey in an acidic stomach is small, soft, easily digestible, and emptied quickly. Table 5–3 compares the essential amino acid compositions of breast milk and a casein-based formula relative to infant requirements.

Other protein sources used in infant formulas include soy-protein isolates and protein hydrolysates. Infant formulas containing soy protein are well received by vegetarian families who wish to avoid cow milk and animal products. Soy proteins contain trypsin inhibitors that may interfere with absorption. These inhibitors are largely inactivated by heat treatment of the protein isolate. Soy also produces tightly bound protein phytate mineral complexes that may reduce the bioavailability of some minerals. For these reasons, and because of concerns over their phytoestrogen content, soy formulas are not recommended for routine infant feedings.

Between 20% and 80% of infants who are allergic to casein are also allergic to soy, so hydrolyzed casein is the protein of choice for these infants. The enzymatic hydrolysis process results in a mixture of free amino acids and peptides of various chain lengths and diminishes its antigenicity. Free amino acid formulas are also available for infants who fail the hydrolysate formulas. Formulas labeled as hypoallergenic must demonstrate suitability to sustain infant growth and development and failure to provoke reactions in 90% of infants with confirmed cow-milk allergy.

Vitamins

Many vitamins play important roles as cofactors and catalysts for cell function and replication. The content of most commercial infant formulas is adequate to meet the requirements of most healthy infants when they consume approximately 750 mL (26 oz) of formula each day. Vitamin supplementation may be necessary for infants whose intake is less than this, when steatorrhea is present (e.g., from hepatobiliary disease, pancreatic insufficiency, or small intestinal disease causing malabsorption), or when prescribed medications affect vitamin absorption or utilization. Table 5–6 provides guidelines

Table 5-6 GUIDELINES FOR USE OF VITAMINS AND MINERAL SUPPLEMENTS IN HEALTHY INFANTS AND CHILDREN[a,b]

| Group | Multivitamins | Individual Vitamins | | | Minerals | |
		Vitamin D	Vitamin E	Folate	Iron	Fluoride
Preterm infants						
Breastfed[c]	+	+	±	±	+	—
Formula-fed	+	+	±	±	+	—
Term infants (0–6 mo)						
Breastfed	—	+	—	—	—	—
Formula-fed	—	—	—	—	—	—
Infants >6 mo[d]	—	+	—	—	±[e]	±[e]
Children >1 year	—	—	—	—	—	±
Pregnant women	±	—	—	±	+	—
Lactating women	±	—	—	—	±	—

[a]Vitamin K is not shown but should be given to all newborn infants.

[b]Extra calcium for pregnant and lactating women is not shown.

[c]The sodium content of human milk is marginal for preterm infants.

[d]If high risk (poor intake, steatorrhea, or medication use that affects vitamin absorption or utilization), multivitamins and multiminerals (including iron) are preferred.

[e]See discussion in text.

for using vitamin and mineral supplements in healthy infants and children.

Minerals

The mineral content of commercial formulas warrants special consideration. The American Academy of Pediatrics recommends a dietary calcium/phosphorus ratio between 1:1 and 2:1 for optimal calcium absorption. The ratio declines during infancy with the introduction of solid food. There are also minimum and maximum levels for sodium, potassium, and chloride in formulas, which will meet growth needs and leave little residue to be excreted in the urine. The sodium/potassium ratio should not exceed 1, and the (sodium + potassium)/chloride ratio should be at least 1.5.

Iron deficiency is the most common cause of anemia in infants and children. In the healthy term infant there is no need for exogenous iron between birth and 4 months of age. The usually abundant neonatal iron stores gradually decline during this period to provide for the synthesis of hemoglobin, myoglobin, and enzymes, but iron deficiency is rare in the first several months unless there has been substantial loss of iron through perinatal or subsequent blood loss.

There are two forms of iron in food—heme iron and nonheme iron (see Chapter 26). Because infant diets contain little meat, the vast preponderance of iron is in the nonheme form. The extent of nonheme iron absorption depends on how soluble it becomes in the duodenum, and this is determined by the composition of food consumed in a given meal. The most important enhancers of nonheme iron absorption are ascorbic acid (vitamin C) and meat, fish, and poultry. Major inhibitors are bran (whole-grain cereal), oxalates (spinach), polyphenols (tannates in tea), and phosphates (cow milk and egg yolks). Absorption of the small amount of iron in breast milk is uniquely high—50% on average—in contrast to much lower absorption from cow-milk formulas and dry infant cereals. Formula manufacturers offset the lower absorption by fortifying some formulas with

---

BOX 5-5   Optimizing Iron Status in Infants

Unfortified Food

Maintain breastfeeding as the sole feeding for at least
    4–6 months.
Do not give fresh cow milk until after about 12 months.
Use vitamin C-rich foods and fruit juice and/or meat with
    meals of solid food after about 6 months.

Iron- and Vitamin C-Fortified Foods

If cow-milk formula is used, choose one fortified with iron and
    vitamin C.
Use infant cereal or milk-cereal products fortified with iron
    ± vitamin C.
Use vitamin C-fortified fruit juice with meals of solid food.

**Iron Supplementation (Ferrous Sulfate or Similarly
Bioavailable Compounds)**

Supplement low-birth weight infants with the following amounts
    of iron from formula and/or drops, beginning no later than
    2 months of age and continuing through the sixth month:
    Birth weight; supplemental iron dose
    1500–2500 g; 2 mg/kg/day
    1000–1500 g; 3 mg/kg/day
    <1000 g; 4 mg/dg/day
For established iron deficiency: 3 mg/kg/day

---

higher concentrations of iron. Box 5–5 suggests ways to
optimize iron status in infants.

Trace Minerals

Normal volumes of commercial formulas provide
adequate amounts of trace elements for full-term infants.
The fluoride concentration of breast milk ranges from
3 to 10 µg/L. Fluoride is poorly transported from plasma
to milk, and concentrations in milk remain low even if
the mother consumes fluoridated water. There is no
convincing evidence that orally ingested fluoride is
important in preventing dental caries (i.e., by altering
the composition of the dental enamel). However, there

is clear evidence that oral consumption may contribute to fluorosis of the permanent dentition. Therefore *no* fluoride supplements are recommended for infants until after teeth have erupted, when it is recommended that fluoridated water be offered (when feasible) several times daily to infants fed by breast milk, cow milk, or formulas prepared with water that contain no more than 0.3 mg/L.

REFERENCES

1. United States Department of Health and Human Services: Healthy People 2010. Available at http://www.healthypeople.gov.
2. Ostrea EM, Mantaring JB, Silvestre MA: Drugs that affect the fetus and newborn infant via the placenta or breast milk. Pediatr Clin North Am 51:539–579, 2004.

SUGGESTED READINGS

American Academy of Pediatrics, Committee on Nutrition: Breastfeeding and the use of human milk. Pediatrics 115:496–605, 2005; available at http://pediatrics.aappublications.org/cgi/content/full/115/2/496.
Kleinman RE (ed): Pediatric Nutrition Handbook, 5th ed. Elk Grove, Ill, American Academy of Pediatrics, 2003.
Meek JY (ed): New Mother's Guide to Breastfeeding. Elk Grove, Ill, American Academy of Pediatrics, 2002.

WEB SITES

American Association of Pediatrics, http://www.aap.org/
Infant formula manufacturers, http://www.ross.com; http://www.meadjohnson.com; http://www.novartis.com; http://www.nestleusa.com

6

Childhood and Adolescence

BONNIE A. SPEAR, PhD •
REINALDO FIGUEROA, MD

The nutritional requirements of children and adolescents change as they grow and develop. Nutrient needs vary somewhat depending on the growth rate and total body size. Toddlers have a slower growth rate that continues through childhood until the growth spurt of adolescence. Healthy food habits help ensure that children obtain enough nutrients from their diet.

By planning early food experiences, parents can guide the development of a child's personal food preferences and choices. Children move from being dependent on parents to provide healthy food choices to making their own food choices when they are in late adolescence. An important role for parents and other caregivers is to provide a wide variety of healthy foods, letting children decide the amounts and types of foods to eat.

Normal Growth Rates

Growth rates are predictable in normal children. A child's weight usually triples by 12 months of age and quadruples by 2 years of age. Thereafter, weight gain slows to a relatively steady yearly increase of 2 to 3 kg until the adolescent growth spurt begins. Between 3 and 10 years of age, the height gained by girls and boys remains consistently between 5 and 8 cm per year. A normal 2-year-old has reached 50% of adult height, and a normal 10-year-old has reached about 80% of height potential. The head circumference of a newborn in the

United States is about 34 cm. The brain normally doubles in size during the first year of life, and by 3 years of age the head circumference has increased to approximately 50 cm. Thereafter, head circumference does not change markedly.

Growth assessment is the best way to determine whether children are well nourished. When they are getting enough to eat and have no health problems, children should grow normally. Plotting height (or length for children less than 24 months old) and weight on the CDC standardized growth charts can help determine if a child's growth is appropriate (Figs. 6–1 through 6–8).

Weight and height can be plotted on growth grids to determine whether individuals are maintaining their growth pattern or staying within a growth channel. For children older than 2 years of age, the relationship between weight and height can be evaluated by using growth charts for body mass index (BMI) by age (see Figs. 6–6 and 6–8). BMI is calculated by dividing body weight (in kilograms) by the square of height (in meters), or kg/m^2. Appropriate weights for height, according to age and sex, lie between the 5th and 85th percentiles, allowing for individual differences in body build. Children with BMIs below the 5th percentile should be assessed for organic diseases or eating disorders. Children with BMIs between the 85th and 95th percentiles are considered at risk of becoming overweight, and additional evaluations should be performed to determine causes and health risks. Children with BMIs greater than or equal to the 95th percentile for age and gender are overweight and should have an in-depth medical assessment that includes data on family history, blood pressure, total cholesterol level, any major change in BMI, and concern about weight.

Anthropometric measurements yield further precision by distinguishing between fat and lean body mass (see Chapter 10). For example, a low triceps skinfold measurement in an individual who is above the 85th percentile for BMI indicates that the child is overweight but not overfat. Assessment of midarm muscle circumference should confirm a muscular composition.

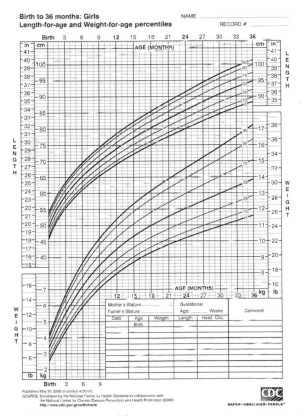

Figure 6–1. GIRLS, BIRTH TO 36 MONTHS, LENGTH-FOR-AGE AND WEIGHT-FOR-AGE. Developed by the National Center for Health Statistics in collaboration with the National Center for Chronic Disease Prevention and Health Promotion (2000); http://www.cdc.gov/growthcharts.

A skinfold in the 90th percentile or greater with a BMI greater than the 95th percentile suggests overfat status, or true overweight.

Figure 6–9 shows growth velocity curves, which are calculated by dividing the difference between two height measurements as near to one year apart as possible by the exact time elapsed between them. Growth velocity is plotted at the midpoint of the time interval. There are

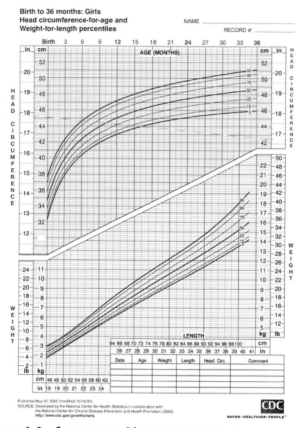

Birth to 36 months: Girls
Head circumference-for-age and
Weight-for-length percentiles

Figure 6–2. GIRLS, BIRTH TO 36 MONTHS, HEAD CIRCUMFERENCE-FOR-AGE AND WEIGHT-FOR-LENGTH. Developed by the National Center for Health Statistics in collaboration with the National Center for Chronic Disease Prevention and Health Promotion (2000); http://www.cdc.gov/growthcharts.

three epochs of growth: early, rather fast growth before the age of 2; a relatively unchanging pattern of growth during preschool and primary school years; and an adolescent growth spurt. There is little difference between boys and girls before 10 years of age, but then the typical girl starts her adolescent growth spurt and for a few years

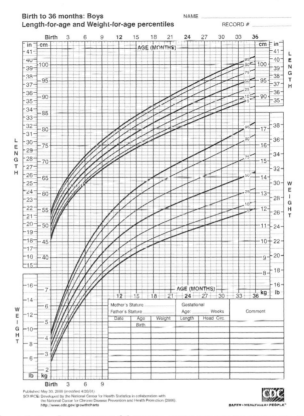

Figure 6-3. BOYS, BIRTH TO 36 MONTHS, LENGTH-FOR-AGE AND WEIGHT-FOR-AGE. Developed by the National Center for Health Statistics in collaboration with the National Center for Chronic Disease Prevention and Health Promotion (2000); http://www.cdc.gov/growthcharts.

is taller than a boy of the same age. About 2 years later, the boy starts his spurt and by the age of 14 is the taller. The mean difference in mature height between men and women in the United States is 12.5 cm. Inadequate or excessive growth can be detected by plotting height changes on the CDC growth charts. The major cause of short stature during adolescence is genetically late initiation of puberty, although other conditions such as

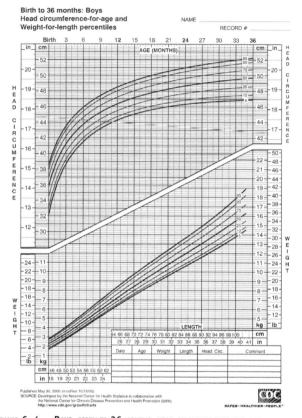

Figure 6–4. BOYS, BIRTH TO 36 MONTHS, HEAD CIRCUMFERENCE-FOR-AGE AND WEIGHT-FOR-LENGTH. Developed by the National Center for Health Statistics in collaboration with the National Center for Chronic Disease Prevention and Health Promotion (2000); http://www.cdc.gov/growthcharts.

chronic disease or skeletal and chromosomal abnormalities can account for certain children being shorter than normal. Hormonal imbalances leading to abnormal growth are rare.

Puberty, the process of physically developing from a child to an adult, is initiated by physiologic factors and includes maturation of the total body. Adolescence is the

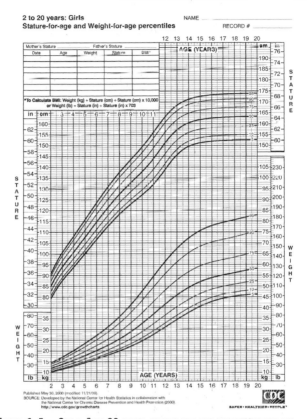

Figure 6–5. Girls, 2 to 20 years, stature-for-age and weight-for-age.
Developed by the National Center for Health Statistics in collaboration
with the National Center for Chronic Disease Prevention and Health
Promotion (2000); http://www.cdc.gov/growthcharts.

only time following birth when the velocity of growth
actually increases (see Fig. 6–9). The adolescent gains
about 20% of adult height and 50% of adult weight
during this period. Because adolescents of the same age
often differ markedly in size, it is impossible to use age
alone in evaluating pubertal growth. An assessment of
the degree of maturation of secondary sexual characteristics is useful both for evaluating physical growth and

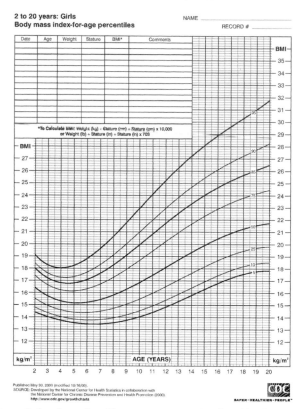

2 to 20 years: Girls
Body mass index-for-age percentiles

NAME

RECORD #

Figure 6–6. **Girls, 2 to 20 years, bmi-for-age.** Developed by the National Center for Health Statistics in collaboration with the National Center for Chronic Disease Prevention and Health Promotion (2000); http://www.cdc.gov/growthcharts.

for detecting certain diseases and disorders associated with adolescence. Sexual maturity ratings (SMRs), often called Tanner stages, are widely used to evaluate growth and developmental age during adolescence.[1,2] Figure 6–10 shows the interrelationships between maturity stages and the adolescent growth spurt together with testicular volume in boys and the mean age of menarche in girls. The development of breasts and male

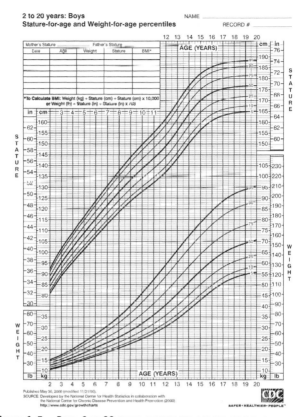

2 to 20 years: Boys
Stature-for-age and Weight-for-age percentiles

NAME

RECORD #

Figure 6–7. Boys, 2 to 20 years, stature-for-age and weight-for-age.
Developed by the National Center for Health Statistics in collaboration
with the National Center for Chronic Disease Prevention and Health
Promotion (2000); http://www.cdc.gov/growthcharts.

genitalia and the growth of pubic hair in both genders
are graded in stages 1 (prepubertal) through 5 (mature),
and utilize convenient and reasonably objective
anatomic criteria. In general, girls experience adolescence earlier than boys, but this is most striking in
terms of the growth spurt. In girls, puberty has begun
when breast stage 2 is reached, although in a small percentage the adolescent growth spurt has already started.

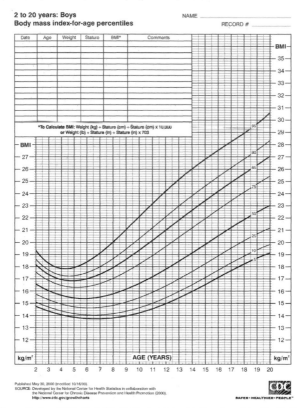

Figure 6–8. Boys, 2 to 20 years, bmi-for-age. Developed by the National Center for Health Statistics in collaboration with the National Center for Chronic Disease Prevention and Health Promotion (2000); http://www.cdc.gov/growthcharts.

The peak of the growth spurt is usually reached by breast stage 3, and by the time a girl is menstruating, her growth spurt is virtually always on the wane. In boys, testicular enlargement to 4 mL capacity, from a prepubertal 2 to 3 mL, is usually the first evidence of puberty, although this small change is not evident on a cursory examination. The adolescent growth spurt is a

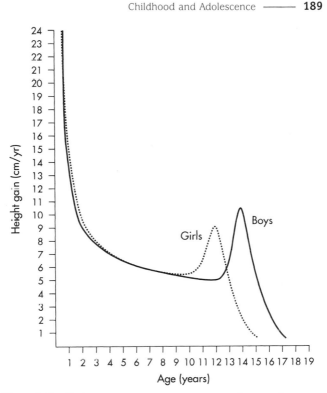

Figure 6–9. Height-velocity curves for a typical boy (*SOLID LINE*) and girl (*BROKEN LINE*). From Tanner JM, Whitehouse RH, Takaishi M: Standards from birth to maturity for height, weight, height velocity, and weight velocity: British children, 1965. Arch Dis Child 41:454, 1966.

late event, seldom starting before genitalia stage 3 and peaking between genitalia stages 4 and 5.

Nutrient Requirements

Adequate intakes of energy, protein, and all other essential nutrients are required for the rapid growth and development of the young child and adolescent. Children who

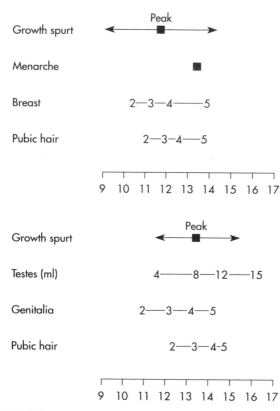

Figure 6–10. INTERRELATIONSHIPS AMONG EVENTS AT PUBERTY (GIRLS, *UPPER PANEL;* BOYS, *LOWER PANEL*). The mean attainment ages of the breast, genitalia, and pubic hair stages are indicated by the *numbers 2 to 5*. For testes, the numbers indicate the volume in ml of a single testis at the mean attainment age. The peaks for growth spurt and menarche are at the mean age and are indicated by *solid blocks*. The *horizontal arrows* represent the typical span of the growth spurt for an average child. From Falkner F, Tanner JM (eds): Human Growth, vol 2. New York, Plenum Press, 1978.

limit energy intake or have food insecurity that limits it may achieve lower adult heights.

Energy

Energy intake recommendations are intended to maintain health, promote optimal growth and maturation, and support a desirable level of physical activity. Equations for determining energy requirements are included in the Dietary Reference Intakes (DRIs) as Estimated Energy Requirements (EERs; Box 6-1). EERs are calculated using age, gender, weight, height, and one of four physical activity levels (sedentary, low active, active, and

---

BOX 6-1   Estimated Energy Requirements (EERs) for Infants, Children, and Adolescents

EER = *Total Energy Expenditure* (TEE) + *Energy Deposition*

Infants

  0 to 3 months
  EER = (89 × weight of infant [kg] − 100) + 175 (kcal for Energy Deposition)
  4 to 6 months
  EER = (89 × weight of infant [kg] − 100) + 56 (kcal for Energy Deposition)
  7 to 12 months
  EER = (89 × weight of infant [kg] − 100) + 22 (kcal for Energy Deposition)
  13 to 35 months
  EER = (89 × weight of infant [kg] − 100) + 20 (kcal for Energy Deposition)

Boys 3 to 8 years of age

  EER = 88.5 − 61.9 × Age [y] + Physical Activity (PA) × (26.7 × Weight [kg] + 903 × height [m])+ 20 (kcal for Energy Deposition)

Girls 3 to 8 years of age

  EER = 135.3 − 30.8 × Age [y] + Physical Activity (PA) × (10.0 × Weight [kg] + 934 × height [m]) + 20 (kcal for Energy Deposition)

Box continued on following page

BOX 6-1   Estimated Energy Requirements (EERs) for Infants, Children, and Adolescents *(Continued)*

Boys 9 to 18 years of age

EER = 88.5 − 61.9 × Age [y] + Physical Activity (PA) × (26.7 × Weight [kg] + 903 × height [m]) + 25 (kcal for Energy Deposition)

Girls 9 to 18 years of age

EER = 135.3 − 30.8 × Age [y] + Physical Activity (PA) × (10.0 × Weight [kg] + 934 × height [m]) + 25 (kcal for Energy Deposition)

Where PA is the physical activity coefficient (PAL = Physical Activity Level):

For boys and girls 3 to 8 and boys 9 to 18

PA = 1.00 if PAL is estimated to be ≥1.0 and <1.4 (sedentary)
PA = 1.13 if PAL is estimated to be ≥1.4 and <1.6 (low active)
PA = 1.26 if PAL is estimated to be ≥1.6 and <1.9 (active)
PA = 1.42 if PAL is estimated to be ≥1.9 and <2.5 (very active)

For girls 9 to 18

PA = 1.00 if PAL is estimated to be ≥1.0 and <1.4 (sedentary)
PA = 1.16 if PAL is estimated to be ≥1.4 and <1.6 (low active)
PA = 1.31 if PAL is estimated to be ≥1.6 and <1.9 (active)
PA = 1.56 if PAL is estimated to be ≥1.9 and <2.5 (very active)

Example physical activities for PAL categories (miles walked at 2 to 4 mph)

Sedentary	None
Low active	1.5–2.2 mi/d
Active	3.0–4.4 mi/d
Very active	7.5–10.3 mi/d

From Food and Nutrition Board, Institute of Medicine: Dietary Reference Intakes for Energy, Carbohydrate, Fiber, Fat, Fatty Acids, Cholesterol, Protein, and Amino Acids (Macronutrients). Washington, DC, Institute of Medicine, National Academy Press, 2002; available at http:// www.nap.edu/books/ 0309085373/html/index.html.

very active) reflecting energy expended beyond that required for the activities of daily living.[3] For children and adolescents, an additional factor is included for energy deposition (growth). Variability in EERs between girls and boys arises from variations in growth rates and physical activity. For example, differences in energy requirements from sedentary to very active range from 600 calories in 3-year-olds to 1200 calories in 18-year-olds.

Protein

Protein needs, like those for energy, correlate more closely with a child's growth pattern than with chronologic age. The DRIs for protein are based on the amount of protein needed for growth and positive nitrogen balance (see Table 3–1).[3] Average protein intakes of U.S. children are well above the RDA for all age groups. However, if energy intake is inadequate for any reason (e.g., food insecurity, chronic illness, or attempts to lose weight), dietary protein may be used to meet energy needs, making it unavailable for synthesis of new tissue or for tissue repair. This may lead to a reduction in growth rate and a decrease in lean body mass. Current dieting patterns in some adolescent females can result in restricted energy intakes that are potentially harmful, especially when protein sources are used to meet energy needs. Excess protein consumption, whether from food or supplements, can also be harmful, leading to dehydration, weight gain, and calcium loss, and potentially affecting renal function.

Micronutrients

Micronutrients (vitamins and minerals) play an important role in the growth and health of children and adolescents. The majority of children do not eat adequate amounts of micronutrient-rich fruits and vegetables, potentially increasing risk for chronic disease in later years. Because of the many health benefits associated with fruits and vegetables, the U.S. *Dietary Guidelines* recommend 2 cups of fruit and 2½ cups of vegetables per day for persons consuming 2000 calories. Unfortunately, surveys show that actual intakes are far below these recommendations; in 2003, it was estimated that only about 22% of adolescents ate 5 or more servings of fruits or vegetables per day.[4]

Despite low levels of fruit and vegetable intake, most children get sufficient amounts of vitamins and minerals until they reach adolescence, when requirements increase dramatically due to growth demands. Because of increased energy demands during this period, higher intakes of thiamin, riboflavin, and niacin are required for the release of energy from carbohydrates. With tissue synthesis, there is an increased demand for vitamin B_6, folic acid, and vitamin B_{12}. There is also an increased requirement for vitamin D (for rapid skeletal growth), and vitamins A, C, and E are needed for new cell growth. Although there are few reports of low serum vitamin C levels in teens, those who habitually avoid fruits and vegetables and those who smoke cigarettes may be at increased risk for deficiency.

Because of accelerated muscular, skeletal, and endocrine development, calcium needs are greater during puberty and adolescence than in the childhood and adult years. At the peak of the growth spurt, the daily deposition of calcium can be twice that of the average during the rest of the adolescent period. In fact, 45% of the skeletal mass is added during adolescence. The DRI for calcium is 1300 mg for all adolescents. Dietary survey data indicate that adolescents, particularly females, are at risk for inadequate calcium intake.

Developmental Stages

Toddlers (1 to 3 years)

A toddler's developmental stages, behavioral characteristics, and food preferences must be considered when providing food. Between years 1 and 3, the annual weight gain decreases from 6.5 kg to 2.5 kg, and height gain declines from 25 cm to 7 cm per year. The growth in head circumference also slows to 0.5 to 1.2 cm per year by age 3. There is a concurrent decrease in energy and protein needs to approximately 100 kcal/kg and 1.2 g protein/kg.

Feeding behavior develops progressively during the toddler years, as shown in Table 6–1. Oral and neuromuscular development improves the ability to eat. Increased refinement of hand and finger movement occurs, and the appearance of most of the primary teeth leads toddlers to self-feeding. As children gain proficiency in coordinating arm, wrist, and hand movements, they demand increased responsibility in feeding themselves and may reject offers of assistance. Use of finger foods, spoons, and cups should be encouraged to help continue development of manual dexterity and coordination.

Parents should offer three meals and two snacks each day, but food intake will vary. Avoid foods likely to be aspirated, such as hot dogs, nuts, grapes, hard candies, popcorn, and raw carrots. Limits should be set so that

Table 6–1	DEVELOPMENT OF FEEDING BEHAVIOR
Age	**Typical Feeding Behavior**
12 months	Chews solid food
	Begins to use spoon but turns it before reaching mouth
	May hold cup; likely to tilt cup, causing spilling
18 months	Uses spoon well with frequent spilling
	Turns spoon in mouth
	Holds glass with both hands
24 months	Feeds self without inverting spoon
	Uses spoon well with moderate spilling
	Holds glass with one hand
	Plays with food
	Distinguishes between food and inedible materials
36 months	Self feeding complete with occasional spilling
	Can manage knife and fork with some help with hard foods
	Obtains drink of water from faucet
	Pours from pitcher

demands for food and drink do not become attention-getting devices that might lead to inappropriate intake.

The eating patterns of most toddlers are characterized by decreased food intake relative to body size. This change in food consumption after infancy, often worrisome to parents, is normal and related to the dramatic reduction in growth rate. Needless conflicts often occur because of discrepancies between the child's food intake and the parents' expectations of what the child should eat. Box 6–2 lists suggestions to facilitate the feeding of toddlers. They should be offered a variety of foods from each of the six basic food groups, at regular intervals. Food preferences may be erratic, with foods readily accepted one day being totally rejected the next day. Milk consumption usually decreases as solid food intake

---

BOX 6–2   Hints to Give Parents on Feeding Toddlers

1. Try to relax; feeding/eating and meal times should be pleasant for everyone.
2. Avoid battles over eating. Encourage your child, but avoid forced feeding or punitive approaches.
3. You are responsible for deciding when, where, and what foods your child is offered (with consideration for your child's preferences); your child should decide how much to eat.
4. Use positive reinforcement (e.g., praise for eating well).
5. Withholding food is not an appropriate form of punishment.
6. Accept your child's desire to feed himself or herself. Accept that messes will occur and be prepared (e.g., newspaper on the floor).
7. Try to eat together as a family. Good eating behavior can be modeled, and young children like to mimic older siblings and parents.
8. Allow about 1 hour without food or drink (except water) before a meal to stimulate the appetite.
9. Consumption of excessive fluids reduces the intake of solid foods; offer solids first and limit juices to 4 to 8 oz per day.
10. Establish a routine of meals and snacks at set times, with some flexibility; avoid snacks right after an unfinished meal.
11. Recognize your child's cues indicating hunger, satiety, and food preferences.
12. Limit possible distractions (e.g., television) during meals.

increases. In order to foster sound eating habits, the child's environment should be pleasant and enjoyable during meals. The child should be allowed to eat with other family members when possible and should not be punished for spilling milk or making messes. Quiet surroundings (e.g., television turned off) decrease distractions and enhance food intake.

Early Childhood (4 to 6 years)

In this age group, the child poses fewer nutritional problems. Mealtime is more pleasant for all family members. The preschool child is developmentally able to self-feed without assistance, has more coordinated gross motor skills, and has varied and changing interests. The appetite tends to be sporadic and parallels weight gain. Food becomes a secondary interest. More time is spent away from home at day care centers, school, or friends' homes, and food consumption between meals increases. To promote sound nutritional habits and prevent nutritional deficiencies or excesses, parents should be informed of the basic principles of nutrition and meal planning and serve as role models for the preschool child. The quality of foods from all food groups should be emphasized. In order to prevent obesity and dental caries, as well as promote sound nutritional habits, snacks or desserts high in concentrated sweets or of low nutritional value should be consumed infrequently. Skim or low-fat milk may be substituted for whole milk, especially if the child is at risk of becoming overweight.

Middle Childhood (7 to 10 years)

This age group is characterized by a moderate growth rate, about 2 to 4 kg/year in weight and 5 to 6 cm/year in height. Nutrient and energy intakes are important, as children in middle childhood are laying down reserves in preparation for the adolescent growth spurt. However, excessive weight gain in anticipation of this growth spurt may result in childhood weight problems. The eating habits of preadolescents are often influenced more by peer pressure than by parents' actions. Adaptation to school may likewise present nutritional problems. Breakfast may be eaten alone or skipped altogether, and snacks after school may be unsupervised. These adaptations may be less of a problem if sound eating habits are established earlier in life.

Nutrition education should be integrated into the school curriculum to encourage children to learn basic nutrition principles related to their physiologic needs and to incorporate them into their daily lives. This training will allow children to accept more responsibility for their health and hopefully optimize their dietary habits in adulthood.

Adolescents (11 to 18 years)

Nutrient requirements increase markedly during adolescence because of the virtual doubling of body mass. EERs are based on energy expenditure, requirements for growth, and level of physical activity. Adolescents often show marked variation in energy expenditure, and the EERs represent average, rather than individual, requirements. Dietary proteins are essential to provide amino acids for growth, but they will be oxidized for energy and unavailable for growth if energy needs are not met by carbohydrates and fats in the diet. The greatest demand for calcium occurs during the adolescent growth spurt, and increased intake should allow for variation in the timing of this event. The adolescent requirement for iron is related to increases in blood volume and hemoglobin and myoglobin synthesis, and in girls, menstrual losses. The timing of the increased iron requirement is subject to enormous variations in the pace of puberty. Iron losses before menarche are approximately the same as in adults, approximately 0.5 to 1.0 mg/day, and the recommendations assume that 10% of dietary iron is absorbed.

The food habits of the adolescent differ from those of any other age group. They are characterized by an increasing tendency to skip meals, snack, inappropriately consume fast foods, diet, and practice fad diets. This behavior can be explained by the teen's newfound independence, questioning of existing values, poor body image, and search for self-identity, peer acceptance, and conformity of lifestyle. It is necessary to understand these factors to counsel teenagers properly regarding diet. Particular care should be taken to provide adequate calcium, iron, and zinc, which are frequently marginal in adolescents' diets. Vegetarian teenagers who do not eat eggs or drink milk may develop deficiencies of vitamins D and B_{12}, calcium, iron, zinc, and other trace elements. A careful review of the dietary intake is needed to ensure that it meets nutrient needs. On occasion, dietary supplements may be considered.

REFERENCES

1. Tanner JM, Whitehouse RH, Takaishi M: Standards from birth to maturity for height, weight, height velocity, and weight velocity: British children, 1965 Arch Dis Child 41:454, 1966.
2. Falkner F, Tanner JM (eds): Human Growth, vol 2. New York, Plenum Press, 1978.
3. Food and Nutrition Board, Institute of Medicine: Dietary Reference Intakes for Energy, Carbohydrate, Fiber, Fat, Fatty Acids, Cholesterol, Protein, and Amino Acids (Macronutrients). Washington, DC, Institute of Medicine, National Academy Press, 2002; available at http://www.nap.edu/books/0309085373/html/index.html.
4. Grunbaum JA, Kann L, Kinchen S, et al: Youth Risk Behavior Surveillance—United States, 2003. MMWR 53(SS02):1-96, 2004; available at http://www.cdc.gov/mmwr/preview/mmwrhtml/ss5302a1.htm.

SUGGESTED READING

Samora, PQ, King K. *Handbook of Pediatric Nutrition,* 3rd edition. Jones and Bartlett, Sudbury, MA. 2005.

WEBSITES

NCHS/CDC Growth Charts, http://www.cdc/gov/growthcharts
Institute of Medicine, http://www.iom.edu (Child Health link)
Guidelines for Adolescent Nutrition Services, http://www.epi.umn.edu/let/pubs

7

Aging

CHRISTINE S. RITCHIE, MD

Since 1900, when there were 3 million people age 65 or older in the United States (4% of the total population), the number of older Americans has increased more than 10-fold as a result of the convergence of "successful aging" and declining birth rates. In 2000, the 65-and-older population was 35 million, or about 13% of the total population. By 2030, an estimated 20% of the population will be 65 years or older. This same trend is occurring worldwide; the global average lifespan has increased from 49.5 years in 1972 to higher than 63 years at present. As a consequence of increasing lifespan, older adults as a group have increased susceptibility to a number of age-related chronic diseases—including cardiovascular disease (CVD), neurologic disease, hypertension, diabetes, and some cancers—that may be ameliorated by nutritional intervention.

Epidemiologic studies have found undernutrition to be a problem in 1% to 20% of elderly people living at home and up to 70% in persons living in institutions. Conversely, about 48% of adults between ages 65 and 74 and 40% older than age 75 are overweight; 19% and 10% are obese, respectively (see Chapter 17).

Dietary intake studies of the elderly have shown that 10% of men and 20% of women have intakes of protein below the Recommended Dietary Allowance (RDA); one third consume less than the RDA of calories. Fifty percent of older adults who live at or near the poverty line have intakes of minerals and vitamins below the RDA. Approximately 10% to 30% of all older adults have subnormal levels of minerals and vitamins.

Major nutritional deficits are rarely seen among healthy community-dwelling older adults. However, it is likely that subclinical alterations in nutrition contribute to an older adult's increased vulnerability to stressors. In acutely ill, hospitalized older adults, intakes of both calories and protein are frequently so low that up to 60% are undernourished at admission or develop serious nutritional deficits prior to discharge.

Aging Changes that Increase Nutritional Risk

Much of the variation in nutritional status results from the heterogeneity of the older adult population and physiologic changes associated with aging. Normal aging involves a steady erosion of certain organ system reserves and homeostatic controls. The loss of homeostatic reserves is most evident during periods of maximal exertion or physiologic stress. For example, in many instances, after weight loss during an illness, older patients may have difficulty increasing their intake to the point necessary to return to their baseline weight.

Physiologic Factors

Changes in Body Composition

As humans age, their ratio of fat to muscle increases. Compared to adults in their 20s, older adults who are 65 to 75 often have a positive energy balance and decreased activity, resulting in an increase in body weight and centralized adiposity along with a moderate decrease in muscle and bone compartments of lean tissue. In contrast, adults older than 75 begin to exhibit lower weight mostly because of large losses of lean body mass from disuse and inadequate intake of protein and energy. The loss of muscle mass and strength that inevitably occurs with aging is known as sarcopenia. Activity of growth hormone and testosterone, which promote lean tissue growth, appears reduced in the very old and may contribute to these changes. Along with chronic diseases, neuroendocrine dysregulation, and chronic inflammation, sarcopenia contributes significantly to the development of frailty and functional impairment in older age.

Exercise programs may prevent or reverse some of the decrease in lean body mass.

These changes in body composition have several important implications. As muscle mass decreases, resting energy expenditure decreases and energy requirements decline. Protein reserves available during periods of stress are diminished. Because body water is associated with muscle mass, there is a decrease in total body water and an increased susceptibility to dehydration. Because relative fat mass is increased, the distribution volume of fat-soluble drugs increases and their elimination is delayed. Examples of fat-soluble drugs whose metabolism may be affected by these changes include diazepam and propranolol.

Changes in Endocrine Function

Alterations in endocrine function that affect nutritional status include an increased incidence of insulin resistance and a change in water metabolism. Insulin resistance may be due in part to the proportional increase in body fat. This contributes to higher fasting blood glucose levels with increasing age and higher incidence of Type 2 diabetes mellitus. The renin-angiotensin-aldosterone axis, the response to vasopressin, and the thirst response are less sensitive to volume depletion, placing older adults at greater risk for dehydration.

Gastrointestinal Changes

Anorexia of aging describes the physiologic decrease in appetite and food intake that accompanies normal aging and that may produce undesirable weight loss. The etiology of this anorexia is not altogether clear but is influenced by a number of factors including impairment of the receptive relaxation of the gastric fundus with aging and slowing of gastric emptying along with alterations in central mediators of satiety.

One third of individuals older than age 70 have a significantly diminished capacity to secrete stomach acid. In addition, many older adults are treated chronically with histamine-2 antagonists or proton pump inhibitors for gastroesophageal reflux or ulcer disease. In both settings, the lack of gastric acid may lead to decreased absorption of vitamin B_{12}, calcium, iron, folic acid, and possibly zinc, and may account for the increased tendency for depletion of these nutrients with age. The prevalence of lactose intolerance also rises with age and may contribute to a decreased intake of dairy products, a key dietary source of calcium and vitamin D.

Sensory Changes

Sensory changes that occur with aging include decreased ability to smell, alterations in taste, and often a decline in visual and auditory function. Because smell is an important part of food appreciation, decline in olfactory perception can negatively affect appetite and food intake. Many medications also affect smell and may magnify this decline. Whether a decrease in taste sensation occurs with aging is controversial. However, threshold sensitivities to sweet and salty tastes also decrease; this contributes to a relative increase in sweet- and salty-food intake by some to get the same "taste" they experienced when younger. Visual impairment due to cataracts, glaucoma, or macular degeneration may affect the ability to prepare food and remain independent. Hearing impairment interferes with many of the social aspects of eating.

Pathophysiologic Factors

Comorbid conditions with a high prevalence in older populations that can adversely affect nutritional status include depression, oral disease, renal impairment, and diseases that increase metabolic demands. Depression and dysphoria are commonly present in older adults, often remain unrecognized and undertreated, and are a significant cause of weight loss in ambulatory patients, in subacute care, and in the nursing home.

Forty percent of older adults are edentulous. Only 17% to 20% of these individuals have dentures, and many of them do not have ones that fit properly. Between 60% and 90% of older adults with teeth have severe periodontal disease, leading to gum recession, tooth loss, and oral pain, all of which may contribute to poor food intake.

Changes in renal function may include a steady decline in glomerular filtration rate (GFR) and a decreased ability to concentrate urine and conserve sodium. Decreased GFR leads to a reduction in both urinary acidification and renal clearance of many drugs. Hydroxylation of vitamin D to its active form is also diminished.

A number of disease conditions may increase metabolic demands. One half to two thirds of cancer patients present with cachexia, mainly caused by anorexia (see Chapter 21). High prevalence rates of malnutrition (>30%) have also been observed in subgroups of patients with inflammatory bowel diseases, chronic heart failure, and chronic lung diseases. Other hypermetabolic conditions, such as hyperthyroidism, are common in older populations and often present atypically, making them more insidious.

Chronic Disease and Disability Factors

Eighty-five percent of the elderly have multiple chronic diseases, ranging from three to seven per person. Arthritis is the most common, followed by impairments in hearing and vision, heart disease, and hypertension. Almost 60% of persons older than age 75 have some limitation of activity, compared to 8.5% of persons aged 17 to 44. About 3% of men and women ages 65 to 74 have Alzheimer's disease, and nearly half of those age 85 and older have the disease. The net effect of these chronic conditions may be that older adults' ability to acquire, prepare, and enjoy food is limited. Restrictive diets for heart failure, diabetes, or hypertension may also be imposed. When several conditions are present, a diet that has combined restrictions, such as being low in salt, low in fat, and restricted in carbohydrates, may be unpalatable.

Medications

A number of medications can influence food consumption. Drugs may alter appetite, taste, or smell; directly interact with nutrients; or produce side effects such as nausea, vomiting, or diarrhea. Examples of these interactions are listed in Table 7–1.

Socioeconomic Factors

Social factors influencing nutritional status in older adults include isolation at mealtimes and financial limitations affecting food acquisition. One third of persons older than 65, and half older than 85 live alone, which typically decreases food enjoyment and calorie intake. Although the elderly are about as likely as those who are

Table 7–1	IMPACT OF MEDICATIONS ON NUTRITION-RELATED SYMPTOMS IN OLDER ADULTS
Symptoms	**Causative Agents**
Anorexia	Selective serotonin reuptake inhibitors (e.g., sertraline, fluoxetine; paroxetine may cause either anorexia or weight gain); antibiotics (e.g., ciprofloxacin); opioids
Altered taste	Sulfa-containing medications (e.g., furosemide); antibiotics (e.g., clarithromycin)
Nausea	Nonsteroidal anti-inflammatory agents; antibiotics; digoxin; theophylline
Dry mouth	Antihistamines (e.g., chlorpheniramine); anticholinergic agents (e.g., oxybutinin, benztropin)
Confusion/Distraction	Anticholinergics; nonsteroidal anti-inflammatory agents; neuroleptics (e.g., clozapine, risperidone)
Constipation	Anticholinergics; smooth muscle relaxants/antispasmotics; calcium channel blockers (e.g., verapamil); opioids; calcium; iron
Diarrhea	Antibiotics (e.g., amoxicillin); medication elixirs (e.g., containing sorbitol; see Chapter 13)

not elderly to be poor, a greater proportion of the elderly live near the poverty line. Individuals with fixed incomes may use money previously spent on food for medications and other needed items.

Dietary Requirements of Older Adults

Energy

Energy requirements decrease over the lifespan largely because of the decline in metabolically active lean body mass and decreased physical activity. The Dietary Reference Intakes' Estimated Energy Requirements (EERs) equations include a factor for age that deducts about 7 and 10 kcal/year for adult women and men, respectively (see Chapter 3).

Protein

Protein needs do not change with age; therefore, as total energy requirements decline, the percentage of calories from protein must increase to maintain the same level of total protein intake. The current RDA for protein, 0.80 g/kg/d, does not increase with age. It is preferable that this come from good quality protein (i.e., protein from vegetable sources and from animal sources that are low in saturated fat). During periods of stress such as infection or trauma, protein intake should be increased to 1.2 to 1.5 g/kg per day to provide a safeguard against progressive protein depletion.

Fat

Fat serves as a fuel source and aids in the absorption of fat-soluble vitamins and other dietary components. Saturated fatty acids, monounsaturated fatty acids, and cholesterol are not essential nutrients, as they can be synthesized by the body. There is no age-related change in the amount of fat intake recommended, but National Health and Nutrition Examination Survey data demonstrate that adults tend to decrease their percentage of calories from fat after age 60.

Carbohydrate and Fiber

Carbohydrates (sugars, starches) are an important energy source; the RDA for carbohydrates is 130 g/d for adults. Absolute intakes of carbohydrate decrease with age as energy intakes gradually decline. However, due to the reduction in fat intakes with age, the percentage of dietary calories coming from carbohydrates increases slightly.

Fiber intakes are generally lower than recommended in all segments of the population, including elderly persons. While the recommended Adequate Intake (AI) is 20 to 30 grams per day, intakes are substantially lower: 50% of women consume fewer than 13 g/d and 50% of men consume fewer than 17 g/d. The AI is achievable with 5 servings of fruits or vegetables and a supplement of bran. Adequate fluid intake is essential, as a high-fiber diet without additional fluids can cause dehydration and constipation. Abdominal discomfort and flatulence are common when adapting to a higher fiber intake.

Water

Changes in thirst mechanisms, decreased ability to concentrate the urine, and the reduction in total body water that occurs with aging put older adults at high risk for dehydration. Fluid intake prescriptions should be written for at-risk patients, particularly those who are institutionalized, with a goal of six glasses of fluid a day except during stressful situations likely to increase fluid loss (e.g., severely hot weather or heavy exertion). Potential negative effects of excessive water consumption have also been noted in older adults, including dilutional hyponatremia (water intoxication) and increased nocturia (nocturnal need to urinate). Therefore, any recommendation regarding fluid intake should be tailored to the patient's overall condition.

Vitamins

In general, vitamin requirements are the same in older adults as in younger adults. Exceptions include vitamins D and B_{12}, for which some elderly people need higher intakes. Lack of sun exposure, impaired skin synthesis of pre-vitamin D, and decreased hydroxylation in the kidney with advancing age contribute to marginal vitamin D status in many older adults. Inadequate vitamin D status has been linked to muscle weakness, functional impairment, and increased risk of falls and fractures. For this reason, the recommended AI (10 to 15 µg/day) is higher for adults 50 years and older than for younger adults (see Table 3–1). Even this amount of vitamin D may not be sufficient for some individuals, particularly if they do not have sun exposure or if they are at high risk for osteoporosis. All older adults should be encouraged to consume increased quantities of dietary sources of vitamin D. Daily supplements of 20 µg (800 IU) of vitamin D should be considered for older adults who are not exposed to sunlight.

The prevalence of B_{12} deficiency in older adults ranges between 10 % and 20 %. Some persons with mild deficiencies including neurologic signs have normal serum B_{12} levels, in which case an elevated serum methylmalonic acid level is diagnostic. In the past a majority of B_{12} deficiencies were thought to result from intrinsic factor deficiency, but it is now known that many older adults are B_{12} deficient due to food-cobalamin malabsorption. This is characterized by the inability to release cobalamin from food or a deficiency of intestinal cobalamin transport proteins. It is often related to the presence of atrophic gastritis, bacterial overgrowth, and treatment with histamine-2 receptor blocker and proton-pump inhibitor drugs. Patients can generally be treated with oral B_{12} supplements rather than injections, and may benefit from increasing the intake of B_{12} in food to overwhelm the binding capacity of the bacteria. The current RDA for vitamin B_{12}, 2.4 µg/d, is the same for older as for younger adults. However, because it is usually unknown whether an older adult has impaired B_{12} absorption and because B_{12} malabsorption is so common in older adults, it is recommended that for individuals older than 50, most of the requirement should be met by taking supplements containing vitamin B_{12}

or by eating fortified food products. Given the potentially significant effects of vitamin B_{12} deficiency on the nervous system, it is prudent to advocate a daily intake of 3 µg or more.

Folate, along with vitamins B_{12} and B_6, is involved in the metabolism of homocysteine (Hcy). Numerous reports indicate that Hcy concentration increases as a function of age and is associated with occlusive vascular diseases, osteoporosis, presbyopia, and cognitive impairment. Mechanisms for this effect may include LDL cholesterol oxidation, toxicity to endothelial cells, impaired platelet function, the toxic effect of Hcy on connective tissues and its contribution to increased proliferation of smooth muscle. The current adult RDA for folate is 400 µg/d; in older adults with known vascular disease, doses up to 5 mg/d may be beneficial.

Although the absorption and metabolism of vitamin C are not changed with aging, many studies have shown low serum levels in some older adults, attributed to low intakes, chronic disease, smoking, or acute illness. While there is no direct evidence of an increased need for vitamin C with aging, benefits of maintaining generous stores may include protection against cataracts, heart disease, and oxidative stress.

In addition to vitamin deficiencies, hypervitaminosis is seen in older adults who consume megadoses of vitamins. Malaise, liver dysfunction, headaches, hypercalcemia, and leukopenia may be seen with high doses of vitamin A. Diarrhea, false-negative fecal occult blood tests, renal stones, and higher mortality can occur with megadoses of vitamin C. Peripheral neuropathy can result from excessive use of vitamin B_6.

Minerals and Trace Elements

Except for iron, calcium, and zinc, aging probably does not significantly alter the requirements for minerals and trace elements. The iron RDA for older men and women is 8 mg/d. When iron deficiency occurs in older adults, it is usually from gastrointestinal blood loss rather than poor diet.

Calcium nutrition is strongly influenced by age. The efficiency of calcium absorption from the gastrointestinal tract decreases significantly after age 60 in both sexes. Individuals between 70 and 90 years of age absorb about one third less calcium than do younger adults. Osteoporosis affects 25% of white women older than 50, causing more than 1.5 million fractures in that population each year, and is thus a major detriment to health quality in older adults. Given the impact of calcium deficiency on cortical bone loss, the AI for calcium for persons 51 years of age and older is now 1200 mg/d. These levels may also help prevent colon cancer and hypertension.

Marginal zinc status is common in older adults. Institutionalized and hospitalized persons are at particularly high risk for zinc deficiency, especially those stressed by infection, trauma, or surgery. Deficiency may impair wound healing, immune function, taste, and smell. Zinc supplementation accelerates wound healing only in zinc-deficient patients, and excessive zinc supplementation may interfere with immune function and copper metabolism.

Factors Affecting Dietary Prescriptions in Older Adults

Dental State

Many older adults have periodontal disease and poor dentition. Pay close attention to the patient's oral status so that appropriate diets will be prescribed. In persons with oral pain, a soft-mechanical or dental-soft diet may be preferred over a regular diet.

Changes in Taste Sensitivity

As previously mentioned, sensitivity to salty and sweet tastes decreases with age, so older persons tend to over-compensate with a higher intake of salty and sweet foods. Diets restricting these may thus result in decreased food consumption. Much of the flavor in food results from its fat content. When fats are restricted, energy consumption may fall to unacceptable levels because of decreased energy density and decreased palatability.

Swallowing Disorders

Disorders of swallowing usually result from disease, the most common being neurodegenerative disorders. The loss of voluntary initiation of swallowing is a frequent finding in late-stage dementia. Because 60% of long-term care residents have dementia, difficulties with oral feeding are common in this setting. Many individuals with oropharyngeal dysphagia benefit from specific dysphagia diets and chewing protocols (such as use of the chin tuck when swallowing to minimize aspiration) designed in collaboration with a speech pathologist and a dietitian. Most patients can receive adequate intake with assisted feeding and should not require the placement of a gastrostomy tube.

Weight Maintenance

The Longitudinal Study of Aging found that body mass indices in the mildly obese or overweight range (30 to 35 kg/m² for women and 27 to 30 kg/m² for men) were associated with the lowest mortality rates in adults older than 70.[1] The Cardiovascular Health Study also found that the association between higher BMI and mortality seen in middle aged adults was not a risk factor for 5-year mortality in persons older than 70.[2] These findings may be influenced by survival selection and events such as hip fractures that are more common and more catastrophic in thinner older adults. What may be more important is whether the older adult has adequate lean body mass and the extent to which body fatness in younger adulthood influences the development of subsequent disease, such as atherosclerosis, in the elderly years. When plotted against body weight, mortality rates appear to be lowest with lean weight in the 20s and moderately higher weights in middle age and older ages.

The involuntary loss of more than 5% to 10% of an older person's usual weight during one year is an ominous clinical sign associated with increased risk for mortality. Unintentional weight loss should thus be met with concern and prompt a search for the cause. Causes of unintended weight loss in the elderly are shown in Table 7-2.

Cultural and Societal Habits

Most people, old or young, define food culturally rather than nutritionally. Food is a cultural symbol of love, status, hospitality, and friendship and is also strongly associated with emotional states. Foods can be a link to the past for elderly persons and provide security in unfamiliar surroundings. Under stress, people often

Table 7-2	COMMON CAUSES OF WEIGHT LOSS IN OLDER ADULTS
Social Factors	Poverty, social isolation, substance abuse (especially alcohol)
Sensory Factors	Visual impairment, altered taste and smell
Physical Factors	Functional impairment due to disability, frailty, chronic illnesses
Mechanical Barriers	Oral disease, swallowing disorders
Iatrogenic Factors	Medications (see Table 7-1)
	Overly restricted diets
Neuropsychiatric Conditions	Depression (often occurs concurrently with heart disease, stroke, and dementia)
	Dementia
	Late-life paranoia
Medical Conditions Leading to Increased Energy Requirements	Infections
	Chronic obstructive pulmonary disease
	Hyperthyroidism
	Wounds, burns, fractures
Medical Conditions Leading to Interference with Eating	Congestive heart failure
	Diabetic gastroparesis
	Malabsorption
	Cholelithiasis

regress to eating foods familiar from childhood. Specific cultural factors including religion, ethnic origin, and social pressures influence food selections. When menus are planned centrally, as in institutional settings, malnutrition may result. Breakfast is the meal most enjoyed and most completely eaten by elderly people.

Adherence

Adherence with drug and dietary therapy tends to be higher in older populations. Even so, about one third of medication prescriptions are never filled by this group, and nonadherence with dietary restrictions may be even higher. Diets prescribed for older persons are less likely to be followed unless cultural, ethnic, and socioeconomic factors are considered. Adherence to dietary prescriptions can be improved by a clinician taking a dietary history, considering cultural preferences, and evaluating the economic resources available. On the whole, foods that are restricted in salt, fat, or carbohydrates are more expensive than unrestricted foods.

REFERENCES

1. Allison DB, Gallagher D, Heo M, et al: Body mass index and all-cause mortality among people age 70 and over: The Longitudinal Study of Aging. Int J Obes 21:424–431, 1997.
2. Diehr P, Bild DE, Harris TB, et al: Body mass index and mortality in nonsmoking older adults: The Cardiovascular Health Study. Am J Public Health 88:623–629, 1998.

SUGGESTED READINGS

Akner G, Cederholm T: Treatment of protein-energy malnutrition in chronic nonmalignant disorders. Am J Clin Nutr 74:6–24, 2001.

Bales CW, Ritchie CR: Nutritional Needs and Assessment During the Life Cycle: The Elderly. In Shils ME, Shike M, Ross AC, et al (eds): Modern Nutrition in Health and Disease, 10th ed. Baltimore, Lippincott Williams & Wilkins, 2005.

Bales CW, Ritchie CS: Handbook of Clinical Nutrition and Aging. Totowa, NJ, Humana Press, 2004.

Fiatarone MA, O'Neill EF, Ryan ND, et al: Exercise training and nutritional supplementation for physical frailty in very elderly people. N Engl J Med 330:1769–1775, 1994.

Lesourd B, Mazari L: Nutrition and immunity in the elderly. Proc Nutr Soc 58:685–695, 1999.

Morley JE: Pathophysiology of anorexia. Clin Geriatr Med 18:661–673, 2002.

Li I: Feeding tubes in patients with severe dementia. Am Fam Physician 65: 1515, 1605–1610, 2002.

Sullivan DH, Liu L, Roberson PK, et al: Body weight change and mortality in a cohort of elderly patients recently discharged from the hospital. J Am Geriatr Soc 52:1696–1701, 2004.

Thomas DR: Vitamins in health and aging. Clin Geriatr Med 20: 259–274, 2004.

WEBSITES

American Geriatrics Society, http://www.americangeriatrics.org/

Mini-Nutritional Assessment for geriatric patients, http://www.mna-elderly.com

Merck Manual of Geriatrics, http://www.merck.com/mrkshared/mmg/home.jsp

8

Complementary and Alternative Nutritional Therapies

JEFFREY MECHANICK, MD

The practice of medicine encompasses activities intended to promote health and heal diseases. This practice is influenced by prevailing resources, technologies, cultural mores, economics, and idiosyncratic preferences on the part of the health care practitioner and patient. In today's medically pluralistic environment, this spans the spectrum from disciplined scientific investigation and intervention to an impressionistic philosophy of health. Ideally, all these should be considered as clinical problems and subjected to creative solutions incorporating science and humanism. Though many well-accepted medical interventions lack conclusive proof, this does not justify supplanting scientifically proven standards of care with unproven and potentially dangerous interventions. Such is the case for many, but not all, of the published and purported uses for dietary supplements (DSs).

Complementary and alternative medicine (CAM) is a group of diverse medical and health care systems, practices, and products explicitly used for the purposes of medical intervention, health promotion, or disease prevention that are not routinely taught at U.S. medical schools nor routinely underwritten by third-party payers within the existing U.S. health care system. *Complementary* therapies are used *together* with conventional medicine and *alternative* therapies are used *in place of* conventional medicine. The term *integrative medicine* is sometimes used to denote the integration of healing concepts and therapies that are native to traditional cultures and that may have credible scientific evidence for efficacy and safety.

Individuals seek CAM for assistance with a wide range of conditions and interests, including weight control, heart disease, cancer, menopausal symptoms, arthritis and other aches and pains, sexual function, athletic performance, fatigue, anxiety, stress, depression, prostate hypertrophy, memory loss and Alzheimer disease, Parkinson disease, and the common cold. Patients typically seek CAM when their complaints or conditions are not relieved by conventional medical cures. CAM use is fueled by the news media, word of mouth, distrust of traditional physicians and the pharmaceutical industry, and a preference for "natural" products. CAM practitioners are motivated by beliefs, economic rewards, and sometimes sheer fanaticism. Thus, CAM practices span a spectrum from well-intended and healthful to the utterly fraudulent. CAM is typically covered lightly, if at all, in U.S. medical school curricula, is often based on weak or no clinical evidence, and targets symptoms rather than disease-specific diagnoses. Box 8–1 outlines levels of scientific evidence and grades of recommendations that utilize them.

In response to growing health care costs, a perceived need for Americans to "self-treat" to save costs, and a public frustrated with the unavailability of many DSs on the market, Congress passed the Dietary Supplement Health and Education Act (DSHEA) in 1994. Its features are shown in Box 8–2. The act limits the ability of the Food and Drug Administration (FDA) to regulate DSs since it stipulates that manufacturers do not need to provide complete safety and efficacy data for products unless they make a disease claim. It does not provide safeguards against manufacturing shortcomings such as inaccurate labeling of quantities of the active ingredient(s) and potentially dangerous contaminants that could create a public hazard. As a result of the more liberal availability of DSs afforded by DSHEA, CAM expenditures have skyrocketed; it is estimated that perhaps 29,000 unique formulations are available in about 75,000

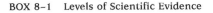

BOX 8–1   Levels of Scientific Evidence

1   Well-controlled, adequately powered, generalizable prospective randomized controlled trials; well-controlled multicenter trial; large meta-analysis with quality ratings; "all-or-none" evidence
2   Limited prospective randomized controlled trials; well conducted prospective cohort study; well conducted meta-analysis of cohort studies
3   Flawed randomized trials; observational studies; case reports or series; conflicting evidence predominantly supporting conclusion
4   No evidence; expert consensus or opinion; theory-driven conclusions

Grades of Recommendations

A   First-line treatment
One or more conclusive level 1 reports demonstrating that benefits outweigh risk

B   Second-line treatment
No conclusive level 1 evidence demonstrating that benefits outweigh risk
　　One or more conclusive level 2 reports demonstrating that benefits outweigh risk

C   No objection to use
No conclusive level 1 or level 2 evidence demonstrating that benefits outweigh risk
　　One or more conclusive level 3 reports demonstrating that benefits outweigh risk
　　Level 1 to level 3 evidence demonstrating no risk even without benefit

D   Do not use
No conclusive level 1 to level 3 evidence demonstrating that benefits outweigh risk
　　Conclusive level 1 to level 3 evidence demonstrating that risks outweigh benefits

From Mechanick JI, Brett EM, Chausmer AB, et al: American Association of Clinical Endocrinologists medical guidelines for the clinical use of dietary supplements and nutraceuticals. Endocr Pract 9:417–470, 2003; available at http://www.aace.com/clin/guidelines/Nutraceuticals2003.pdf.

BOX 8-2   Features of the 1994 Dietary Supplement Health and Education Act

Mandated creation of NIH Office of Dietary Supplements
Mandated more studies of dietary supplements and nutraceuticals by the Cochrane Controlled Trials Register
Defined dietary supplements as:
- Vitamins or minerals
- Herbs or other botanicals
- Amino acids
- Dietary substances that increase the total dietary intake
  - Enzymes
  - Organ tissue
  - Glandular tissue
- Concentrates, metabolites, constituents, extracts, or combinations of the above
- Intended for ingestion in pills, capsules, tablets, or liquid form; they are not foods in their natural forms
- Not meal substitutes

Exempted dietary supplements from the requirements and regulations involved in drug development. Proof of efficacy, safety, and purity are not required.
Defined allowable labeling claims
- Nutrient-content claims allowed, e.g., "high in calcium"
- Structure-function or nutrition support claims allowed, e.g., "builds strong bones" or "supports healthy prostate function"
- Disease claims, e.g., "calcium treats osteoporosis" allowed only with FDA authorization based on strong evidence

Permits FDA to sue for misleading advertisements
Permits FDA to issue warnings, intervene, and regulate based on adverse event reports. To remove a product from the market, FDA must prove that it presents a significant unreasonable risk of illness and injury.

distinctly labeled products. Many patients taking DSs fail to disclose the practice to their physicians. This increases the potential for harm, such as what occurred from ephedra use. Ephedra was the first CAM product removed from the market by the FDA, fully 10 years after DSHEA was enacted.

Selected Disease-Specific Interventions

Dietary supplements are defined by DSHEA. *Nutraceuticals* are DSs containing a concentrated form of a presumed bioactive substance, originally derived from a food, but now in a nonfood matrix, and used to promote health in dosages exceeding those obtainable from natural foods. Examples include ipriflavone, contained in soy, promoted for treating osteoporosis, and n-3 fatty acids or fish oils, for hypertriglyceridemia. *Functional foods* are natural, whole foods that may confer health benefits beyond their basic nutritional content. Examples of functional foods include red wine consumed to obtain polyphenols like epigallocatechin gallate, oat bran for fiber, nuts or fish oils or plant sterols or stanols to reduce serum cholesterol levels, and fresh garlic for the antioxidant diallyl disulfide or allicin. A list of dietary supplements with evidence-based efficacy and safety is given in Table 8-1. Other DSs with lesser degrees of evidentiary proof for obesity and diabetes are shown in Boxes 8-3 and 8-4.

Functional medicine is a branch of CAM that focuses on chronic diseases and symptoms, preventive medicine, and healthy aging. It attempts to integrate elements of conventional medicine and CAM, though the latter is overtly favored. Dietary supplements commonly used in functional medicine are shown in Table 8-2. Arguments defending its use are buttressed by intricate physiologic theory with, so far, a paucity of strong clinical data. However, the emergence of "nutrigenomics" has validated many functional medicine assertions. Specifically, gene arrays and proteomic and metabolomic analyses identify individual nutritional requirements during periods of stress and disease that can potentially lead to successful tailored therapies. This futuristic, personalized approach to critical illness, cancer, heart disease, metabolic syndrome, and aging may allow the integration of functional medicine and nutrigenomics into mainstream medical practice in the coming years.

Table 8–1	SOME EVIDENCE-BASED USES FOR DIETARY SUPPLEMENTS	
Clinical Problem	**Dietary Supplement**	**Recommendation Grade**
Alcoholism	Taurine	B
Atherosclerosis prevention	Phytosterols	A
	Flavonoids	A
Benign prostatic hypertrophy	Saw palmetto	B
Cardiac disease	Carnitine	C
	Coenzyme Q10	C
	n-3 Fatty acids	A
Colitis (*C.difficile*)	Probiotics	C
Critical illness	Glutamine	A
Diabetic neuropathy	α-Lipoic acid	B
	γ-Linolenic acid	B
Hypercholesterolemia	Phytosterols	A
Hypertriglyceridemia	n-3 Fatty acids	B
McArdle's disease	Creatine	C
Osteoarthritis	Chondroitin	B
	Glucosamine	B
Osteoporosis	Calcium	A
	Flavonoids	B
	Vitamin D	A
Pouchitis	Probiotics	B
Pregnancy	Choline	A
Sleep disorders	Melatonin	C
TPN-induced hepatopathy	Choline	C
	Taurine	C

TPN, total parenteral nutrition.
From Mechanick JI, Brett EM, Chausmer AB, et al: American Association of Clinical Endocrinologists medical guidelines for the clinical use of dietary supplements and nutraceuticals. Endocr Pract 9:417–470, 2003; available at http://www.aace.com/clin/guidelines/Nutraceuticals2003.pdf.

Recommendations

The following guidelines are recommended for integrating CAM practices into medical practice.
- CAM recommendations should be subjected to the same evidentiary standards required of other medical therapies.
- If no evidence of benefit is available after a diligent effort but the literature supports safety (no risk), CAM need not be resisted.

Text continued on p. 225

BOX 8–3   Dietary Supplements Promoted for Treating Obesity with Insufficient Evidence of Efficacy or With Evidence of Harm

Alisma root, *Angelica dahuricae* root, *Angelica sinensis* root, Arabinose, Arginine, Benzocaine, Bitter orange, Caffeine (guarana), *Capsicum,* Carnitine, Cayenne, Chitosan, Chromium picolinate, *Codonopsis* root, Coleus, Dehydroepiandrosterone, Docosahexanoic acid, Eicosapentanoic acid, Ephedra (Ma Huang), *Eucommia* bark, Fiber, Folic acid, *Garcinia cambogia* (hydroxycitrate), Garlic, Ginseng, Glucomannan, Glycine, Green tea (catechins), *Griffonia* seed extract (L-5-hydroxytryptophan), Guggul, Gymnemic acid, Hawthorn berry, Hibiscus acid, β-hydroxy-β-methylbutyrate, Inulin, Jujube seed, Leucine, Linoleic acid, Magnesium, n-3 Fatty acid, Niacin, *Nomame herba,* Notoginseng, Phenylalanine, Phenylpropanolamine, Prebiotics and probiotics, Psyllium, Pyridoxine, Pyruvate, Rehmannia root, Riboflavin, *Schizandrae* berry, Spirulina (blue-green algae), St. John's wort, Thiamine, Vanadium, Vitamin B$_{12}$, Vitamin C, Vitamin D, Yohimbe, Zinc

BOX 8–4   Dietary Supplements Promoted for Treating Diabetes Based on Weak Clinical Evidence (Grade C) or Preclinical Evidence Alone (Grade D)

Grade C Dietary Supplements

Aloe vera, American ginseng, Asian ginseng, Basil, Bilberry, Bitter melon, Burma cutch, Cinnamon, Cranberry juice, Curry, Fenugreek, Fig leaf, Flaxseed, Garlic, Green tea, Oolong tea, Gudmar, Indian Malabar, Ivy guard, Jangli amia, Milk thistle, Onion, Prickly pear cactus, Salt bush

Grade D Dietary Supplements

Alfalfa, Alpine ragwort, Allspice, Amarta, Anjani, Athalaki, Banana, Bay leaf, Bean pod, Behen, Betelnut, Bitter apple, Blackberry, Black catnip, Black tea, Buckwheat, Caper plant, Caturang, Centaury, Chirata, Clove, Cocoa, Cowitch, Cumin, Dandelion, Davana, Divi-divi, Eucalyptus, European goldenrod, Fever nut, Garden beet, German sarsaparilla, Ginger, Goat's rue,

Box continued on following page

BOX 8–4   Dietary Supplements Promoted for Treating
Diabetes Based on Weak Clinical Evidence (Grade C) or
Preclinical Evidence Alone (Grade D) *(Continued)*

Greek sage, Guar gum, Holy fruit tree, Indian banyan tree,
Indian gum Arabic tree, Jambolan, Kutki, Laksmana, Lotus,
Madagascar periwinkle, Mango, Mountain ash berry,
Mushroom (shitake), Mushroom (white), Mustard, Neem, Noni,
Nutmeg, Oats, Oregano, Papaya, Phtica, Plantain, Poley,
Pomegranate, Ponkoranti, Red silk cotton tree, Red gram, Reed
herb, Sage, Sakkargand, Shoe flower, Stevia, Stinging nettle,
Surinam cherry, Triticum, Turmeric, White mulberry, Wild serv-
ice tree, Witch hazel

Table 8–2	DIETARY SUPPLEMENTS USED IN FUNCTIONAL MEDICINE
Purported Physiologic Function	**Dietary Supplement**
Adrenal	Dehydroepiandrosterone (DHEA)
	Holy basil leaf
	Licorice root
	5-Methyltetrahydrofolate
	Pregnenolone
	Vitamins B_5, B_6, B_{12}, and C
Antioxidant	B-complex vitamins, vitamins C, and E
	Coenzyme Q10
	Lipoic acid
	Quercetin
Diabetes	Chromium
	Magnesium
	n-3 Fatty acid
	Vitamin E
	Zinc
Lipid-lowering	Coenzyme Q10
	Policosanol
	Red yeast rice
Menopause	*Acorus calamus*
	Bacopa monniera
	Betaine
	Centella asiatica (Gotu Kola)
	Cimicifuga racemosa (black cohash)
	Enterolactone and enterodiol
	Folic acid and 5-Methyltetrahydrofolate

Table 8–2	DIETARY SUPPLEMENTS USED IN FUNCTIONAL MEDICINE—Cont'd
Purported Physiologic Function	**Dietary Supplement**
	Hypericum perforatum (St.John's wort flowering tops)
	Indole-3-carbinol
	Lavandula angustifolia (Lavender flower)
	Linum usitatissimum (Flax)
	Matricaria recutita (chamomile flower)
	Panax ginseng
	Pueraria lobata (Kudzu vine root)
	Soy isoflavones
	Trifolium pretense (red clover)
	Vitamins B_{12} and B_6
Polycystic ovary syndrome	*D-chiro*-inositol
	Chromium
	Magnesium
	n-3 Fatty acid
	Vitamin E
Prostate	Quercetin
	Saw palmetto
	Soy isoflavones
	Vitamin E
Stress	*Cordyceps sinensis* (caterpillar fungus)
	Eleutherococcus senticosus (Siberian ginseng)
	Panax ginseng (Asian ginseng root)
	Rhodiola crenulata (Arctic root; goldenroot)
	Withania somnifera (ashwagandha; Indian ginseng)
Thyroid	Carsonic acid
	Dessicated animal thyroid extract
	Iodide
	Linoleic acid
	Myrrh
	n-3 Fatty acid
	Selenium-methionine
	Tiratricol (TRIAC: 3,5,3'-triiodothyroacetic acid)
	Tyrosine
	Vitamins A, D, E
	Withania somnifera
	Zinc

From Mechanick JI, Brett EM, Chausmer AB, et al: American Association of Clinical Endocrinologists medical guidelines for the clinical use of dietary supplements and nutraceuticals. Endocr Pract 9:417–470, 2003; available at http://www.aace.com/clin/guidelines/Nutraceuticals2003.pdf.

Table 8-3	INTERACTIONS BETWEEN DIETARY SUPPLEMENTS AND PHARMACEUTICAL AGENTS
Pharmaceuticals	**Dietary Supplements**
Anticonvulsants	Borage oil, evening primrose oil, shankapulshpi, biotin, folate, vitamins B_6 and D
Barbiturates	Valerian
Benzodiazepines	Valerian, kava root, grapefruit juice
Bisphosphonates	Bonemeal, calcium, ipriflavone, iron, magnesium
Corticosteroids	Aloe, buckthorn bark and berry, cascara, fenugreek, licorice root, ephedra, echinacea, zinc
Cyclosporine	St. John's wort
Digoxin	Digitalis, ephedra, guar gum, hawthorn, licorice root, pectin, psyllium, plantain, ginseng
Estrogen	Androstenedione, grapefruit juice, fenugreek, licorice root, ginseng, saw palmetto
Glitazones (thiazolidinediones)	Inositol, niacin
Heparin	Goldenseal
Insulin	Chromium, ginseng
Iron	St. John's wort, saw palmetto
Lithium	Caffeine, coffee, guarana, psyllium
Metoclopramide	Chasteberry
Oral contraceptives	St. John's wort
Oral hypoglycemics	α-Lipoic acid, ephedra, fenugreek, feverfew, garlic, ginger, Gotu Kola, licorice root, ginseng, psyllium, karela, inositol, niacin
Proton pump inhibitors	Bonemeal, calcium, indole-3-carbinol, iron, vitamin B_{12}
Spironolactone	Licorice root
Selective serotonin reuptake inhibitors (SSRIs)	St. John's wort
Statins	Red yeast rice, grapefruit juice, pectin, coenzyme Q10, vitamin C
Tetracycline	Calcium, iron, manganese, magnesium, pectin
Theophylline	Ipriflavone, vitamin B_{12}

Table 8-3	INTERACTIONS BETWEEN DIETARY SUPPLEMENTS AND PHARMACEUTICAL AGENTS—Cont'd
Pharmaceuticals	**Dietary Supplements**
Thiazides	*Gingko biloba*
Thyroid hormone	Bugleweed, red yeast, kelp, calcium, iron, bonemeal
Warfarin	Garlic, ginger, *gingko biloba*, *ginseng*, guar gum ("5-G's" cause bleeding), borage oil, chondroitin, coenzyme Q10, evening primrose oil, flaxseed oil, feverfew, inositol, iodine, niacin, psyllium, tiratricol, wheat and barley grass, vitamin E

From Mechanick JI, Brett EM, Chausmer AB, et al: American Association of Clinical Endocrinologists medical guidelines for the clinical use of dietary supplements and nutraceuticals. Endocr Pract 9:417–470, 2003; available at http://www.aace.com/clin/guidelines/Nutraceuticals2003.pdf.

- If there is no benefit and safety cannot be demonstrated with clinical evidence, or if harm is demonstrated with clinical evidence, patients must be informed and the CAM should not be recommended.
- Even if a CAM therapy is deemed safe and effective, it still cannot be recommended unless a properly manufactured product is available; there are no adverse reactions with other foods, drugs, or DSs (Table 8-3); and patient monitoring is provided.

These recommendations are in accordance with the American Association of Clinical Endocrinologists' Clinical Practice Guidelines on the use of CAM.[1] The American Heart Association does not recommend any DS to prevent heart disease or stroke, with the exception of n-3 fatty acids in certain patients, and advises that patients consume a variety of whole foods to obtain all necessary nutrients.[2] Many other credible scientific and consumer organizations provide up-to-date CAM information on their web sites, which are listed below. Because the popularity of specific CAM therapies and the evidence regarding them evolves rapidly, health care practitioners should regularly consult these web sites.

REFERENCES

1. Mechanick JI, Brett EM, Chausmer AB, et al: American Association of Clinical Endocrinologists medical guidelines for the clinical use of dietary supplements and nutraceuticals. Endocr Pract 9: 417–470, 2003; available at http://www.aace.com/clin/guidelines/Nutraceuticals2003.pdf.
2. AHA Scientific Statement: AHA Dietary Guidelines, Revision 2000, #71-0193. Circulation 102:2284–2299, 2000; Stroke 31:2751–2766, 2000.

SUGGESTED READINGS

Hendler SS, Rorvik D (eds): PDR for Nutritional Supplements. Montvale, NJ, Medical Economics, Thomson Healthcare, 2001.
LaGow B (ed): PDR for Herbal Medicines, 3rd ed. Montvale, NJ, Thomson PDR, 2004.
Jellin JM (ed): Natural Medicines Comprehensive Database. Stockton, Calif, Therapeutic Research Faculty, 1999; available at http://www.naturaldatabase.com.

WEBSITES

American Botanical Council, http://www.herbalgram.org
American Nutraceutical Association, http://www.americanutra.com
The Cochrane Library, http://www.thecochranelibrary.com
ConsumerLab.com, http://www.consumerlab.com
FDA Overview of Dietary Supplements, http://www.cfsan.fda.gov/~dms/ds-oview.html
Food and Nutrition Information Center, http://www.nal.usda.gov/fnic/etext/000015.html
HerbMed, http://www.herbmed.org/
The Institute for Functional Medicine, http://www.functionalmedicine.org
MD Anderson Complementary/Integrative Medicine, http://www.mdanderson.org/departments/cimer/
Mayo Clinic, http://www.mayoclinic.com/
National Center for Complementary and Alternative Medicine, http://nccam.nih.gov/
National Institutes of Health Office of Dietary Supplements, http://www.ods.od.nih.gov/
Natural Database, http://www.naturaldatabase.com
Natural Standard, http://www.naturalstandard.com (requires individual or institutional subscription).
Office of Cancer Complementary Alternative Medicine, http://www3.cancer.gov/occam/
Phytochemical and Ethnobotanical Databases, http://www.ars-grin.gov/duke/
Quackwatch, http://www.quackwatch.com/

PART II

Nutritional Support in Patient Management

9

Illness-Associated Malnutrition

DOUGLAS C. HEIMBURGER, MD

Prevalence

Malnutrition can arise from primary or secondary causes, with the former resulting from inadequate or poor-quality food intake and the latter from diseases that alter food intake or nutrient requirements, metabolism, or absorption. Primary malnutrition, which occurs mainly in developing countries and is unusual in the United States, will not be discussed here. Secondary malnutrition, the main form encountered in developed countries, was largely unrecognized until the late 1960s or early 1970s, probably because of a narrow concept of nutrition. It was not well appreciated that persons with adequate food supplies can become malnourished as a result of acute or chronic diseases that alter nutrient intake or metabolism.

At the University of Alabama at Birmingham (UAB) in 1974, Charles E. Butterworth called attention to the "skeleton in the hospital closet," focusing on iatrogenic (physician-induced) malnutrition in the United States.[1] Since that time, various studies have shown that protein-energy malnutrition (PEM) affects one third to one half of the patients on general medical and surgical wards in U.S. teaching hospitals. In a study of consecutive admissions to a UAB general medical ward in 1976, 48% of patients had a high likelihood of malnutrition, and nutritional parameters tended to deteriorate in those hospitalized for 2 weeks or longer.[2] A follow-up study in the same institution found a slightly lower likelihood of malnutrition on admission (38%) and a slight improvement in nutritional status in patients hospitalized for 2 or more weeks.[3] These and many other studies have shown that patients with evidence of malnutrition have significantly longer hospital stays and higher mortality and morbidity rates, such as surgical complications.

The questions whether treating illness-associated malnutrition improves patient outcomes, and the potential for doing greater harm by feeding too aggressively, are discussed in Chapter 11. However, the consistent finding that nutritional status influences patient prognosis underlines the importance of preventing malnutrition as well as detecting and treating it. The term *iatrogenic* used in connection with malnutrition does not imply malicious intent or disregard for a patient's welfare. However, malnutrition can occur as a result of physicians' actions. To a considerable extent, iatrogenic malnutrition is caused by emphasis on complex treatments while fundamental principles of nutrition remain in the background. Physicians can lose sight of the facts that antibiotics cannot replace host defenses, sutures and dressings cannot heal wounds, and the most advanced, sophisticated life-support systems cannot revitalize the malnourished patient. It is paradoxical that nutritional failure in hospitalized patients can result from spectacular successes in other fields. Patients can be kept alive longer only to exhaust their nutritional reserves and succumb to nutritional deprivation. Whatever the cause, the end result is the same: Patients sometimes fail to receive the full benefit of current nutritional knowledge and technology.

Protein-Energy Malnutrition

The two major types of PEM are marasmus and kwashiorkor. These conditions are compared in Table 9–1, and the criteria for diagnosing them are listed in Table 9–2. Marasmus and kwashiorkor can occur singly or in combination, as marasmic kwashiorkor. Kwashiorkor can occur rapidly, whereas marasmus is the end result of a gradual wasting process that passes through stages of

Table 9–1	COMPARISON OF MARASMUS AND KWASHIORKOR	
	Marasmus	**Kwashiorkor**
Clinical Setting	↓ Energy intake	↓ Protein intake during stress state
Time Course to Develop	Months or years	Weeks
Clinical Features	Starved appearance Weight <80% standard for height Triceps skinfold <3mm Midarm muscle circumference <15cm	Well-nourished appearance Easy hair pluckability Edema
Laboratory Findings	Creatinine-height index <60% standard	Serum albumin <2.8 g/dL Total iron binding capacity <200 μg/dL Lymphocytes <1500/mm^3 Anergy
Clinical Course	Reasonably preserved responsiveness to short-term stress	Infections Poor wound healing, decubitus ulcers, skin breakdown
Mortality	Low, unless related to underlying disease	High

Table 9–2	MINIMUM CRITERIA FOR THE DIAGNOSIS OF MARASMUS AND KWASHIORKOR	
Marasmus		**Kwashiorkor***
Triceps skinfold <3 mm and mid-arm muscle circumference <15 cm		Serum albumin <2.8 g dL At least one of the following: Poor wound healing, decubitus ulcers, or skin breakdown Easy hair pluckability† Edema

*The findings used to diagnose kwashiorkor must be unexplained by others causes.
†Tested by *firmly* pulling a lock of hair from the top (not the sides or back) of the head, grasping with the thumb and forefinger. An average of three or more hairs removed easily and painlessly is considered abnormal hair pluckability.

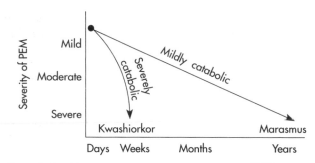

Figure 9–1. Time course of protein-energy malnutrition (PEM).
Marasmus, end-stage energy deficiency; kwashiorkor, maladaptive state
during catabolic stress with protein deficiency.

underweight, then mild, moderate, and severe cachexia
(Fig. 9–1).

Marasmus

The most severe or "end stage" of the process of cachexia,
marasmus is the state in which virtually all available
body fat stores have been exhausted due to starvation.
Conditions that produce marasmus in developed countries tend to be chronic and indolent, such as cancer,
chronic pulmonary disease, and anorexia nervosa.
Marasmus is easy to detect because of the patient's
starved appearance. The diagnosis is based on severe
fat and muscle wastage resulting from prolonged calorie
deficiency. Diminished skinfold thickness reflects the
loss of fat reserves; reduced arm muscle circumference
with temporal and interosseous muscle wasting reflects
the catabolism of protein throughout the body, including
vital organs such as the heart, liver, and kidneys.

The laboratory picture in marasmus is relatively unre-
markable. The creatinine-height index (the 24-hour
urinary creatinine excretion compared with normal values
based on height) is low, reflecting the loss of muscle mass
noted on clinical examination. Occasionally, the serum
albumin level is reduced, but it may not drop below
2.8 g/dL in uncomplicated cases. Despite a morbid

appearance, immunocompetence, wound healing, and the ability to handle short-term stress are reasonably well preserved in most patients with marasmus.

Marasmus is a chronic, fairly well-adapted form of starvation rather than an acute illness; it should be treated cautiously, in an attempt to reverse the downward trend gradually. Although nutritional support is necessary, overly aggressive repletion can result in severe, even life-threatening metabolic imbalances such as hypophosphatemia and cardiorespiratory failure (see Chapter 11). When possible, enteral nutritional support is preferred; treatment started slowly allows readaptation of metabolic and intestinal functions.

Kwashiorkor

In contrast to marasmus, kwashiorkor in developed countries occurs mainly in connection with acute, life-threatening illnesses such as trauma and sepsis, and chronic illnesses that involve an acute-phase inflammatory response. The physiologic stress produced by these illnesses increases protein and energy requirements at a time when intake is often limited. A classic scenario for kwashiorkor is the acutely stressed patient who receives only 5% dextrose solutions for periods as short as 2 weeks. Although the etiologic mechanisms are not clear, the fact that the adaptive response of protein sparing normally seen in starvation is blocked by the stress state and by carbohydrate infusion may be an important factor. It has been argued that this state differs enough from kwashiorkor seen in developing countries that it should be given a different label such as "hypoalbuminemic stress state," but we believe the distinction is immaterial. The two conditions are substantially similar in physiology, clinical findings, and prognosis.

In its early stages, the physical findings of kwashiorkor are few and subtle. Fat reserves and muscle mass may be normal or even above normal, giving the deceptive appearance of adequate nutrition. Signs that support the diagnosis of kwashiorkor include easy hair pluckability, edema, skin breakdown, and poor wound healing. The major *sine qua non* in the diagnosis is severe reduction of levels of serum proteins such as albumin (less than 2.8 g/dL) and transferrin (less than 150 mg/dL) or iron-binding capacity (less than 200 µg/dL). Cellular immune function is depressed, reflected by lymphopenia (less than 1500 lymphocytes/mm^3 in adults and older children) and lack of response to "recall" skin test antigens (anergy).

The prognosis of adult patients with full-blown kwashiorkor is not good, even with aggressive nutritional support. Surgical wounds often dehisce (fail to heal), pressure sores develop, gastroparesis and diarrhea can occur with enteral feeding, the risk of gastrointestinal bleeding from stress ulcers is increased, host defenses are compromised, and death from overwhelming infection may occur despite antibiotic therapy. Unlike treatment in marasmus, aggressive nutritional support is indicated to restore better metabolic balance rapidly. Although kwashiorkor in children can be less foreboding, perhaps because of the lower degree of stress required to precipitate the disorder, it is still a serious condition.

Marasmic Kwashiorkor

Marasmic kwashiorkor, the combined form of PEM, develops when the cachectic or marasmic patient is subjected to an acute stress such as surgery, trauma, or sepsis, superimposing kwashiorkor onto chronic starvation. An extremely serious, life-threatening situation can occur because of the high risk of infection and other complications. It is important to determine the major component of PEM so that the appropriate nutritional plan can be developed. If kwashiorkor predominates, the need for vigorous nutritional therapy is urgent; if marasmus predominates, feeding should be more cautious. The stressed, hypermetabolic patient is more likely to suffer the consequences of underfeeding, and the starved, unstressed hypometabolic patient is at risk for the complications of overfeeding. See Chapter 11 for more details.

Body Defenses in Protein-Energy Malnutrition

The body has three main types of defenses against infection: mechanical, cellular, and humoral. Mechanical defenses include epithelial surfaces, mucous barriers, and digestive enzymes. Cellular defenses are mediated by lymphocytes, plasma cells, and polymorphonuclear leukocytes, which ingest and destroy bacteria and foreign bodies. Humoral defenses include immunoglobulins and other plasma proteins involved in destruction of microorganisms. Some antibodies appear in secretions such as tears, colostrum, and intestinal mucus.

Evidence is ample that all of these defense systems are impaired in PEM. Epithelial cells, like all other cells, require adequate nutrients for growth, turnover, and function. Kwashiorkor is commonly associated with low lymphocyte counts and non-reactivity to skin recall antigens (impaired cellular immunity), and low circulating protein levels that usually include immunoglobulins (humoral immunity). With nutritional repletion, immunocompetence can often be restored. However, tests of immune function cannot always be directly related to nutritional status, and the use of skin tests to demonstrate anergy adds little to the diagnosis or treatment of kwashiorkor.

Physiologic Characteristics of Hypometabolic and Hypermetabolic States

The metabolic characteristics and nutritional needs of hypermetabolic patients who are stressed from injury, infection, or chronic inflammatory illness differ from those of hypometabolic patients who are unstressed but chronically starved. In both cases, nutritional support is important, but misjudgments in selecting the appropriate approach may have disastrous consequences.

The hypometabolic patient is typified by the relatively unstressed but mildly catabolic and chronically starved individual who, with time, will develop marasmus (see Fig. 9–1). The hypermetabolic patient stressed from injury or infection is catabolic (experiencing rapid breakdown of body mass), and is at high risk for developing kwashiorkor if nutritional needs are not met and the illness does not resolve quickly. As shown in Table 9–3, the two states are distinguished by differing alterations in metabolic rate, rates of protein breakdown (proteolysis), and rates of gluconeogenesis. These differences are mediated by proinflammatory cytokines and counterregulatory hormones—tumor necrosis factor, interleukins 1 and 6, C-reactive protein, catecholamines (epinephrine and norepinephrine), glucagon, and cortisol—that are relatively reduced in hypometabolic patients and increased in hypermetabolic patients. Although insulin levels are also elevated in stressed patients, insulin resistance in the target tissues prevents the expression of insulin's anabolic properties.

Metabolic Rate

In starvation and semistarvation the resting metabolic rate falls between 10% and 30% as an adaptive response to energy restriction, slowing the rate of weight loss. By contrast, resting metabolic rate rises in the presence of

Table 9–3	PHYSIOLOGIC CHRACTERISTICS OF HYPOMETABOLIC AND HYPERMETABOLIC STATES	
Physiologic Characterstics	Hypometabolic, Non-stressed Patient (Cachectic, Marasmic)	Hypermetabolic, Stressed Patient (Kwashiorkor-risk*)
Cytokines, catecholamines, glucagon, cortisol, insulin	↓	↑
Metabolic rate, O_2 consumption	↓	↑
Proteolysis, gluconeogenesis	↓	↑
Ureagenesis, urea excretion	↓	↑
Fat catabolism, fatty acid utilization	↑	↑
Adaptation to starvation	Normal	Abnormal

*These changes characterize the stressed, kwashiorkor-risk patient seen in developed countries, and differ in some respects from primary kwashiorkor seen in developing countries.

physiologic stress in proportion to the degree of the insult. For example, the rise may be about 10% after elective surgery, 20% to 30% after bone fractures, 30% to 60% with severe infections such as peritonitis or gram-negative septicemia, and as much as 110% after major burns (Fig. 9–2, *upper graph*). Because the rise in metabolic rate is a generalized response and is not isolated to any one organ system or injury site, the accompanying increase in oxygen consumption affects the entire body.

In either state, if the metabolic rate (energy requirement) is not matched by energy intake, weight loss results—slowly in hypometabolism and quickly in hypermetabolism. Losses of up to 10% of body weight are unlikely to have an adverse effect; however, in acutely ill hypermetabolic patients losses greater than that may be associated with rapid deterioration in body function.

Protein Catabolism

The rate of endogenous protein breakdown (catabolism) to supply energy needs normally falls during uncomplicated energy deprivation. After about 10 days of total starvation, the unstressed individual will have protein losses amounting to only 12 to 18 g/day (equivalent to approximately 2 oz of muscle tissue or 2 to 3 g of nitrogen). By contrast, in injury and sepsis, protein breakdown accelerates in proportion to the degree of stress, to 30 to 60 g/day after elective surgery, 60 to 90 g/day with infection, 100 to 130 g/day with severe sepsis or skeletal trauma, and at times, over 175 g/day with major burns or head injuries. These losses are reflected by proportional increases in the excretion of urea nitrogen, the major by-product of protein breakdown (Table 10–4; see Fig. 9–2).

Protein catabolism occurs throughout the body and not solely at the site of injury. Because protein represents approximately 25% of the weight of muscle tissue, if protein losses are not offset by intake, the amount of muscle wasted each day can be estimated as four times the amount of protein catabolized. Consider this example: A patient with multiple traumas, without any protein intake, had a 24-hour urinary urea nitrogen (UUN) excretion

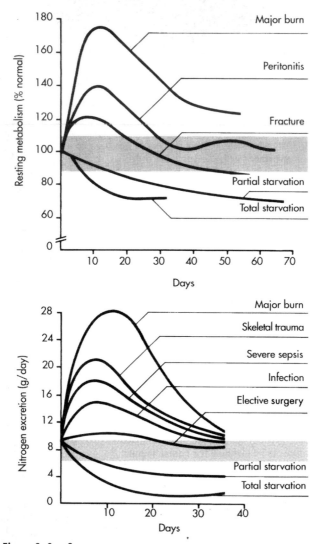

Figure 9-2. CHANGES IN METABOLIC RATE AND NITROGEN EXCRETION WITH VARIOUS TYPES OF PHYSIOLOGIC STRESS. Normal ranges are indicated by *shaded areas*. From Long CL, Schaffel N, Geiger JW, et al: Metabolic response to injury and illness: Estimation of energy and protein needs from indirect calorimetry and nitrogen balance. JPEN 3:452–456, 1979.

of 17 g. As described in Chapter 10, estimated protein losses are calculated as follows:

$$\text{Protein Catabolic Rate (g/day)} = (24\text{-hour UUN} + 4)$$
$$\times 6.25$$
$$= (17 + 4) \times 6.25$$
$$= 131 \text{ g/day}$$

The breakdown of 131 g protein per day is equivalent to about 4 times that amount of muscle mass, i.e., with this degree of stress and protein catabolism, 524 g or over 1 lb of muscle tissue will be wasted each day if not offset by protein intake.

Gluconeogenesis

The major aim of protein catabolism during a state of starvation is to provide the glucogenic amino acids (especially alanine and glutamine) that serve as substrates for endogenous glucose production (gluconeogenesis) in the liver. In the hypometabolic/starved state, protein breakdown for gluconeogenesis is minimized, especially as ketones become the substrate preferred by certain tissues. In the hypermetabolic/stress state, gluconeogenesis increases dramatically and in proportion to the degree of the insult to increase the supply of glucose (the major fuel of reparation). Glucose is the only fuel that can be utilized by hypoxic tissues (anaerobic glycolysis), by phagocytosing (bacteria-killing) white cells, and by young fibroblasts.

Infusions of glucose partially offset a negative energy balance but do not significantly suppress the high rates of gluconeogenesis in the catabolic patient. Hence, adequate supplies of protein are needed to replace the amino acids utilized for this metabolic response.

In summary, the two physiologic states represent different responses to starvation. The hypometabolic patient, who conserves body mass by reducing the metabolic rate and using fat as the primary fuel (rather than glucose and its precursor amino acids), is adapted to starvation. The hypermetabolic patient also uses fat as a fuel but rapidly breaks down body protein to produce glucose, the fuel of reparation, thereby causing loss of muscle and organ tissue and endangering vital body functions.

Micronutrient Malnutrition

PEM is not the only type of malnutrition found in sick patients. The same illnesses and reductions in nutrient intake that lead to PEM can produce deficiencies of vitamins and minerals. Deficiencies of nutrients that are only stored in small amounts (such as the water-soluble vitamins) or are lost through external secretions (such as zinc in diarrhea fluid or burn exudate) are probably quite common.

Deficiencies of vitamin C, folic acid, and zinc are reasonably common in sick patients. For instance, signs of scurvy such as corkscrew hairs on the lower extremities are frequently found in chronically ill and alcoholic patients. The diagnosis can be confirmed with plasma vitamin C levels. Folic acid intakes and blood levels are often less than optimal even among healthy persons; when factors such as illness, alcoholism, poverty, or poor dentition are present, deficiencies are common. Low blood zinc levels are prevalent in patients with malabsorption syndromes such as inflammatory bowel disease. Patients with zinc deficiency often exhibit poor wound healing, pressure ulcer formation, and impaired immunity. Thiamin deficiency is a common complication of alcoholism, but it may be seen less commonly than the previously mentioned deficiencies because of the frequent use of therapeutic doses of thiamin after patients are admitted for alcohol abuse.

Patients with low plasma vitamin C levels usually respond to the doses found in multivitamin preparations, but patients with deficiencies should be supplemented with 250 to 500 mg per day. Folic acid is absent from some oral multivitamin preparations; patients with deficiencies should be supplemented with about 1 mg per day. Patients with zinc deficiencies resulting from large external losses sometimes require oral daily supplementation with 220 mg of zinc sulfate 1 to 3 times daily.

For these reasons, laboratory assessments of the micronutrient status of patients at high risk are desirable.

Hypophosphatemia (low serum phosphorus level) develops in hospitalized patients with remarkable frequency and generally results from rapid intracellular shifts of phosphate in cachectic or alcoholic patients receiving intravenous glucose. The adverse clinical sequelae are numerous, and some such as acute cardiopulmonary failure can be life-threatening (see Table 11-1).

For more information on the functions of these micronutrients, and common causes and physical findings of their deficiencies, see Tables 3-6 and 10-2. Appendix C (Vitamin and Mineral Supplements) lists recommended daily dose ranges of the vitamins for prevention and treatment of various diseases.

REFERENCES

1. Butterworth CE: The skeleton in the hospital closet. Nutr Today 9:4, 1974.
2. Weinsier RL, Hunker EM, Krumdieck CL, Butterworth CEJr.: Hospital malnutrition: A prospective evaluation of general medical patients during the course of hospitalization Am J Clin Nutr 32:418 426, 1979.
3. Coats KG, Morgan SL, Bartolucci AA, Weinsier RL.: Hospital-associated malnutrition: A reevaluation 12 years later. J Am Dietetic Assoc 93:27-33, 1993.

SUGGESTED READINGS

Kotler DP: Cachexia. Ann Intern Med 133:622, 2000.
ASPEN: The science and practice of nutrition support: A case-based core curriculum. Dubuque, IA, Kendall/Hunt, 2001.
Shils ME, Shike M, Ross AC, et al (eds): Modern nutrition in health and disease, 10th ed. Baltimore, Lippincott Williams & Wilkins, 2005.

10

Nutritional Assessment

DOUGLAS C. HEIMBURGER, MD

Because the interaction between illness and nutritional status is complex, many physical and laboratory findings reflect underlying disease as well as nutritional status. Therefore, the nutritional evaluation of a patient requires an integration of the patient's nutritional history, a physical examination, anthropometrics, and laboratory studies. This approach helps to detect nutritional problems and to avoid concluding that isolated findings indicate nutritional problems when they actually may not. For example, hypoalbuminemia caused by an underlying illness does not necessarily indicate malnutrition.

Nutritional History

Taking a nutritional history helps to identify underlying mechanisms that put patients at risk for nutritional depletion or excess. These mechanisms include inadequate intake, impaired absorption, decreased utilization, increased losses, and increased requirements of nutrients (Table 10–1). Individuals with the characteristics listed in Box 10–1 are at particular risk for nutritional deficiencies.

The major types of diet histories are dietary recalls generally covering 24 hours; food records in which patients write down everything consumed during a 1- to 7-day period; and food frequency questionnaires, in which patients estimate how often they ate the foods identified on a list during the previous 6 to 12 months.

Table 10-1 NUTRITIONAL HISTORY SCREEN, BY MECHANISMS OF DEFICIENCY AND MEDICAL CONDITIONS

Mechanism of Deficiency	History	Conditions	Deficiencies to Suspect
Inadequate Intake	Weight loss	AIDS, cancer, depression, gastrointestinal obstruction or dysmotility (e.g., gastroparesis), aging neurologic disease, hyperemesis gravidarum	Calories, protein, multiple nutrients
	Alcohol abuse, substance abuse		Calories, protein, thiamin, niacin, folate, pyridoxine, riboflavin
	Avoidance of fruits, vegetables, grains		Vitamin C, thiamin, niacin, folate
	Avoidance of meat, dairy products, eggs		Protein, vitamin B$_{12}$
	Isolation, poverty, food idiosyncrasies		Various nutrients
	Eating disorder	Anorexia or bulimia nervosa	Calories, protein, multiple nutrients
		Constipation, hemorrhoids, diverticulosis	Dietary fiber
		Hospitalization, NPO status	Calories, protein, multiple nutrients
Inadequate Digestion and/or Absorption	Maldigestion (diarrhea, steatorrhea, weight loss)	Pancreatic insufficiency, cystic fibrosis, cholestasis, intestinal bacterial stasis or overgrowth	Calories, protein, Vitamins A, D, K, calcium, magnesium, zinc
		Disaccharidase deficiency (e.g., lactase)	Calories, protein

Table continued on following page

Table 10-1	NUTRITIONAL HISTORY SCREEN, BY MECHANISMS OF DEFICIENCY AND MEDICAL CONDITIONS *(Continued)*		
Mechanism of Deficiency	History	Conditions	Deficiencies to Suspect
	Malabsorption (diarrhea, steatorrhea, weight loss)	Short bowel syndrome, radiation enteritis, inflammatory bowel disease, Whipple's disease, AIDS, gluten enteropathy (celiac sprue), tropical sprue, intestinal lymphoma	Vitamins A, D, K, protein, calcium magnesium, zinc

Calories, protein, iron, various nutrients |
		Parasites (fish tapeworm)	Iron, vitamin B_{12}
		Pernicious anemia	Vitamin B_{12}
		Surgery:	
		Gastrectomy	Vitamin B_{12}, iron, folate
		Intestinal resection	Vitamin B_{12}, iron, others as in malabsorption
	Drugs (antacids, anticonvulsants, cholestyramine, laxatives, neomycin, alcohol)		See Chapter 15
Decreased Utilization, Impaired Metabolism		Chronic liver disease	Calories, protein, vitamins A, D, E, K, B_{12}, thiamin, folate, pyridoxine
		Chronic renal disease	Calories, vitamin D, water-soluble vitamins
		Inborn errors of metabolism	Various nutrients

	Drugs (corticosteroids, anticonvulsants, antimetabolites, oral contraceptives, isoniazid, alcohol)	See Chapter 15
Abnormal Losses	Alcohol abuse	Magnesium, zinc
	Blood loss	Iron
	Centesis (ascitic, pleural fluid)	Protein
	Diarrhea	Protein, zinc, magnesium, electrolytes
	Peritoneal or hemodialysis	Protein, water-soluble vitamins, zinc
	Diabetes, uncontrolled	Calories (glycosuria)
	Draining abscesses, wounds	Protein, zinc
	Protein-losing enteropathy	Protein
	Nephrotic syndrome	Protein, zinc
Increased Requirements	Fever	Calories
	Physiologic demands (infancy, adolescence, pregnancy, lactation)	Various nutrients
	Cigarette smoking	Vitamin C and E, folate, β-carotene
	Hyperthyroidism	Calories
	Surgery, trauma, burns, infection	Calories, protein, vitamin C, zinc
	Chronic lung disease	Calories

BOX 10-1 The High-Risk Patient

- Underweight (BMI <18.5) and/or recent loss of 10% or more of usual body weight
- Poor intake: anorexia, food avoidance (e.g., psychiatric condition), or NPO (nothing by mouth) status for more than about 5 days
- Protracted nutrient losses: malabsorption, enteric fistulae, draining abscesses or wounds, renal dialysis
- Hypermetabolic states: sepsis, protracted fever, extensive trauma or burns
- Alcohol abuse or use of drugs with antinutrient or catabolic properties: steroids, antimetabolites (e.g., methotrexate), immunosuppressants, antitumor agents
- Impoverishment, isolation, advanced age

A variety of computer programs permit rapid estimation of nutrient intake from these questionnaires or records. Some of these are available free on the Internet (see http://www.usda.gov/cnpp/ihei.html and http://nat.crgq.com/). Each method has advantages and disadvantages, involving factors such as labor intensity, cost, and accuracy. For instance, a 24-hour dietary recall may significantly underestimate usual intakes, but can be easily elicited from most patients. Three-day food records provide a reasonable way to obtain a qualitative estimate of nutrient intakes, but food choices often change during recording periods, and may be unrepresentative. Sometimes combinations of the various methods work best. For a routine nutritional assessment in the hospital or clinic setting, a 24-hour dietary recall provides an overview of the patient's dietary pattern that is adequate to determine if further detailed evaluation is necessary. However, in the course of taking the entire medical history, it is important to obtain information about all of the areas noted in Table 10-1 (e.g., presence of alcohol abuse, dental disease, drug use, malabsorption) to determine potential nutrient deficiencies not easily identified by dietary recall.

Physical Examination

Physical findings that suggest vitamin, mineral, and protein-energy deficiencies and excesses are outlined in Table 10-2. Most of the physical findings are not specific for individual nutrient deficiencies and must be integrated with the historical, anthropometric, and laboratory findings to make a diagnosis. For example, the finding of follicular hyperkeratosis isolated to the back of one's arms is a fairly common, normal finding. On the other hand, if it is widespread on a person who consumes little fruit and vegetables and smokes regularly (increasing ascorbic acid requirements), vitamin C deficiency is a very possible cause. Similarly, easily pluckable hair may be a consequence of recent chemotherapy. On the other hand, in a hospitalized patient who has poorly healing surgical wounds and hypoalbuminemia, easily pluckable hair strongly suggests kwashiorkor.

It is noteworthy that tissues with the fastest turnover rates are those most likely to show signs of nutrient deficiencies or excesses. Thus the hair, skin, and lingual papillae (an indirect reflection of the status of the villae of the gastrointestinal tract) are particularly likely to reveal nutritional problems and should be examined closely.

Anthropometrics

Anthropometric measurements provide information on body muscle mass and fat reserves. The most practical and commonly used measurements are body weight, height, triceps skinfold, and midarm muscle circumference.

Body weight is one of the most useful nutritional factors to study in patients who are acutely or chronically ill. Unintentional weight loss during illness often reflects loss of lean body mass (muscle and organ tissue), especially if rapid and not caused by diuresis. This can be an ominous sign since it indicates use of vital body protein stores as a metabolic fuel. The reference standard for normal body weight, body mass index (BMI, or weight in kg divided by height, in meters, squared), is discussed

Table 10-2   PHYSICAL FINDINGS OF NUTRITIONAL DEFICIENCIES

Clinical Findings	Deficiency to Consider*	Excess to Consider	Frequency†
Hair, Nails			
Corkscrew hairs and unemerged coiled hairs	Vitamin C		Common
Easily pluckable hair	Protein		Common
Flag sign (transverse depigmentation of hair)	Protein		Rare
Sparse hair	Protein, biotin, zinc	Vitamin A	Occasional
Transverse ridging of nails	Protein		Occasional
Skin			
Cellophane appearance	Protein		Occasional
Cracking (flaky paint or crazy pavement dermatosis)	Protein		Rare
Follicular hyperkeratosis	Vitamins A, C		Occasional
Petechiae (especially perifollicular)	Vitamin C		Occasional
Purpura	Vitamins C, K		Common
Pigmentation, scaling of sun-exposed areas	Niacin		Rare
Poor wound healing, decubitus ulcers	Protein, vitamin C, zinc		Common
Scaling	Vitamin A, essential fatty acids, biotin	Vitamin A	Occasional
	Zinc (hyperpigmented)		
Yellow pigmentation sparing sclerae (benign)		Carotene	Common

Eyes		
Night blindness	Vitamin A	Rare
Papilledema		Rare
Perioral		
Angular stomatitis	Riboflavin, pyridoxine, niacin	Occasional
Cheilosis (dry, cracking, ulcerated lips)	Riboflavin, pyridoxine, niacin	Rare
Oral		
Atrophic lingual papillae (slick tongue)	Riboflavin, niacin, folate, vitamin B$_{12}$, protein, iron	Common
Glossitis (scarlet, raw tongue)	Riboflavin, niacin, pyridoxine, folate, vitamin B$_{12}$	Occasional
Hypogeusesthesia, hyposmia	Zinc	Occasional
Swollen, retracted, bleeding gums (if teeth present)	Vitamin C	Occasional
Bones, Joints		
Beading of ribs, epiphyseal swelling, bowlegs	Vitamin D	Rare
Tenderness (subperiosteal hemorrhage in children)	Vitamin C	Rare
Neurologic		
Confabulation, disorientation	Thiamin (Korsakoff's psychosis)	Occasional
Drowsiness, lethargy, vomiting	Vitamins A, D	Rare

Table continued on following page

Table 10-2	PHYSICAL FINDINGS OF NUTRITIONAL DEFICIENCIES (Continued)		
Clinical Findings	Deficiency to Consider*	Excess to Consider	Frequency†
Dementia	Niacin, vitamin B12, folate		Rare
Headache		Vitamin A	Rare
Ophthalmoplegia	Thiamin, phosphorus		Occasional
Peripheral neuropathy (e.g., weakness, paresthesias, ataxia, foot drop, and decreased tendon reflexes, fine tactile sense, vibratory sense, and position sense)	Thiamin, pyridoxine, vitamin B12	Pyridoxine	Occasional
Tetany	Calcium, magnesium		Occasional
Other			
Edema	Protein, thiamin		Common
Heart failure	Thiamin ("wet" beriberi), phosphorus		Occasional
Hepatomegaly	Protein	Vitamin A	Rare
Parotid enlargement	Protein (consider also bulimia)		Occasional
Sudden heart failure, death	Vitamin C		Rare

*In this table, "protein deficiency" is used to signify kwashiorkor.
†These frequencies are an attempt to reflect our experience in the setting of a U.S. medical practice. Findings common in other countries but virtually unseen in usual medical practice settings in the United States (e.g., xerophthalmia and endemic goiter) are not listed.

in Chapter 17. People with BMIs <18.5 are considered underweight, 18.5 to 24.9 are normal, 25 to 29.9 are overweight, and ≥30 are obese.

Measurement of skinfold thickness is useful for estimating body fat stores, because about 50% of body fat is normally located in the subcutaneous region. Skinfold thicknesses can also permit discrimination of fat mass from muscle mass. The triceps skinfold (TSF) is a convenient site that is generally representative of the fatness of the entire body's fat level. The TSF measurement is taken with calipers on the upper arm at the midpoint between the acromion and olecranon processes with the arm relaxed and the elbow flexed at 90° (Fig. 10–1). A fold of skin on the posterior aspect of the arm is grasped and pulled away from the underlying muscle. Calipers are applied and the fold is still held with the hand to release skin tension from the calipers. The reading is taken after about 3 seconds. Clinically useful values for TSF are listed in Table 10–3. A thickness of less than 3 mm (equivalent to about three dimes) suggests virtually complete exhaustion of fat stores.

The midarm muscle circumference (MAMC) is often used to estimate skeletal muscle mass. A tape measure is used to determine the upper arm circumference of a

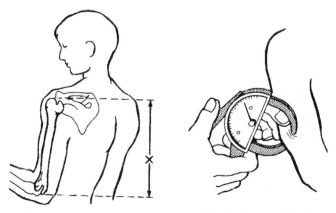

Figure 10-1. Technique for measurement of triceps skinfold (TSF).

relaxed, extended arm at the same midpoint used for the TSF. The MAMC is calculated using the following equation and is compared with reference values in Table 10–3.

$$\text{MAMC (cm)} = \text{upper arm circumference (cm)} - [0.314 \times \text{TSF (mm)}]$$

Because they can distinguish fat from lean body mass, which BMI cannot do, TSF and MAMC are useful supplements to measurements of BMI. Underweight and cachectic patients usually lose both lean and fat mass (see Chapter 9), but weight loss can sometimes affect one compartment more than the other. Conversely, elevated BMI levels can sometimes be caused by large muscle mass rather than fat mass; TSF and MAMC can help make this distinction. Also, persons who are healthy and

Table 10–3	**TRICEPS SKINFOLD THICKNESS AND MIDARM MUSCLE CIRCUMFERENCE IN ADULTS**		
Percent of Reference Value	**Men (mm)**	**Women (mm)**	**Calorie Reserves**
Triceps Skinfold Thickness			
100	12.5	16.5	
90	11	15	
80	10	13	Adequate
70	9	11.5	
60	7.5	10	
50	6	8	
40	5	6.5	Borderline
30	4	5	
20	2.5	3	Severely depleted
Percent of Reference Value	**Men (cm)**	**Women (cm)**	**Muscle Mass**
Midarm Muscle Circumference			
100	25.5	23	Adequate
90	23	21	
80	20	18.5	Borderline
70	18	16	
60	15	14	
50	12.5	11.5	Severely depleted
40	10	9	

fit may have TSF measurements in the low-adequate or borderline ranges.

As with BMI, there is wide variation in values of TSF and MAMC among healthy people, and they vary according to age. For these reasons, TSF and MAMC are often more useful for tracking body composition changes in patients over a period of time than as single measurements. Additionally, they are not accurate in patients with edema of the upper extremities.

Laboratory Studies

A number of laboratory tests used routinely in clinical medicine can yield valuable information about a patient's nutritional status if a slightly different approach to the interpretation of laboratory results is used. For example, abnormally low levels of serum albumin and total iron-binding capacity and anergy may each have a separate explanation. However, collectively they may represent kwashiorkor. In the clinical setting of a hypermetabolic, acutely ill patient who is edematous, has easily pluckable hair, and has inadequate protein intake, the diagnosis of kwashiorkor is clear-cut. Commonly used laboratory tests for assessment of nutritional status are outlined in Table 10–4. Because none of them is specific to a nutritional problem, the table provides tips to help avoid assigning nutritional significance to tests that may be abnormal for other than nutritional reasons.

Assessment of Body Composition

The serum creatinine level reflects muscle mass to a certain extent: a value of less than 0.6 suggests muscle wasting. The creatinine-height index—a better measure for estimating and tracking skeletal muscle mass—is determined by comparing a patient's 24-hour urinary creatinine excretion with reference values from normal weight persons of the same height. Because the rate of formation of creatinine from creatine phosphate in skeletal muscle is constant, the amount of creatinine excreted in the urine every 24 hours reflects skeletal

Table 10–4 LABORATORY TESTS FOR NUTRITIONAL ASSESSMENT

Test (Normal Values)	Nutritional Use	Causes of Normal Value Despite Malnutrition	Other Causes of Abnormal Value
Serum albumin (3.5–5.5 g/dL)	2.8–3.5 (compromised protein status) <2.8 (possible kwashiorkor) Increasing value reflects positive protein balance	Dehydration Infusion of albumin, fresh frozen plasma, or whole blood	LOW Common— Infection and other stress, especially with poor protein intake Bu·ns, trauma Congestive heart failure Fluid overload Severe liver disease Uncommon— Nephrotic syndrome Zirc deficiency Bacterial stasis/overgrowth of small intestine
Serum prealbumin, also called transthyretin (20–40 mg/dL; lower in prepubertal children)	10–15 mg/dL (mild protein depletion) 5–10 mg/dL (moderate protein depletion) <5 mg/dL (severe protein depletion) Increasing value reflects positive protein balance	Chronic renal failure	Similar to serum albumin
Serum total iron binding capacity (TIBC) 240–450 mg/dL	<200 (compromised protein status, possible kwashiorkor) Increasing value reflects positive protein balance More labile than albumin	Iron deficiency	LOW Similar to serum albumin

Prothrombin time 12.0–15.5 sec	Prolongation (vitamin K deficiency)	HIGH Iron deficiency PROLONGED Anticoagulant therapy (warfarin) Severe liver disease
Serum creatinine 0.6–1.6 mg/dL	<0.6 (muscle wasting due to prolonged energy deficit) Reflects muscle mass	HIGH Despite muscle wasting— Renal failure Severe dehydration
24-hour urinary creatinine 500–200 mg/d (standardized for height and sex)	Low value (muscle wasting due to prolonged energy deficit) >24-hour collection Decreasing serum creatinine	LOW Incomplete urine collection Increasing serum creatinine Neuromuscular wasting
24-hour urinary urea nitrogen (UUN) <5 g/d (depends on level of protein intake)	Determine level of catabolism (as long as protein intake is ≥10 g below calculated protein loss or <20 g total, but at least 100g carbohydrate is provided) 5–10 g/d = mild catabolism or normal fed state 10–15 g/d = moderate catabolism >15 g/d = severe catabolism	

Table continued on following page

Table 10-4	LABORATORY TESTS FOR NUTRITIONAL ASSESSMENT (Continued)		
Test (Normal Values)	**Nutritional Use**	**Causes of Normal Value Despite Malnutrition**	**Other Causes of Abnormal Value**
	Estimate protein balance Protein balance = protein intake − protein loss where protein loss (protein catabolic rate) = [24-hr UUN (g) + 4] × 6.25 Adjustments required in burn patients and others with large non-urinary nitrogen losses and in patients with fluctuating BUN levels (e.g., renal failure)		
Blood urea nitrogen (BUN) 8–23 mg/dl	<8 (possibly inadequate protein intake) 12–23 (possibly adequate protein intake) >23 (possibly excessive protein intake) If serum creatinine is normal, use BUN If serum creatinine is elevated, use BUN/creatinine ratio (normal range is essentially the same as for BUN)		LOW Severe liver disease Anabolic state Syndrome of inappropriate antidiuretic hormone Despite poor protein intake— HIGH Renal failure (use BUN/creatinine ratio) Congestive heart failure Gastrointestinal hemorrhage

muscle mass. Women excrete approximately 18 mg/kg per day, and men excrete approximately 23 mg/kg per day. Table 10-5 shows more detailed predicted urinary creatinine values for adult men and women. Values of 80% to 100% of those predicted indicate adequate muscle mass, values of 60% to 80% indicate a moderate deficit, and values less than 60% indicate a severe deficit of muscle mass. More sophisticated procedures for assessing body composition include dual-energy x-ray absorptiometry (DXA), whole body air-displacement plethysmography, and underwater weighing (hydrodensitometry).

Assessment of Circulating (Visceral) Proteins

The visceral compartment is composed of proteins that act as carriers, binders, and immunologically active proteins.

Table 10-5	PREDICATED URINARY CREATININE VALUES FOR ADULTS		
Men*		**Women†**	
Height	Predicted Creatinine‡ (mg/24 hr)	Height	Predicted Creatinine‡ (mg/24 hr)
5'2" (157.5 cm)	1288	4'10" (147.3 cm)	830
5'3" (160 cm)	1325	4'11" (149.9 cm)	851
5'4" (162.6 cm)	1359	5'0" (152.4 cm)	875
5'5" (165.1 cm)	1386	5'1" (154.9 cm)	900
5'6" (167.6 cm)	1426	5'2" (157.5 cm)	925
5'7" (170.2 cm)	1467	5'3" (160 cm)	949
5'8" (172.7 cm)	1513	5'4" (162.6 cm)	977
5'9" (175.3 cm)	1555	5'5" (165.1 cm)	1006
5'10" (177.8 cm)	1596	5'6" (167.6 cm)	1044
5'11" (180.3 cm)	1642	5'7" (170.2 cm)	1076
6'0" (182.9 cm)	1691	5'8" (172.7 cm)	1109
6'1" (185.4 cm)	1739	5'9" (175.3 cm)	1141
6'2" (188 cm)	1785	5'10" (177.8 cm)	1174
6'3" (190.5 cm)	1831	5'11" (180.3 cm)	1206
6'4" (193 cm)	1891	6'0" (182.9 cm)	1240

*Creatinine coefficient (men) = 23 mg/kg of ideal body weight/24 hours
†Creatinine coefficient (women) = 18 mg/kg of ideal body weight/24 hours
‡80% to 100% of predicted = acceptable; 60% to 80% = moderate depletion; <60% = severe depletion.
From Blackburn GL, Bistrian BR, Maini BS, et al: Nutritional and metabolic assessment of the hospitalized patient. J Parent Ent Nutr 1:11–22, 1977.

The serum proteins that may be used to assess nutritional status include albumin, total iron-binding capacity (or transferrin), thyroxine-binding prealbumin (or transthyretin), and retinol-binding protein. Because they have differing synthesis rates and half-lives—the half-life of serum albumin is about 21 days whereas those of prealbumin and retinol-binding protein are about 2 days and 12 hours, respectively—some of these parameters reflect changes in nutritional status more quickly than others. Rapid flucutations can also make shorter half-life proteins less reliable, however.

Levels of circulating proteins are influenced by their rates of synthesis and catabolism, "third spacing" (loss in interstitial spaces), and in some cases external loss. Although an adequate intake of calories and protein is necessary to achieve optimal circulating protein levels, serum protein levels generally do not reflect protein intake. For example, a drop in the serum level of albumin or transferrin often accompanies significant physiologic stress (e.g., from infection or injury) and is not necessarily an indication of malnutrition or poor intake. A low serum albumin level in a burned patient with both hypermetabolism and increased dermal losses of protein may not indicate malnutrition. On the other hand, adequate nutritional support of the patient's calorie and protein needs is critical for returning circulating proteins to normal levels as stress resolves. Thus, low values by themselves do not define malnutrition but often point to an increased risk of malnutrition because of the hypermetabolic stress state. It is not unusual for protein levels to remain low despite aggressive nutritional support as long as significant physiologic stress persists; if the levels do not rise after the underlying illness improves, the patient's protein and calorie needs should be reassessed to insure that intake is sufficient.

Assessment of Protein Catabolic Rate Using Urinary Urea Nitrogen

Because urea is a major byproduct of protein catabolism, the amount of urea nitrogen excreted each day can be used to estimate the rate of protein catabolism and determine if protein intake is adequate to offset it. Total protein loss and protein balance can be calculated from the urinary urea nitrogen (UUN) as follows:

$$\text{Protein catabolic rate (g/day)} = [\text{24-hour UUN (g)} + 4] \times 6.25$$

The value of 4 g added to the UUN represents a liberal estimate of the unmeasured nitrogen lost in the urine (e.g., creatinine and uric acid), sweat, hair, skin, and feces. The factor 6.25 estimates the amount of protein represented by the nitrogen excreted because, on average, nitrogen accounts for about one sixth the weight of dietary protein. When protein intake is small (e.g., less than about 20 g/day), the equation indicates both the patient's protein requirement and the severity of the catabolic state (see Table 10–4). More substantial protein intakes can raise the UUN because some of the ingested (or infused) protein is catabolized and converted to UUN. Thus, at lower protein intakes the equation is useful for estimating *requirements*, and at higher protein intakes it is useful for assessing protein *balance* (the difference between intake and catabolism; see Chapter 11).

$$\text{Protein balance (g/day)} = \text{Protein intake} - \text{Protein catabolic rate}$$

As noted in Table 10–4, changes in the concentration of blood urea nitrogen (BUN) or body-water content during the 24-hour period of urine collection can confound interpretation of the UUN. Misleading results are particularly likely in patients who are receiving intermittent renal dialysis and have rapid changes in BUN during the UUN collection, and in those undergoing rapid diuresis. If changes in BUN and body weight (as a reflection of changes in fluid status) are determined from measurements taken at the beginning and the end of the urine collection, the UUN can be corrected with the calculation that follows. This calculation yields a more accurate estimation of the protein catabolic rate, the urea nitrogen appearance (UNA).

$$UNA\ (g) = UUN\ (g) + \frac{(\Delta BUN \times 10)(W_m)(BW) + (BUN_m \times 10)(\Delta W)}{1000}$$

where

ΔBUN = Change in BUN (mg/dl) during the urine collection (Final BUN − Initial BUN)

BUN_m = Mean BUN (mg/dl) during the urine collection [(Final BUN + Initial BUN)/2]

ΔW = Change in weight (kg) during the urine collection (Final weight − Initial weight)

W_m = Mean weight (kg) during the urine collection [(Final weight + Initial weight)/2]

BW = Assumed body water as a proportion of body weight (normal value = 0.5 for women and 0.6 for men; 0.05 is subtracted for marked obesity or dehydration; 0.05 is added for leanness or edema)

To make a corrected calculation of the patient's rate of protein breakdown, the value for UNA is substituted for UUN in the protein catabolic rate equation provided previously. In most situations the standard UUN calculation is reliable as long as both BUN and body-water content are stable during the urine collection (even if they are abnormal). Under these circumstances, ΔBUN and ΔW equal zero, and UNA equals UUN.

Another common cause of a spuriously high UUN is gastrointestinal hemorrhage. There is no accurate way to correct for this in calculating the protein catabolic rate; it should simply be taken into account qualitatively when the results of the UUN are interpreted.

Assessment of Protein Intake Using Blood Urea Nitrogen

As dietary protein intake increases, the BUN level generally rises unless the patient is unusually anabolic and using all available amino acids for protein synthesis. The converse is also true; BUN levels generally fall when protein intake is reduced. Thus, in instances where the

BUN is high and there are no other causes, such as renal insufficiency, dehydration, or gastrointestinal bleed, dietary protein intake is likely to be excessive. If the BUN is low (e.g., less than 8 mg/dL), it suggests a low and possibly inadequate protein intake. Nondietary causes of low and high BUN levels are outlined in Table 10–4.

Assessment of Vitamin and Mineral Status

The use of laboratory tests to confirm suspected micronutrient deficiencies is desirable because the physical findings for these are often equivocal and nonspecific. Low blood-micronutrient levels can pre-date more serious clinical manifestations and may also indicate drug-nutrient interactions. Assays typically used for micronutrient assessment, with normal values, are outlined in Table 3–2. There are three general approaches to the measurement of vitamin levels:

- Direct measurement of the vitamin or its derivative in body fluids by chemical or biological means (e.g., plasma ascorbic acid level); the same method is used for measurement of many trace elements
- Indirect assessment of vitamin function as reflected in enzymatic reactions under controlled conditions (e.g., erythrocyte activity coefficients for thiamin, riboflavin, and pyridoxine)
- Measurement of abnormal metabolic end products that occur as a result of deficiency (e.g., homocysteine for folic acid or methylmalonic acid for vitamin B_{12})

SUGGESTED READINGS

ASPEN: The Science and Practice of Nutrition Support: A Case-Based Core Curriculum. Dubuque, IA, Kendall/Hunt, 2001.

Shils ME, Shike M, Ross AC, et al (eds): Modern Nutrition in Health and Disease, 10th ed. Baltimore, Lippincott Williams & Wilkins, 2005.

11

Nutritional Support: General Approach and Complications

DOUGLAS C. HEIMBURGER, MD

Feeding Approaches

There are four approaches to supplying nutrients, using two major routes (Fig. 11–1): The enteral routes include oral and tube feeding, and the parenteral routes include central and peripheral parenteral nutrition. Central parenteral nutrition can be infused through a centrally inserted catheter or a peripherally inserted central catheter (PICC), which reaches from an arm vein to the superior vena cava or right atrium of the heart. Every patient can be nourished by at least one of these approaches. Because they are not mutually exclusive, in many cases two or more complementary approaches can be used. Patients should not be completely unfed for more than 5 to 7 days before tube feeding or total parenteral nutrition (TPN) is instituted. Clinical judgment regarding when to intervene must be exercised if there

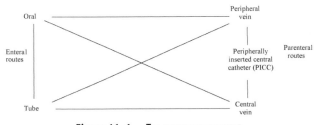

Figure 11–1. THE FEEDING QUADRANGLE.

is food intake but it is insufficient to meet the patient's needs.

The most feasible physiologic feeding approach should always be used. This means that enteral feeding, whether oral or by tube, is always preferred over parenteral feeding unless a contraindication is present. (*If the gut works, use it.*) The reasons for preferring the enteral route (Box 11–1) go beyond the obvious fact that it is the most "normal" way to ingest nutrients. The physiologic responses to enteral feeding differ significantly from those of parenteral nutrition because the latter bypasses the intestinal tract and portal circulation through the liver. Among other things, enteral feeding stimulates gut hormones, subjects nutrients to the absorptive and metabolic controls of the intestinal tract and liver, and produces less hyperglycemia, which allows for better immune function and decreases the risk of systemic infection. The buffering capacity of enteral feeding can improve resistance against stress ulcers. The cost of enteral feeding is only a fraction of that of parenteral. Finally, there is evidence that the intestinal mucosa undergoes atrophy during parenteral nutrition, whereas enteral feeding maintains a healthier mucosa. Although not established in humans, this may enhance mucosal resistance to the translocation of bacteria and endotoxins and reduce the risk of sepsis, multiple organ system failure, and gastrointestinal bleeding. Although it is sometimes tempting to feed a patient parenterally when a central venous catheter is already present,

---

BOX 11–1   Advantages of Enteral Feeding over Parenteral Feeding

Physiologic superiority (e.g., gut hormones, blood glucose levels, buffering capacity)
Maintenance of intestinal structure and function
Protection against sepsis and multiple organ system failure
Lower cost (1/10 to 1/3 that of parenteral nutrition)
Safety (e.g., lower risk of sepsis and other central venous catheter complications)

convenience alone does not justify this route. Because of the benefits of enteral feeding, aggression in gaining enteral access for feeding is warranted (Chapter 13).

Of the enteral options, oral feeding is preferred over tube feeding. Nasogastric or nasointestinal tube feeding is effective in many patients who have inadequate nutrient intake as a result of depressed appetite or the inability to eat. However, if the gastrointestinal tract is not able to be used or is unreliable for more than 5 to 7 days, parenteral nutrition should be used.

Energy Requirements

Goals for feeding patients are derived from estimates or measurements of their energy expenditure and protein utilization.

Estimating Energy Expenditure

A patient's basal energy expenditure (BEE [kcal per day]) can be estimated from his or her height, weight, age, and gender using the Harris-Benedict equations:

$$\text{Men: BEE} = 66.47 + 13.75W + 5.00H - 6.76A$$
$$\text{Women: BEE} = 655.10 + 9.56W + 1.85H - 4.68A$$
$$\text{where } W = \text{weight in kg, } H = \text{height in cm,}$$
$$A = \text{age in years}$$

These equations can be solved with a calculator or the nomograms in Figure 11–2; popular personal digital assistant programs (e.g., MedMath) include the equations as well. Actual energy requirements are then estimated by multiplying the BEE by a factor that accounts for the stress of illness. Multiplying by 1.1 to 1.4 yields a range (10% to 50% above basal) that estimates the 24-hour energy expenditure of the majority of patients.[1] The lower value is used for patients without evidence of significant physiologic stress; the higher value may be appropriate for patients with marked stress such as sepsis or trauma. The result is used as a 24-hour goal for feeding.

There are exceptions to the "1.1 to 1.4 rule." Patients with burns covering more than 40% of the body surface

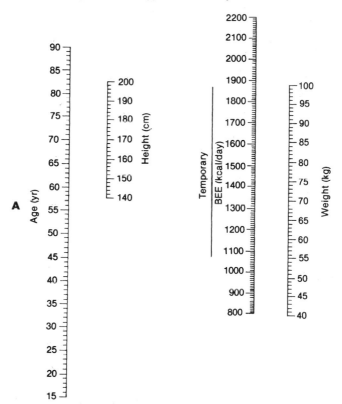

Figure 11-2. NOMOGRAMS FOR CALCULATING BASAL ENERGY EXPENDITURE (BEE) FOR (A) MEN AND (B) WOMEN. Directions: 1. Locate the height and weight on the scales and place a straight-edge (e.g., ruler) between these points, intersecting the temporary variable line. 2. Holding a pencil at the point of intersection (on the temporary variable line), locate the age, and pivot the ruler to this point on the age scale. The point of intersection on the BEE scale is the predicted BEE. (From the Harris-Benedict equations, from Rainey-MacDonald CG, Holliday RL, Wells GA: Nomograms for predicting resting energy expenditure of hospitalized patients. Parent Ent Nutr 6:59–60, 1982, with permission.)

may expend up to 1.6 times the BEE. For unstressed patients in whom weight gain rather than weight maintenance is desired, the BEE may be multiplied by 2. It is not appropriate to provide *excessive* calorie loads to stressed patients because doing so may cause hyperglycemia

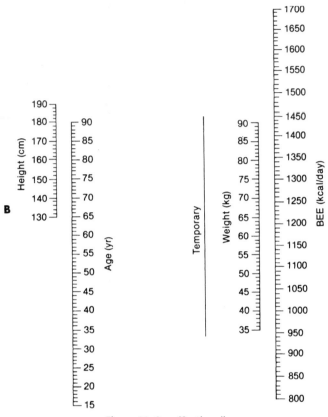

Figure 11-2. *(Continued)*

and fat deposition in the liver. By contrast, such calorie levels are appropriate for weight gain in *stable, unstressed* cachectic patients who have become *well adapted* to feeding. (See later section on Complications of Nutritional Support.)

When calculating the BEE, current body weight should be used rather than ideal weight. In markedly underweight patients the calculated BEE is very low, but this reflects the patient's adaptation to starvation (see Chapter 9). Using the patient's actual body weight also assists in avoiding the complications of rapid refeeding, which will be discussed in this chapter. Estimating energy expenditure in obese patients is more difficult and, given the prevalence of obesity in the United States, is a significant challenge. The Harris-Benedict equations assume a linear relationship between body weight and energy expenditure. However, as weight increases in the obese range, energy expenditure increases more slowly with additional weight. Investigators have proposed different methods of estimating BEE in obese subjects, but none has been shown to be clearly superior. Because there is greater risk from overfeeding critically ill patients than from slightly underfeeding them, it is probably better to underestimate energy expenditure than to overestimate it. In obese patients, the best method may be to include 50% of the excess weight in the Harris-Benedict equation, as shown in Box 11–2.[1] Alternatively, intentional hypocaloric feeding of obese patients (12 to 15 kcal/kg per day) with high protein intakes (2 g protein/kg per day) may be sufficient, and there is no evidence that such feeding worsens outcomes.[2]

Measuring Energy Expenditure: Indirect Calorimetry

When it is important to have a more accurate assessment of energy needs, they can be measured at the bedside using indirect calorimetry. This technique is useful for patients who are believed to be hypermetabolic from

---

BOX 11–2   Adjusting Body Weight to Estimate Basal Energy Expenditure in Obese Patients

Adjusted Weight = [0.5 × (actual weight − ideal weight) + ideal weight]
Where ideal weight is calculated as:
Women: 100 lb (45.5 kg) for the first 5 feet (152 cm) of height, plus 5 lb (2.3 kg) for each additional inch of height
Men: 106 lb (48 kg) for the first 5 feet (152 cm) of height, plus 6 lb (2.7 kg) for each additional inch of height

sepsis or trauma and whose body weights cannot be obtained accurately or patients having difficulty weaning from a ventilator whose energy needs should not be exceeded to avoid excessive CO_2 production. Patients at the extremes of weight or age are good candidates as well, because the Harris-Benedict equations were developed in adults with roughly normal body weights.

Indirect calorimetry is based on the principle that energy expenditure is proportional to O_2 consumption and CO_2 production and the proportion of fuels being utilized is reflected in their ratio, the respiratory quotient (RQ). The test involves using a mobile metabolic cart with a clear plastic hood that is placed over the patient's head or tubing that is connected to the patient's ventilator to measure respiratory gas exchange for 20 to 30 minutes. The protocol for indirect calorimetry is provided in Box 11–3.

If the patient is not agitated and a steady state of gas exchange can be achieved (even for as short a period as 5 minutes) during which he or she is not hyperventilating or hypoventilating, the results are likely to be a valid reflection of resting energy expenditure (REE) when extrapolated to 24 hours. If the patient is being chronically overfed, the measured energy expenditure may be falsely high. For example, if a patient has been regularly receiving 3000 kcal per day before and during the procedure and the measured energy expenditure is 2000 kcal per day, feeding can be reduced to 2000 kcal to better meet the patient's needs. To fine-tune treatment and more accurately estimate the patient's true energy requirements, the test can then be repeated. Conversely, starving or underfeeding a patient who is without significant physiologic stress may give a spuriously low estimate (by about 7% to 15%) of the patient's true energy needs. Repeating the calorimetry study after several days of feeding can yield a more accurate assessment of true energy needs.

The RQ (the ratio of CO_2 produced divided by O_2 consumed) provides information on substrate utilization. Each of the three major substrates has a unique RQ

BOX 11-3   Preparation for Indirect Calorimetry

30 Hours Before Test

24-hour urine urea nitrogen (UUN) collection (with sufficient
 time to receive result) if determination of carbohydrate, fat,
 and protein utilization desired

10 Hours Before Test

Patient fasting if measurement of energy *requirement* desired;
 may continue enteral or parenteral feeding, recognizing that
 results will reflect the patient's energy expenditure in
 response to feeding and may be spuriously high if the
 patient is being overfed

4 Hours Before Test

Patient resting and avoiding physical activity, physical therapy,
 dressing changes

2 Hours Before Test

Endotracheal tube suctioned for the last time before test;
 further ventilator changes or suctioning avoided

1 Hour Before Test

Supine position, complete rest; analgesic or sedative
 administered if needed

(0.7 for fat, 0.8 for protein, and 1.0 for carbohydrate),
and the RQ obtained from the test reflects the proportions being utilized. For example, an RQ of 0.75 suggests that the patient is relying heavily on fat as a fuel
(e.g., when energy intake is insufficient), whereas
0.90 indicates largely carbohydrate oxidation. However,
each of the three substrates is inevitably being used to
some extent. A value of greater than 1.0 suggests that
the patient is receiving excess calories and is synthesizing fat from carbohydrates. Measurement of the urinary
urea nitrogen (UUN) allows estimation of the amount of
protein being catabolized; combining it with the RQ
allows relatively accurate estimates of the amounts of

each of the fuels the patient is utilizing. See Chapter 14 for a discussion of the relative merits of the two forms of nonprotein calories (carbohydrate and fat) in the hospitalized patient.

Protein Requirements

The stress of illness, particularly acute illnesses, usually increases protein catabolism. For this reason, protein requirements are frequently elevated twofold or more above usual levels, often to levels of 1.5 g/kg/day and sometimes as high as 3 g/kg/day. The 24-hour UUN measurement is the most practical method for estimating a patient's protein catabolic rate, which is related to protein requirements (Chapter 10). An estimate of protein intake provided by a dietitian or calculated from enteral and parenteral feeding is compared with the protein catabolic rate to calculate protein balance:

$$\text{Protein balance (g/day)} = \text{Protein intake} - \text{Protein catabolic rate}$$

A cushion of about 10 g/day above the estimated level of protein catabolism is useful to increase the certainty of positive protein balance.

Protein and energy requirements are interrelated. Healthy individuals need about 10% to 12% of energy as protein, but as physiologic stress increases, the body derives an increasing proportion (15%, 20%, or even 25%) of its energy from protein. Therefore to avoid negative protein balance, hypermetabolic patients need a commensurate increase in protein intake relative to energy intake.

Other patient groups that may benefit from relative protein intakes of ≥20% are cachectic patients, who accrue lean body mass more rapidly at these levels, and elderly patients, especially those suffering from infections and other illnesses. However, when high protein intakes are used, the patient should be monitored for progressive azotemia (increasing BUN level). When this occurs, it may be necessary to reduce the protein intake.

The relative protein content of a diet or feeding regimen is calculated as follows:

$$\text{Relative protein content (\% of kcal)} = \frac{\text{protein content (g)} \times 4 \text{ kcal/g} \times 100}{\text{energy content}}$$

For example,

$$\frac{100 \text{ g protein} \times 4 \text{ kcal/g protein} \times 100}{2000 \text{ kcal}} = 20\% \text{ protein}$$

Relating the energy and protein requirements calculated separately from BEE and UUN in this way provides a cross-check to insure that the relative protein content is in an acceptable range. When a UUN is not available, the equation can be rearranged to arrive at a desired protein intake:

$$\text{Desired protein intake (g)} = \frac{\text{energy requirement} \times \% \text{ protein desired}}{4 \text{ kcal/g} \times 100}$$

For example,

$$\frac{2000 \text{ kcal/d} \times 20\% \text{ protein desired}}{4 \text{ kcal/g protein} \times 100} = 100 \text{ g/d}$$

Although adequate protein intake is required to support protein synthesis and prevent unnecessary wastage of muscle mass, high protein intakes do not force the body to synthesize proteins (such as albumin) or muscle tissue. Inactive muscles cannot make full use of available amino acids, so exercise should be encouraged to maintain and possibly build muscle mass.

Serum proteins such as albumin do not reflect changes in protein intake, and cannot be used to guide intake (see Chapter 10). However, if the serum albumin level falls during aggressive nutritional support, the patient's protein balance should be reassessed to ensure that it is positive.

Vitamin and Mineral Allowances

The micronutrient needs of many ill patients are higher than those listed in the DRIs (see Table 3–1), but there are few clear guidelines for appropriate doses of micronutrients in individual patients. The principles discussed in Chapters 1, 3, and 10 are helpful, but blood levels of vitamins, minerals, and trace elements must sometimes be measured to verify that doses are adequate. Even though blood levels are generally the best measures available, they do not always indicate sufficient levels in target tissues. Additional amounts of vitamins and minerals can be admixed with parenteral nutrition, but supplements in enterally fed patients should be provided separately from the formula via an oral, tube, or intravenous route.

Complications of Nutritional Support

The general complications of nutritional support are outlined in this chapter. The specific complications of enteral and parenteral nutrition will be dealt with in Chapters 13 and 14.

The Hypometabolic, Starved Patient

Because chronically starved but otherwise unstressed patients are relatively well adapted to energy-deprived states, they are generally at greater immediate risk of death from inappropriate refeeding than from continued semistarvation. Hypophosphatemia and repletion heart failure are two consequences of refeeding that deserve special attention. Their pathophysiologic components are outlined in Table 11–1.

Hypophosphatemia

Potentially, the most serious complication of refeeding, hypophosphatemia usually results from aggressive feeding using carbohydrate as the predominant energy source. This is especially true in parenteral nutrition.

Table 11–1	COMPONENTS OF HEART FAILURE IN THE REFEEDING SYNDROME IN CACHECTIC PATIENTS		
Underlying Low Cardiac Output	+	Superimposed Demand for Increased Cardiac Output →	Heart Failure
Cardiac atrophy		Fluid challenge	Fluid overload
Low stroke volume		↑Plasma volume	
Low metabolic rate		↑Catecholamines	Cardiac and respiratory decompensation
Low O$_2$ consumption		↑Metabolic rate	
Bradycardia		↑O$_2$ consumption	
Low blood pressure		↑Blood pressure	
Low afterload		↑Afterload	
Predominantly fatty acid utilization		Glucose challenge	
Low phosphorus requirement		↑Insulin	
		Sodium retention	
		↓Phosphorus levels	
		↓Glycolysis	
		↑Blood glucose	
		↓ATP production	
		↓Cardiac contractility	
		↓Minute ventilation	

Because the metabolic rate and glucose oxidation are low during starvation, the need for phosphorus (used in glycolysis and ATP production) is relatively low. When glucose is infused, the demand for phosphorus increases dramatically and can exceed the body's ability to mobilize it from bone. When phosphate levels fall below 1.0 mg/dL, the risk of adverse clinical effects is high, especially (in the authors' experience) if there is concurrent hyperglycemia, which may reflect intracellular phosphate depletion. The complications of severe hypophosphatemia include weakness, muscle paralysis, decreased cardiac output, respiratory failure, decreased oxygen release from red blood cells, and decreased white blood cell bactericidal activity. Refeeding hypophosphatemia has caused cardiorespiratory failure and death within several days in patients who were chronically starved but otherwise stable.[3]

Repletion Heart Failure

Repletion heart failure is another avoidable complication of refeeding starved patients. During starvation, the metabolic rate and oxygen requirements fall, as do cardiac output, blood pressure, and heart rate. During repletion, the metabolic rate rises, demand for cardiac output increases, plasma volume expands, and blood pressure rises—all potentially leading to repletion heart failure (see Table 11–1).

The Hypermetabolic, Stressed Patient

As noted in Chapter 10, energy requirements are increased in physiologically stressed patients. However overfeeding, especially from TPN, can induce hyperglycemia, which impairs immune function and wound healing, increases risk for infections, and increases mortality.[4] It may also promote fat deposition in the liver and cause abnormal liver function tests. Further, if nutritional support exceeds the patient's energy needs, especially through the use of intravenous glucose, the already elevated REE and oxygen consumption may be further increased, perhaps through increased catecholamine and cytokine production.

This increases demand for cardiac output and for oxygen, which may have consequences in patients with congestive heart failure or hypoxic lung disease. In addition, excessive calories can increase carbon dioxide production significantly, possibly requiring a significant increase in minute ventilation. In this setting, patients with ventilatory compromise such as chronic lung disease can develop carbon dioxide retention and respiratory acidosis; overfeeding those on artificial ventilator support could hamper efforts to wean as a result of increased carbon dioxide production. Thus, in hypermetabolic patients the aim of nutritional support should be to meet, but not exceed, energy needs.

The Selective Approach to Nutritional Support

Formulating an appropriate feeding approach requires distinguishing whether the patient is hypometabolic or hypermetabolic (Table 11–2). Although only nutritional support considerations are covered here, pharmacologic interventions may eventually prove to be appropriate complements to nutritional support.[5]

The Hypometabolic, Starved Patient

The absence of significant physiologic stress in the hypometabolic, starved patient can be documented with indirect calorimetry (measured REE should not be greater than calculated BEE) or a 24-hour UUN (nitrogen excretion should be ≤5 g per day if protein intake is low). Because the major risk in this situation is excessively rapid refeeding, nutritional support of these patients should be initiated and increased cautiously, taking up to a week to reach the final calorie goal (Table 11–3). This is the main means of preventing both hypophosphatemia and heart failure because it allows the patient time to adapt to new energy and glucose loads.

The enteral feeding route should be used whenever possible, and the diet or formula should be relatively high in protein as discussed previously. If the intravenous route

Table 11–2	SELECTIVE APPROACHES TO NUTRITIONAL SUPPORT			
Patient Type	Goal	Nutritional Support	Risks	Error to Avoid
Hypometabolic, starved	Rebuild	Cautious and gradual, with portion of fuel as fat and adequate phosphorus	Hypophosphatemia, repletion heart failure	Commission (overzealous, excessive nutritional support)
Hypermetabolic, stressed	Replace	Aggressive but not excessive	Excessive O_2 consumption and CO_2 production	Omission (inadequate nutritional support)

Table 11-3	ENERGY GOALS IN REFEEDING A HYPOMETABOLIC, STARVED PATIENT

Days	Energy Goal
1–2	BEE × 0.8
3–4	BEE × 1
4–6	BEE × 1.1 to 1.4
6+	BEE × 2 if patient is stable and weight gain is desired

is required, initially one third or more of the energy should be provided as fat in order to minimize the glucose load. With either type of feeding, normal phosphorus levels should be documented before repletion and monitored daily during the initial period of refeeding. When parenteral feeding is used, the need for fairly high doses of phosphorus (up to 1 mmol/kg/day) should be anticipated, and phosphorus should be included especially in the first few bags of parenteral solution.

The Hypermetabolic, Stressed Patient

Calorimetry and UUN results in critically ill patients differ from those in hypometabolic, starved patients. REE levels 20% to 50% greater than calculated BEE and UUN values greater than approximately 10 g/day, when protein intake is relatively low, indicate significant stress. Underfeeding a hypermetabolic patient increases risk for developing kwashiorkor. In these situations, nutritional support should be approached aggressively, with the intention to meet but not *exceed* the patient's requirements. It is often possible to reach the goal for energy and protein intake within 24 to 36 hours of initiating enteral or parenteral support. Even if the patient is cachectic, documentation of a hypermetabolic state should prompt aggressive nutritional support, reaching the energy and protein goals within 2 to 3 days.

Effects of Nutritional Support on Patient Outcome

Documenting the effects of nutritional support on patient care outcomes has been difficult and controversial.

In part, the difficulty relates to ethical problems in randomizing patients to feeding and nonfeeding groups. Therefore, most randomized trials have studied patients in whom aggressive nutritional support is discretionary, such as those facing elective surgery. Many of these trials have used parenteral nutrition as the study treatment. Some studies have shown less mortality and intra-abdominal abscesses, peritonitis, anastomotic leaks, and ileus in patients treated with parenteral nutrition. However, others have documented significantly higher rates of sepsis in these patients. In a cooperative study conducted in Veterans Affairs hospitals, preoperative TPN only benefited patients with significant protein-energy malnutrition (PEM); the types of PEM were not distinguished.[6] In the less severely malnourished patients, TPN was associated with *net harm* in the form of higher sepsis rates.

Using these results, some observers have argued that parenteral feeding should be avoided even at the expense of allowing patients to go unfed for up to 3 weeks.[7] However, a more reasonable response is to make aggressive efforts to access the gastrointestinal tract for feeding after 5 to 7 days of insufficient intake. The indications for using TPN should be fairly restrictive (Chapter 13), but it should not be avoided when the only alternative is protracted underfeeding.

Nutrition Support Teams

Many hospitals have established nutrition support teams (NSTs) to provide a coordinated and systematic approach to nutritional support, especially when nutritional support is being introduced or its use expanded within the hospital. Typically, NSTs consist of a dietitian, nurse, pharmacist, and physician. Each member has a valuable role in the overall mission of the NST, which is to assure that nutrition services are delivered in an appropriate, safe, efficient, and cost-effective manner. Box 11–4 outlines typical roles of each member of the NST.

The potential benefits of NSTs are listed in Box 11–5. Having an NST could result in decreased infectious and

BOX 11–4   Typical Duties of Nutrition Support Team Members

Physician

Provides leadership and directs the nutrition support team (NST)

Interprets medical information relative to nutritional support

Performs nutritional assessment –confirms history, performs physical examination, reviews laboratory data

Integrates information from other team members to develop a management plan

Assumes final responsibility for recommendations and patient care

Dietitian

Performs nutrition screening and identifies high-risk patients

Performs nutritional assessment

Estimates energy and protein needs

Translates dietary prescription into food and/or tube feeding selections

Monitors and records energy and protein intake

Monitors transitions in feeding

Serves as a resource for dietary issues including enteral nutrition products and costs and enternal feeding formulary

Nurse

Monitors nursing issues related to administration of nutritional support

Monitors care of feeding access devices (catheters, feeding tubes, etc.)

Teaches and serves as a resource for patients, families, and other nurses

Pharmacist

Participates in formulating and compounding total parenteral nutrition (TPN) solutions

Monitors quality control of TPN solutions

Acts as a resource for drug-related issues (drug-nutrient interactions, appropriateness of medications, compatibility of medications with TPN or enteral feedings)

Monitors hospital-wide usage of TPN

Participates in developing and maintaining a cost-effective nutritional support formulary

Box continued on following page

BOX 11-4   Typical Duties of Nutrition Support Team Members *(Continued)*

Any Member of the NST

Ensures Joint Commission on Accreditation of Healthcare Organizations (JCAHO) standards are met

Conducts research

Provides educational programs

Deals with administrative issues

Participates in designing, implementing, and managing nutrition care plans

Provides discharge planning and outpatient management of nutritional care plans

Monitors laboratory data

Collects continuous quality improvement data

Develops materials for patient instruction and institutional procedures and guidelines

Serves as NST liaison with own or other departments

Writes procedural guidelines related to nutritional support for own department

---

BOX 11-5   Potential Benefits of a Nutrition Support Team

Decreased Complications

Septic

Metabolic

Mechanical (catheter-related)

Drug-nutrient interactions

Decreased Costs

Use of enteral feeding instead of total parenteral nutrition (TPN) whenever possible

Decreased number of days on TPN

Use of individualized goals to avoid overfeeding

Restricted use of expensive nonstandard TPN or enteral formulas to instances when clear indications are present

Decreased errors in ordering and decreased wastage of TPN

Potential decrease in length of hospital stay

Research

Education

Improved Patient Care, Nutritional Status, and Other Outcomes

metabolic complications because of close monitoring and expertise in the use of TPN. By using appropriate amounts of parenteral nutrition only when indicated, an NST might reduce a hospital's overall costs of nutritional support. Members of an NST can participate in research studies and in the education of residents, physicians, and other health care professionals. These factors may translate into improved outcomes in patient care.

REFERENCES

1. Barak N, Wall-Alonso E, Sitrin MD: Evaluation of stress factors and body weight adjustments currently used to estimate energy expenditure in hospitalized patients. J Parent Ent Nutr 26:231, 2002.
2. Dickerson RN: Specialized nutrition support in the hospitalized obese patient. Nutr Clin Pract 19:245, 2004.
3. Weinsier RL, Krumdieck CL: Death resulting from overzealous total parenteral nutrition: The refeeding syndrome revisited. Am J Clin Nutr 34:393, 1981.
4. Van den Berghe F, Wouters P, Weekers F, et al: Intensive insulin therapy in critically ill patients. N Engl J Med 345:1359, 2001.
5. Kotler DP: Cachexia. Ann Intern Med 133:622, 2000.
6. Veterans Affairs Total Parenteral Nutrition Cooperative Study Group: Perioperative total parenteral nutrition in surgical patients. N Engl J Med 325:525, 1991.
7. Koretz RL: Nutritional supplementation in the ICU: How critical is nutrition for the critically ill? Am J Resp Crit Care Med 151:570, 1995.

SUGGESTED READINGS

American Society for Parenteral and Enteral Nutrition: ASPEN Nutrition Support Practice Manual, 2006. Available at http://www.clinnutr.org/
American Society for Parenteral and Enteral Nutrition: The Science and Practice of Nutrition Support: A Case-based Core Curriculum. Dubuque, Iowa, Kendall/Hunt, 2001.
American Society for Parenteral and Enteral Nutrition, Shikora SA, Martindale RG, Schwaitzberg SB (eds): Nutritional Considerations in the Intensive Care Unit: Science, Rationale, and Practice. Dubuque, Iowa, Kendall/Hunt, 2002.
Rombeau JL, Rolandelli RH (eds): Clinical Nutrition: Parenteral Nutrition, 3rd ed. Philadelphia, WB Saunders, 2000.
Rolandelli RH, Bankhead R, Boullata JI, Compher CW (eds): Clinical Nutrition: Enteral and Tube Feeding, 4th ed. Philadelphia, WB Saunders, 2005.

WEB SITES

American Society for Parenteral and Enteral Nutrition (ASPEN), http://www.clinnutr.org/

12

Therapeutic Diets

SARAH L. MORGAN, MD • LAURA E. NEWTON, MA, RD

Diet is a very important aspect of the therapy for many disease states, complementing and even replacing drug therapy in some cases. Therapeutic diets represent permutations of the general dietary guidelines described in Chapters 1 and 3. A useful schema of therapeutic diets breaks the general diet into its basic components (water, carbohydrate, fiber, protein, fat, vitamins, minerals, and other substances such as alcohol) and consistencies (liquid, soft, or solid). It is possible to alter (restrict or increase) each of these to form therapeutic diets as shown by the following examples:

- Fluid-modified diets: restricted fluid intake for treating heart or kidney disease
- Carbohydrate-modified diets: for treating diabetes or hypertriglyceridemia
- Protein-modified diets: low protein for unstressed patients with chronic kidney disease; high protein for stressed patients
- Fat-modified diets: low total and saturated fat for treating hypercholesterolemia; low total fat for treating malabsorption syndromes
- Mineral-modified diets: low sodium, potassium, and phosphorus for treating kidney disease
- Modified-consistency diets: soft diets for treating patients without teeth; high-fiber diets for treating constipation
- Other substances: restricted alcohol for treating hypertriglyceridemia

Consultation with a registered or licensed dietitian is invaluable for assistance in prescribing and monitoring of therapeutic diets. The American Dietetic Association web site, http://www.eatright.org, can help in finding a nutritional professional. Tables 12–1 through 12–7 outline diets for specific medical conditions and with particular modifications. The rationales for many of the therapeutic diets are explained in subsequent chapters.

Refeeding After Brief Bowel Rest

Patients who have been without oral or enteral feeding for less than 1 or 2 weeks can usually be advanced to a full diet within several days. The commonly used regimen of advancing from clear liquids to full liquids to soft or solid food has two inherent drawbacks: (1) some clear liquids are high in osmolality; and (2) full liquids are often high in fat and lactose. Clear liquids may be most appropriate for testing the patient's swallowing mechanism, but their high osmolalities may not be well tolerated and juice often forms gas. The fat and lactose contents of full liquids can complicate the refeeding of patients with impaired intestinal tracts. The guidelines in Box 12–1 are generally satisfactory.

Because tube feeding maintains the bowel's mucosal surface, it is not necessary for tube-fed patients to follow this regimen. Their adaptation to oral intake is usually determined by their ability to chew and swallow or by the underlying medical or surgical condition.

Refeeding After Prolonged Bowel Rest or Bowel Resection

Patients who have been without enteral feeding for 3 weeks or more or recently had a substantial part of their small intestine removed (short bowel syndrome) usually experience digestive dysfunction and malabsorption when they begin to ingest food orally; refeeding should therefore be approached slowly. If patients have diarrhea at the outset, they may need to be on "nothing by mouth" (NPO) status for 1 or 2 days until the stooling stops; then refeeding can be started. If diarrhea persists after 2 days of NPO status, secretory or inflammatory processes should be ruled out.

Text continued on p. 305.

Table 12–1	DIETARY THERAPIES FOR SPECIFIC DIAGNOSES	
Diagnostic Category	**Dietary Therapy**	**Comments**
Cardiovascular Diseases, Hyperlipidemia (see Chapter 20)		
Congestive heart failure (CHF)	Sodium-restricted	Specify grams sodium:
		2–3 g/day suggested initially for acute CHF.
	Low-saturated fat (see Hypercholesterolemia)	More severe restriction such as 0.5–1 g is occasionally required. Fluid restriction is often necessary.
Hypercholesterolemia	Low-saturated fat, low-cholesterol, high-fiber	Specify percent calories as fat and mg cholesterol.
		Limit saturated fatty acid intake to <10% of energy intake. For individuals with elevated LDL levels, reduce saturated fat to <7% of total energy intake.
		For all individuals, lower total cholesterol intake to <300 mg/day.
		For individuals with elevated LDL levels, lower total cholesterol intake to <200 mg/day.
		Substitute monounsaturated or polyunsaturated fats for saturated fat.
		Include at least 2 servings of fish per week for cardioprotective effects.
		Maintain a healthy eating pattern including a variety of fruits, vegetables, whole grains, low-fat and fat-free dairy products, lean meats, fish, legumes, and poultry.
		Choose 5 or more servings of fruits and vegetables per day.
		Choose whole grains to provide complex carbohydrates, vitamins, minerals, and soluble fiber.
		Include plant sterols, soy protein, and nuts.*
		Maintain energy intake and activity to achieve a desirable body weight.

Hypertension	DASH diet with sodium restriction	Emphasize fruits, vegetables, low-fat dairy products, whole grains, poultry, and nuts. Minimize saturated fat; use small amounts of red meat, sugars, and sweets. Reductions in sodium intake to ≤2.4 g (6 g salt) per day with the DASH diet further reduce blood pressure. Maintain energy intake and activity to achieve a desirable body weight. Limit alcohol to ≤2 drinks/day (1 drink = 12 oz beer, 5 oz wine, or 1.5 oz distilled spirits) for men and ≤1 drink/day for women.
Hypertriglyceridemia	Moderate restriction in total fat; sucrose- and alcohol- restricted; calories to achieve or maintain ideal body weight	Specify percent calories as fat (generally <30% of calories from fat with increased servings of complex carbohydrates such as fruits, vegetables, and starches). Concentrated sweets are restricted. Alcohol is restricted. Maintain energy intake and activity to achieve a desirable body weight.
Myocardial infarction	Sodium- and saturated fat-restricted, or cardiac prudent diet	Specify grams sodium; if CHF is present, fluid restriction may be necessary. Fat similar to that for hypercholesterolemia. In some cases, caffeine may be restricted.

Endocrine and Metabolic Disorders (see Chapters 16 and 18)

Diabetes mellitus, Type 1, insulin-dependent (see Table 12–2 for more details)	Low-fat, low-cholesterol, high-fiber; diet order should specify the calorie level.	Coordinate meals with insulin regimen and blood glucose monitoring schedule. Maintain glucose levels in the normal range or close to normal range to minimize diabetic complications. Include whole grains, fruits, vegetables, and low-fat dairy. For glycemic control, the total amount of carbohydrate is more important than the type of carbohydrate.

Table continued on following page

Table 12-1 DIETARY THERAPIES FOR SPECIFIC DIAGNOSES (*Continued*)

Diagnostic Category	Dietary Therapy	Comments
		Sucrose-containing foods don't increase blood sugar more than isocaloric amounts of starches. However, the intake of high-sucrose foods and beverages may increase calories and fat in the diet and reduce vitamin and mineral intakes compared to isocaloric amounts of fruits and vegetables. These foods should be included in the context of a healthy diet.
		Low glycemic index diets may be considered, but they are cumbersome and additional evidence on their superiority is needed.
		Dietary fiber intakes should be in the range recommended for the general population.
		Maintain a lipid profile that reduces risk for macrovascular disease (see Hypercholesterolemia comments).
		For individuals with microalbuminuria, protein intake may be reduced to 0.8–1 mg/kg/day. For individuals with nephropathy, reduction of protein intake to 0.8 mg/kg/day may slow the progression of nephropathy. Patients on protein restriction should have diets designed and monitored by a registered/licensed dietitian to assure adequacy
		Meal planning methods include diabetic exchanges (see Table 12–2) and carbohydrate counting, where grams of carbohydrate or numbers of carbohydrate exchanges are kept constant.
Diabetes mellitus, Type 2, non-insulin-	Low-fat, low-cholesterol, high-fiber; diet should	As for Type 1 diabetes, with emphasis on achieving glucose, lipid, and blood pressure goals.

depernient (see Table 12-2 for more details) Hypoglycemia, postprandial	specify the calorie level.	In overweight individuals, weight reduction is beneficial even if ideal body weight is not achieved.
	Restricted in refined sugars, 6 small meals daily	Meal planning methods include diabetic exchanges (see Table 12-2). Low in refined carbohydrates and high in complex carbohydrates and protein Encourage fat and/or protein intake with carbohydrates to blunt hyperinsulinemia and subsequent hypoglycemia. The diagnosis of hypoglycemia is often questionable, and should be well documented before being applied.
Gout	Purine-restricted	Because of strong positive correlations between insulin resistance and elevated uric acid levels, maintenance of desirable body weight is important. If weight loss is undertaken, it should be done gradually. Gout patients frequently have metabolic syndrome (dyslipidemia, obesity, diabetes mellitus); therefore dietary therapy may also need to be directed to coexisting conditions. Consume alcohol in moderation or not at all since alcohol intake increases blood uric acid levels. Consume liberal amounts of fluid. Low purine diets (limiting kidney, liver. organ meats, and certain seafcods) have limited usefulness, especially with pharmacological therapies for gout. Low-purine diets may be useful at the time of a gouty flare.
Obesity	Weight-reduction	Specify calories to achieve 1–2 lb of weight loss per week. Less than 1000 kcal/day is generally not recommended because of difficulty in achieving nutritional adequacy. Programs that take into account lifestyle modification and exercise are recommended.

Table continued on following page

Table 12-1 DIETARY THERAPIES FOR SPECIFIC DIAGNOSES (Continued)

Diagnostic Category	Dietary Therapy	Comments
Gastrointestinal Conditions (see Chapter 22)		
Esophageal stricture	Individualized	High-protein, high-calorie full liquid, enteral formulas, or pureed foods
		May progress to ground foods or soft diet as tolerated, with small, frequent feedings.
		Use tube feeding if oral intake is insufficient and enteral access can be established.
Hiatal hernia with esophagitis, gastroesophageal reflux disease, peptic ulcer disease	Individualized, eliminating symptom-causing foods	Foods may be irritating via 3 mechanisms:
		Direct irritation because of osmolality, astringency, or acidity (e.g., citrus juices, spicy foods)
		Increased gastric secretions (e.g., coffee, alcohol)
		Relaxed lower esophageal sphincter (chocolate)
Postgastrectomy	Postgastrectomy diet	Postgastrectomy patients are at risk for weight loss, dumping syndrome, diarrhea, anemia (vitamin B_{12}, folate, and iron deficiencies), metabolic bone disease with calcium and vitamin D deficiencies, and reactive hypoglycemia. Nutritional status should be monitored longitudinally.
		To minimize dumping syndrome (nausea, weakness, sweating, and dizziness from hyperosmolar foods passing rapidly into the small intestine), apply the following.
		Increase the frequency and reduce the volume of feedings (individualize to patient tolerance).
		Fluids and meals should initially be separated, and fluid intake adjusted to tolerance.
		Simple sugars should be omitted initially but can often be included later.
		Lactose intolerance may be present.

Bariatric surgery	Specific to the procedure performed, e.g., post-gastric bypass diet	A low-fiber diet is often helpful initially, and fiber may be added as the patient progresses.
		It is important to understand the anatomy and physiology of the specific procedure in following patients long-term.
		After many bariatric surgeries, deficiencies of iron, vitamin B_{12}, vitamin D, and calcium are common. Long-term supplementation with these is important, including multivitamins and individual supplements. Vitamin B_{12} can be given by monthly injections, nasal gel, or daily oral dose. Blood levels should be monitored periodically for deficiencies.
		Dumping syndrome can occur (see post-gastrectomy diet).
		Patients are typically started on non-caloric clear liquids (broth, sugar-free Jell-o, coffee, tea) on the day after surgery and advanced to soft or pureed foods such as grits, scrambled eggs, mashed potatoes, and mashed vegetables. After 2 weeks, solid foods may be incorporated while continuing to avoid concentrated sweets and sweetened beverages.
		Liquids (calorie-free beverages only) should be taken an hour before or after meals and sipped slowly between meals. Sweetened beverages and juices should be avoided for the long-term.
Celiac disease (gluten-sensitive enteropathy, nontropical sprue) and dermatitis herpetiformis	Gluten-free	Wheat, rye, barley, and foods containing these grains should be omitted from the diet.
		Corn, rice, tapioca, soybean, arrowroot, and potato flours can be used as substitutes.
		Oats are gluten-free and can improve diet diversity and quality of life without adverse effects. However, many sources of oats are contaminated with wheat, rye, or barley, making many patients cautious about using them.

Table continued on following page

Table 12-1 DIETARY THERAPIES FOR SPECIFIC DIAGNOSES *(Continued)*

Diagnostic Category	Dietary Therapy	Comments
Constipation, diverticulosis, hemorrhoids	High-fiber (21–38 g/day, as recommended for all adults)	Web sites such as http://www.celiac.com and the Celiac Sprue Association (http://www.csceliacs.org) are helpful resources for patients. Dietary sources of fiber should be tried before using fiber supplements. Soluble fibers include gums, mucilages, pectins, and hemicelluloses. Food sources include fruits, vegetables, barley, oats, oat bran, and legumes (dried beans and peas). Insoluble fibers include cellulose, lignin, and some hemicelluloses. Food sources include fruits, vegetables, cereals, whole-wheat products, and wheat bran. Excessive intakes of fiber may reduce the absorption of calcium, copper, iron, magnesium, selenium, and zinc.
Acute inflammatory bowel disease	Individualized	A soft, low-fiber diet may be tolerated. Bowel rest with total parental nutrition may be useful if oral intake is not tolerated (e.g., because of strictures or fistulae).
Chronic inflammatory bowel disease Regional enteritis (Crohn's disease of the small intestine)	Individualized	Many patients have no food intolerances (i.e., no clear links between food and symptoms), and should not be restricted. Some patients may benefit from avoiding lactose, highly osmotic fruit juices, alcohol, and caffeine. Patients with significant bowel narrowing benefit from a low-fiber diet that restricts beans, nuts, and seeds. Malabsorption may be present, especially after bowel resection. A low-fat diet with medium-chain triglyceride (MCT) supplementation may be beneficial.

Ulcerative colitis	Individualized	Home parenteral nutrition is helpful or lifesaving in severe malabsorption or short bowel syndrome.
		Pay careful attention to fat-soluble vitamins, folic acid, and vitamin B_{12} status (especially if the ileum is involved).
		Patients with extensive or acute colitis may benefit from avoiding high-fiber foods, but fiber restriction is not recommended or required for all patients.
		Lactose restriction may be helpful.
		Avoiding highly spiced foods, highly osmotic fruit juices, caffeine, and alcohol may help some patients.
Irritable bowel syndrome	High-fiber	High-fiber diets may be useful.
		Consider a trial of restrictions of lactose, caffeine, and spicy foods.
		Remove restrictions that provide no benefit.
Milk/lactose intolerance	Lactose-restricted or lactose-free	Lactose is a disaccharide of glucose and galactose and is found in milk products. Lactase deficiency, which causes lactose intolerance, may be congenital or acquired. Symptoms include nausea, abdominal bloating and cramping, and/or diarrhea after consuming lactose-containing foods.
		Lactose intolerance occurs in degrees.
		Individuals with the most severe lactase deficiencies must avoid all milk-containing products (including products prepared with milk or milk powder as a component).
		Individuals with less severe deficiencies often tolerate cultured dairy products (buttermilk, acidophilus milk, yogurt, cottage cheese), in which bacteria have largely digested the lactose.
		Lactase enzymes are available for pretreatment of foods or consumption before eating lactose-containing foods. Lactase pretreated milk is also available.

Table continued on following page

Table 12-1 **DIETARY THERAPIES FOR SPECIFIC DIAGNOSES** (Continued)

Diagnostic Category	Dietary Therapy	Comments
Malabsorption (from many causes, such as chronic pancreatitis or short bowel syndrome)	Low-fat, individualized, with or without MCTs	Nondairy supplements may be used as milk substitutes. Cocoa and chocolate milk may be better tolerated than plain dairy products. Lactalbumin, lactate, and calcium compounds do not contain lactose. Fat restriction (e.g., 40–50 g/day) is indicated if there is symptomatic steatorrhea or divalent cation (Ca, Mg, Zn) deficiency. Attention must be paid to nutritional adequacy of the diet. Fat-soluble vitamin levels and divalent cation levels should be monitored. MCT and MCT-containing products can be added to fat-restricted diets as a readily absorbed source of calories: MCTs, which are composed of fatty acids only 8 to 10 carbons long, are readily absorbed with minimal digestion; the majority enter the portal system rather than the lymphatic system. MCTs can replace long-chain triglycerides in the diet for energy purposes but do not satisfy essential fatty acid requirements. MCTs are available in oil form for addition to foods and oral and tube feeding formulas. MCTs can be combined in a blender with beverages, used in fried and sautéed foods, and added to cereals, vegetables, and potatoes.
Acute pancreatitis	Progress from nothing by mouth to oral intake as tolerated	Enteral feeding is associated with fewer infections, satisfactory resolution of pancreatitis, and reduced surgical interventions as compared to parenteral nutrition. Feeding tubes are often placed in the jejunum to bypass the duodenum. Parenteral nutrition is indicated for severe cases (if enteral feeding is not tolerated).

Chronic pancreatic insufficiency	Low-fat (see Malabsorption comments)	40–50 g/day, usually with pancreatic enzyme replacement MCT supplementation is useful if additional calories are needed. Monitor fat-soluble vitamin status; vitamin and mineral supplementation if indicated.
Hepatic insufficiency without encephalopathy	Regular with or without sodium restriction	Use high-calorie, high-protein diet if weight gain is desired. Fat restriction is unnecessary unless fat malabsorption is symptomatic. Malnutrition is common in patients with cirrhosis. Aggressive nutrition support is important in patients who are candidates for liver transplantation. Assess vitamin and mineral statuses and use supplementation if indicated. Restrict sodium to 1–3 g/day if ascites or edema is present.
Hepatic encephalopathy	Protein- and sodium-restricted vs. branched-chain amino acid (BCAA) modified	With history or likelihood of encephalopathy, restrict protein to 0.5–0.7 g/kg dry body weight per day. This may be increased according to tolerance, or as encephalopathy improves. Restrict sodium and fluid if edema or ascites is present. BCAA products (e.g., Hepatamine, HepaticAid) are useful if encephalopathy does not respond to other therapies. Use 1.2–1.5 g/kg/day (i.e., protein restriction is removed).
Gallbladder disease	Individualized: calories for desirable weight, restrict fat and alcohol	Consult dietitian to obtain patient preferences and tolerances. Provide small, frequent meals. If the patient has chronic cholecystitis and dyspepsia, restrict fat to 40–50 g/day. If the patient has acute cholecystitis, restrict fat to 25–30 g/day while in hospital only.
Renal Disorders (see Chapter 25)		
Acute renal failure (ARF)	Individualized for the degree of renal failure.	Nutritional therapy is tailored to the degree and chronicity of the renal failure. For ARF without dialysis, 0.8 gm/kg/day of protein is recommended.

Table continued on following page

Table 12-1	DIETARY THERAPIES FOR SPECIFIC DIAGNOSES (Continued)	
Diagnostic Category	**Dietary Therapy**	**Comments**
	If necessary, consider sodium, potassium, phosphorus, and fluid restrictions.	ARF doesn't increase energy expenditure, but the diseases associated with ARF often do. Continuous renal replacement therapy (CRRT), such as continuous venovenous hemodiafiltration (CVVHD), can increase protein needs to 1.5 g/kg/day, so higher protein intake may be needed to obtain positive nitrogen balance.
Chronic kidney disease without dialysis	Individualized for degree of renal impairment; consider protein, sodium, potassium, and fluid restrictions.	Tailor energy intake to the patient. Generally, 20–35 kcal/kg ideal body weight is recommended. If weight loss occurs, energy intake should be increased. If hypertension and edema are present, restrict sodium (1–3 g/day) and fluid. Protein restriction (<0.8–1.0 g/kg/day) may be helpful. Potassium is generally not restricted unless there is hyperkalemia or urine output is <1 liter/day. In advanced kidney disease, potassium, magnesium, and phosphorus are restricted. Phosphorus intake should generally be 8–12 mg/kg ideal body weight per day, and phosphorus binders (antacids) should be used. Calcium supplementation may be required. Supplementation with 1,25-dihydroxy vitamin D (calcitriol) may be required. Avoid vitamin A supplements because of risk of toxicity in patients with kidney disease. Assess trace element needs (e.g., iron, zinc). If diabetes is present, see recommendations for diabetics, above, and Chapter 18.
End-stage renal disease (ESRD) with dialysis	Individualized; restrictions of sodium, potassium, phosphorus, and	Adjust energy for activity level and body weight. For weight maintenance, generally 30–35 kcal/kg/day For weight reduction, 20–25 kcal/kg/day can be used.

	fluids are ofter required.	Protein—*Hemodialysis*, 1.1–1.4 g/kg ideal body weight/day; *Peritoneal dialysis*, 1.2–1.5 g/kg ideal body weight/day Phosphorus—*Hemodialysis and peritoneal dialysis*: ≤17 mg/kg ideal body weight/day Sodium—*Hemodialysis*: 2–3 g/day; *peritoneal dialysis*: 2–4 g/day Potassium—*Hemodialysis*: about 40–70 mEq/day; *Peritoneal dialysis*: typically unrestricted, or >75 mEq/day Fluid restriction needs vary according to urine output and the patient's condition. *Hemodialysis*: generally 500–750 mL + urine output, or 1000 mL/day if the patient is anuric; *Peritoneal dialysis*: generally no fluid restriction is required. Calcium supplementation in hemodialysis and peritoneal dialysis depends on serum level.
Post-transplant	Individualized for organ transplanted, previous problems, post-op recovery	Adjust energy intake to achieve or maintain desirable body weight. Tailor protein intake to the degree of catabolism and function of the graft. For a functioning graft, 1.3–2.0 g/kg/day may be necessary because of hypermetabolism and steroids. Because of corticosteroid therapy and insulin resistance, carbohydrates may need to be limited. Replace saturated fats with polyunsaturated or monounsaturated fats (atherosclerosis is frequent in post-transplant patients). Restrict sodium initially to 2 g/day; if hypertension and edema are minimal it can be liberalized. Calcium and phosphorus intakes may be liberalized to reduce risk for metabolic bone disease, which is common because of vitamin D deficiency, secondary or tertiary hyperparathyroidism, and steroid therapy.

Table continued on following page

Table 12-1 DIETARY THERAPIES FOR SPECIFIC DIAGNOSES *(Continued)*

Diagnostic Category	Dietary Therapy	Comments
Miscellaneous Disorders		
Corticosteroid therapy	Low-sodium, high-protein	Steroid therapy can cause proteolysis, sodium retention, and glucose intolerance. Note recommendations for diabetics, above.
Dental impairment	Ground, pureed, or full liquid	See Box 12-4. Patients with fresh dental sutures should not use straws.
Recalcitrant childhood seizures	Ketogenic diet	Ketogenic diets (80%–90% of kcal as fat) can be helpful in intractable childhood epilepsy. The traditional method uses heavy cream; the MCT oil method provides the majority of fat calories as MCT oil. Insure that the diet is adequate in protein to promote normal growth, development, and physical activity. Vitamins and minerals including calcium should be supplemented. Carnitine supplementation may be necessary to help with long-chain fatty acid utilization. More data on long-term adverse effects (e.g., hyperlipidemia) would be beneficial. Adverse effects have included hypoproteinemia, hyperlipidemia, constipation, renal tubular acidosis, and kidney stones.
Monoamine oxidase inhibitor therapy	Tyramine restriction	Tyramine is formed by the decarboxylation of tyrosine. When monoamine oxidase is inhibited, tyramine can accumulate and precipitate hypertensive crisis, headache, chest pain, and sweating.

Restrict intake of aged, fermented, and non-fresh high-protein foods, cheeses (except cottage cheese and cream cheese), yeast extracts and Brewer's yeast (found in soups, bouillon cubes and protein supplements), meat tenderizers, and Italian green beans.
Caffeine is limited to <500 mg/day.

The diet should contain 80–100 g fat/day for 3 days before and during the stool collection. Intake should be monitored to document adequate fat intake.
Normal fecal fat is <6% of intake.

At least 150 g carbohydrate/day for several days before the test, because carbohydrate restriction can give a falsely abnormal glucose tolerance test.
No food or beverages except water should be consumed for 10–14 hours before the test.

This test is used to detect carcinoid tumors.
The diet is consumed for 3 days, followed by a 24-hour urine sample to measure 5-HIAA.
Avoid bananas, tomatoes, tomato juice, pineapple, pineapple juice, avocados, eggplant, plums, kiwi, walnuts, and pecans.

Diets for Diagnostic Tests

72-hour stool fecal fat measurement	100 g fat	
Glucose tolerance test	Regular	
Serotonin (5-HIAA) test diet	5-HIAA or low serotonin	

5-HIAA, 5-Hydroxyindole Acetic Acid; DASH, Dietary Approaches to Stop Hypertension; LDL, low-density lipoprotein.
*Source: Jenkins DJA, Kendall CWC, Marchie A, et al: Effects of a dietary portfolio of cholesterol-lowering foods vs. lovastatin on serum lipids and C-reactive protein. JAMA 290:502–510, 2003.

| Table 12-2 | DIABETIC EXCHANGES |

| | | Contents per Exchange | | | |
Group/Subgroup/ Serving Size	Example Serving Sizes	Carbohydrate (g)	Protein (g)	Fat (g)	Calories
Carbohydrate Group					
Starch	1 piece of bread, 1/2 hamburger bun, 1/2 cup of plain boiled pasta, 1/3 cup rice, 1/3 cup cooked or canned beans, 1/2 cup cooked cereal. Starchy vegetables include 1/2 cup cooked corn, 1/2 cup peas, a small 3 oz potato, 1 cup of winter squash, 1/2 cup of yam or sweet potato.	15	3	<1	80
Fruit	1 piece of fruit, such as an apple or orange, the size of tennis ball; 1/2 banana, 12–15 grapes, 1/2 cup canned fruit in juice or water, 2T raisins, 1/2 cup apple, orange, or cranberry juice, 1/3 cup cranberry, grape, or prune juice	15			60
Milk	1 cup				
Skim milk		12	8	0–3	90
Low-fat milk		12	8	5	120
Whole milk		12	8	8	150
Vegetables	1 cup raw or 1/2 cup cooked	5	2		25

Meats and Meat Substitutes				
Very lean meat	1 ounce prepared without extra fat—a 3 oz serving is approximately the size of a deck of cards	7	0-1	35
Lean meat	Cheeses with 1–3 gm fat/ounce, chicken with no skin, 1/4 cup cottage cheese, lean beef, turkey with no skin, and 1 oz of shellfish such as clams, crab, lobster, or shrimp	7	5	55
Medium-fat meat		7	8	75
High-fat meat		7	8	100
Fat Group	1 tsp of butter, 1 slice of bacon, 1 T of cream cheese, 1 tsp of margarine, 1 T of nuts or seeds		5	45

Foods or beverages with less then 20 calories are considered free. These include unlimited servings of items such as club soda, coffee, sugar-free drinks, mineral water, tea, fresh or dried herbs, soy sauce, vinegar, sugar-free gelatin, sugar-free gum, sugar-free Popsicles. Some of these may be high in sodium. Free foods to be limited to 2–3 servings per day include 1/2 cup cranberries with no sugar added, 1/2 cup rhubarb with no sugar added, 2 tsp of sugar-free jam or jelly, 2 T of whipped topping, 1 tsp of spreadable fruit, 1 T of ketchup, 2 T of reduced-calorie dressing, 2 T of taco sauce.

Table 12-3 MODIFIED DIETS: FAT

Daily Fat Intake	Food Limitations	Practicality
90–110 g (35%–40% of calories*) 65–80 g (25%–30% of calories*)	Meat is limited to 8–9 oz/day (1 egg = 1 oz meat). Fat is limited to 3–7 tsp butter, mayonnaise, salad dressing, oil. Whole milk intake is limited. All products prepared with fat (biscuits, cornbread, cakes, pastries, fried foods) are excluded unless fat in these products is counted as a part of the total fat allowance.	Typical intake of many Americans Very practical for home use, and recommended for all; easily manipulated according to patient preferences
40–50 g† (15%–20% of calories*)	All fried foods are excluded from the diet. Meats and eggs are limited to 6 oz lean meat, poultry, fish, or egg if 3 tsp of margarine or equivalent is used daily. 8–9 oz of meat and eggs may be used daily if no extra fat is used, such as in whole milk, margarine, butter, mayonnaise, salad dressing, nuts, and gravies.	Fairly practical for home use
20–25 g† (8%–10% of calories*)	Meats and eggs limited to 5–6 oz/day. All other above restrictions apply.	Impractical for home use

*Based upon 2400 calories/day.
†MCT oil may be added to these diets. Generally, start by adding 1 tsp/meal and gradually increase to 2–4 tsp/meal.

Table 12-4	MODIFIED DIETS: PROTEIN	
Daily Protein Intake	Food Limitations*	Practicality
150–200 g	Meats, cheeses, eggs: >10 oz/day (1 egg = 1 oz meat); starches: 5 or more servings/day; vegetables: 4 or more servings/day; fruits: 3 or more servings/day. Milk, shakes, eggnogs, protein supplements added	High-protein, high-fat diet; dietitian supervision is preferable
100–140 g	Meats, cheeses, eggs: 10 oz/day; starches: 5–6 servings/day; vegetables: 4–5 servings/day; fruits 3–4 servings/day; milk included	Typical intake of many Americans; relatively high in fat
60 g (10% of calories)†	Meats, cheeses, eggs: 6 oz/day; starches: 5 servings/day; vegetables: <4 servings/day; fruits: <3 servings/day; milk in limited amounts; calories increased with sugar and fat	Generally acceptable for home use; fairly easily manipulated according to patient preferences
40 g (6% of calories)†	Meats, cheeses, eggs: 4 oz/day; starches: 3 servings/day; vegetables: 4 servings/day; fruits: 3 servings/day; calories increased with sugar and fat	Difficult to follow at home unless patient is unusually cooperative

*Serving sizes: most vegetables = ½ cup; most fruits = 1 piece or ½ cup; starches = 1 slice bread or ⅓ to ½ cup of cooked starch
†Based on 2400 calories/day

Table 12-5   MODIFIED DIETS: SODIUM*

Daily Sodium (Salt) Intake	Food Limitations	Practicality
5-6 g Na+ (12.5-15 g salt) 4 g Na+ (10 g salt) 3 g Na+ (7.5 g salt)	Includes table salt, heavily or visibly salted items No additional salt on tray or at table Food only lightly salted in preparation; heavily or visibly salted items restricted (potato chips, pretzels, crackers, pickles, olives, relishes, sauces, many commercially prepared soups); no salt on tray	Typical intake of many Americans Practical for home use Practical for home use
2 g Na+ (5 g salt)	Above limitations, plus no salt in food preparation; most processed foods avoided (canned foods, luncheon meats, bacon, ham, cheese) unless calculated into diet; regular bread, butter, and milk in limited amounts	Fairly practical for home use with cooperative patients
1 g Na+ (2.5 g salt)	Above limitations plus use of only salt-free bread	Practical for home use only with unusually cooperative patients
0.5 g Na+ (1.25 g salt)	Above limitations plus limitation of meat (4 oz/day), eggs, some vegetables; milk (1 pt/day) and salt-free butter allowed	Not practical for home use

*Also see the box on the following page.

High-Sodium Foods to Omit in Sodium-Restricted Diets*

Condiments

Pickles, olives, relishes, salted nuts, meat tenderizers, commercial salad dressings, monosodium glutamate (e.g., Accent, steak sauces, ketchup, soy sauce, Worcestershire sauce, horseradish sauce, chilli sauce, commercial mustard, onion salt, garlic salt, celery salt, butter salt, seasoned salts. (Note: Salt substitutes often contain substantial amounts of sodium; read labels. Many salt substitutes contain potassium and should be avoided in patients taking spironolactone or ACE inhibitors.)

Breads

Salted crackers and breads

Meats, Fish, Poultry, Cheeses, and Substitutes

Cured, smoked, and processed meats such as ham, bacon, corned beef, chipped beef, wieners, luncheon meats, bologna, salt pork, regular canned salmon and tuna, all cheeses except low sodium and cottage cheese; TV dinners, pizza, frozen Italian entrees, imitation sausage and bacon

Beverages

Commercial buttermilk, instant hot cocoa mixes

Soups

Commercial canned and dehydrated soups (except low-sodium soups), bouillon, consommé

Vegetables

Sauerkraut, hominy, pork and beans, canned tomato and vegetable juices (choose low-sodium varieties)

Fats

Gravy, regular peanut butter

Potato or Potato Substitutes

Potato chips, corn chips, salted popcorn, pretzels, frozen potato casseroles, commercially packaged rice and noodle mixes, dehydrated potatoes and potato mixes, bread stuffing

*For additional nutrient content information, see the USDA Nutrient Data Laboratory web site, http://www.nal.usda.gov/fnic/foodcomp/.

Table 12–6A	MODIFIED DIETS: POTASSIUM	
Potassium Level	**Food Limitations**	**Practicality**
3 g (80 mEq)		Typical intake of many Americans
1.5 g (40 mEq)	Limited meats, vegetables, fruits; milk, potatoes, tea, coffee, chocolate only in minimal amounts	Most common level used in renal diets; not practical to prescribe a low-potassium, high-protein diet

Table 12–6B	FOODS WITH LOW OR HIGH POTASSIUM CONTENTS*
	Amount per 120 mL (1/2 cup)
Low (<2.5 mEq [100 mg])	**High (>5 mEq [200 mg])**
Bean sprouts	Asparagus
Beets	Bran and whole grain cereals
Cabbage, cooked or raw	Broccoli
Carrots	Brussels sprouts
Cauliflower, cooked	Collards
Corn	Dried beans and peas, cooked (including lima beans)
Cucumber	Fruit, dried or cocktail
Eggplant	Fruit, fresh: Apricots, bananas, grapefruit, oranges, peaches, pears, strawberries
Fruit: Apples and applesauce; blueberries; cherries; cranberries; lemons; pears, canned; pineapple, fresh or canned; plums, fresh or canned; raspberries; tangerines	Melons: Cantaloupe, honeydew, watermelon
	Mushrooms
	Potatoes, cooked
	Rhubarb
Green beans and green peas, cooked	Some salt substitutes (read labels)
Lettuce	Spinach, cooked
Onions, cooked	Sweet potatoes, cooked
Radishes	Tomatoes
Summer squash, cooked	Winter squash, cooked

*The primary sources of potassium in the diet are fruits, vegetables, and milk. For additional nutrient content information, see the USDA Nutrient Data Laboratory web site, http://www.nal.usda.gov/fnic/foodcomp/.

Table 12-7	FOODS OF LOW AND HIGH PHOSPHORUS CONTENT*
Low	**High**
Most fruits	Bran
Most vegetables	Carbonated beverages (phosphoric acid added); clear carbonated beverages such as 7-Up and Sprite do not contain added phosphoric acid.
	Dried beans and peas
	Meats (including chicken), fish
	Milk, dairy products

*For additional nutrient content information, see the USDA Nutrient Data Laboratory web site, http://www.nal.usda.gov/fnic/foodcomp/.

Initially, meals should be small and consist of soft, nonfibrous, bland foods. Salt should be used only in small amounts if at all in meal preparation, and fat (e.g., butter, margarine, cooking oil) should be avoided. As refeeding progresses, salt may be added to food at the table, and a medium-chain triglyceride (MCT) oil supplement may be used as needed for calories. Patients should only have minimal amounts of liquid with meals to minimize the transit rate and dilution of gastric juices; the major portion of liquids should be consumed between meals.

BOX 12-1   Refeeding After Brief Bowel Rest

Day 1

Clear liquids to check swallowing, followed by low-lactose full liquids, e.g., oral supplement formulas, as tolerated (see Chapter 13)

Days 2 to 3

Lactose-free oral supplement formulas or six small feedings of a 30 to 40 g fat, low-lactose, soft diet

Days 4 to 5

50 g fat diet, progressing to regular diet as tolerated

BOX 12-2   Refeeding after Prolonged Bowel Rest or Bowel Resection

Days 1 to 5

Eat two foods at each meal, with the total amount being no more than ½ cup.
Combine ½ serving from group A with ½ serving from group B *or* combine ½ serving from group C with 1 serving from group D (see Box 12-3).

Days 6 to 10

Eat three foods at each meal. Combine 1 serving each from groups A + B + E *or* groups B + C + D.

Days 11 to 15

Eat four foods at each meal. Combine 1 serving each from groups A + B + C + D *or* groups A + B + C + E.
If extra calories are needed, add 1 to 2 tsp MCT oil to each meal by cooking vegetables and meat in it or adding it to vegetables, starches, and meats at the table.
If desired, small amounts of salt may be used at the table.

The patient should start by eating only two different foods at each meal to determine which foods can be tolerated. Six small meals per day should be eaten according to the guidelines in Boxes 12-2 and 12-3.

The durations of each of the three phases can be adjusted according to patient tolerance. After the third phase, new foods can be added to the diet about every 2 days to monitor the tolerance of each new food. Tailor the dietary regimen to each patient's needs. For further discussion of the management of malabsorption, see Chapter 22.

Diets of Modified Consistency

Box 12-4 outlines diets of varying consistencies. Foods of altered consistency are useful in refeeding protocols and in patients who have problems with chewing and swallowing. Dysphagia diets often use thickened liquids

BOX 12–3   Preferred Foods for Refeeding

Group A: Starches (serving = $\frac{1}{2}$ cup)

*Potato (boiled, baked, mashed), *white rice, *canned pumpkin, sweet potato, acorn squash, enriched noodles or spaghetti, instant oatmeal, cream of wheat, puffed rice cereal, crisped rice or corn flakes, white bread, graham crackers

Group B: Vegetables (well cooked, serving = $\frac{1}{2}$ cup)

*Carrots, *yellow squash, beets, asparagus tips, green beans

Group C: Fruits (serving = $\frac{1}{2}$ cup)

*Applesauce, *stewed apples or pears without skin, banana, canned peaches, canned pears

Group D: Dairy Products (serving size)

*Buttermilk, skimmed only (4 to 6 oz)
Low-fat cottage cheese ($\frac{1}{3}$ cup)
Plain low-fat yogurt (4 oz)

Group E: Meat (serving = 2 oz boiled, baked, or broiled without added fat)

Skinned poultry, fish

Beverages

Tea, water, tomato juice, homemade vegetable broth (not from bouillon)

---

*Preferred selections for days 1 to 5.

BOX 12–4   Modified Diets: Consistency

Clear Liquid Diet *(nutritionally incomplete)*

This diet provides clear fluids that leave little residue and are adsorbed with a minimum of digestive activity. It includes broth, gelatin, strained fruit juices, clear beverages, and low-residue supplements. Since some of these have high osmolality, they may not be well tolerated by some patients. Clear liquids generally do not provide the RDA for any nutrients, except perhaps vitamin C. They should not be used for more than 2 to 3 days without supplementation.

Box continued on following page

BOX 12–4   Modified Diets: Consistency *(Continued)*

Full Liquid Diet

This diet includes foods that are liquid at room temperature. Many foods such as whole milk, custard, pudding, strained cream soups, eggnog, and ice cream contain fat and lactose, which patients may tolerate poorly. Complete enteral supplements may be preferred in such cases or may be added to increase calories and protein (see Chapter 13). This diet can meet the RDA for all nutrients, except iron for women of childbearing age. Modifications of the full liquid diet can be made, such as high-protein/high-calorie or low fat. To minimize lactose intake, lactose-free oral feeding supplements and lactase-treated dairy products may be used.

Dental Soft Diet/GI Soft Diet

The soft diet contains foods that are tender but are not ground or pureed. Whole meats, cooked vegetables and fruits of moderate fiber content (e.g., canned) are allowed. This generally excludes fried foods, most raw fruits and vegetables, and very coarse breads and cereals, and is fairly low in fiber and residue. The GI soft diet is a modification that omits highly seasoned and spicy foods and foods high in fiber.

Pureed or Ground Diet

This diet includes foods that are especially easy to masticate and swallow and the foods are pureed or ground. It is useful in patients who have dysphagia or dental problems.

Low-Fiber, Low-Residue Diet

This diet is intended to reduce fecal bulk and is restricted in milk, certain vegetables, fruits, and whole-grain breads and cereals.

High-Fiber Diet

This diet includes unrefined starches (whole-grain bread, brown rice, potatoes, corn, beans), raw fruits, and vegetables. Bran and other fibers may be added if desired.

---

in patients with swallowing problems. Evaluation by a speech pathologist can be indispensable in reducing the risk for aspiration. High-fiber diets are useful in managing constipation, dyslipidemia, and diabetes. Fiber can be divided into soluble or viscous fibers (pectins, mucilages, gums, and some hemicelluloses found in fruits, vegetables, oats, and oat bran) and insoluble or poorly fermentable fibers (cellulose, some hemicelluloses, and lignin found in fruits, vegetables, and cereal products such as whole wheat and wheat bran). The Dietary Reference Intakes recommend that adults consume between 21 and 38 g of fiber per day, depending on age and gender (see Table 3–1).

SUGGESTED READINGS

Bray GA, Vollmer WM, Sacks FM, et al: A further subgroup analysis of the effects of the DASH diet and three dietary sodium levels on blood pressure: Results of the DASH-Sodium trial. Am J Cardiol 94:222–227, 2004.

Chan L-N: Nutritional support in acute renal failure. Curr Opin Clin Nutr Metab Care 7:207–212, 2004.

American Diabetes Association: Nutrition principles and recommendations in diabetes. Diabetes Care 27(Suppl 1):S36–S46, 2004.

Fitzgibbons J (ed): Simplified Diet Manual, 9th ed. Ames, Iowa. Iowa State Press, 2002.

Krauss RM, Eckel RH, Howard B, et al: Revision 2000: A statement for healthcare professionals from the nutrition committee of the American Heart Association. J Nutr 131:132–146, 2001.

Marchesini G, Biarchi G, Merli M, et al: Nutritional supplementation with branched-chain amino acids in advanced cirrhosis: A double-blind, randomized trial. Gastroenterology 124:1792–1801, 2003.

Marik PE, Zaloga GP: Meta-analysis of parenteral nutrition versus enteral nutrition in patients with acute pancreatitis. Br Med J 328:1407–1413, 2004.

Monro J: Redefining the glycemic index for dietary management of postprandial glycemia. J Nutr 133:4256–4258, 2003.

Peraaho M, Collin P, Kaukinen K, et al: Oats can diversify a gluten-free diet in celiac disease and dermatitis herpetiformis. J Am Diet Assoc 104:1148–1150, 2004.

Slater GH, Ren CJ, Siegel N, et al: Serum fat-soluble vitamin deficiency and abnormal calcium metabolism after malabsorptive bariatric surgery. J Gastrointest Surg 8:48–55, 2004.

Thiele EA: Assessing the efficacy of antiepileptic treatments: The ketogenic diet. Epilepsia 44:26–29, 2003.

WEB SITES

American Dietetic Association, http://www.eatright.org

13

Enteral Nutrition

DOUGLAS C. HEIMBURGER, MD

Although *enteral nutrition* is technically any nutrient delivery system that uses the gastrointestinal tract, the term is generally used to refer to tube feeding. Tube feeding is indicated when the oral intake of nutrients is insufficient to meet requirements for more than 5 to 7 days, provided the gastrointestinal tract is functional. The advantages of enteral nutrition over parenteral nutrition are reviewed in Chapter 11.

As in any therapeutic feeding situation, before enteral nutrition is begun, definitive objectives must be set. The patient's energy and protein requirements should be estimated or measured as described in Chapter 11, and a goal for weight maintenance or weight gain should be clear.

Gastrointestinal Access

The selection of tubes and pumps specifically designed for feeding is quite broad. Because of their pliability and long-term tolerance, small gauge feeding tubes should virtually always be used for enteral feeding. The main drawback of these tubes is that gastric contents cannot be reliably aspirated through them.

Although many feeding tubes have weighted tips that are intended to prevent retrograde migration or facilitate nasoduodenal intubation, such weights may actually impede passage of the tip into the duodenum. When transpyloric feeding is desired (e.g., to reduce the risk of aspiration or to bypass a gastric ileus), nasoduodenal intubation can be accomplished by several methods. A conservative method involves giving 10 mg of metoclopramide intravenously and inserting an ample length of an *unweighted* tube into the stomach (weighted tips arc less likely to traverse the gastric pylorus spontaneously). Fluoroscopic and endoscopic techniques can be used as well.

Although soft nasogastric tubes have been used safely for years in some patients, long-term tube feeding is best accomplished through a percutaneous endoscopic gastrostomy (PEG) tube. The risk of tube-feeding aspiration is not appreciably lower with gastrostomies than with nasogastric tubes, so in patients at high risk for aspiration, intestinal intubation via a nasoduodenal or nasojejunal tube, a PEG tube extended to the jejunum (PEG-J), or a direct jejunostomy tube is advisable. Jejunostomy tubes can sometimes be placed using a laparoscope, obviating the need for laparotomy.

In patients who are at risk for aspiration, radiographic confirmation of nasogastric tube placement is recommended. Radiographic confirmation is not always necessary in patients who are not at high risk for aspiration (i.e., alert with a normal gag reflex). Insufflation of air and auscultation of the stomach may suffice and allow earlier institution of feeding.

Formula Selection

Enteral feeding formula choices have increased phenomenally in recent decades. Although many new formulas have been designed to meet the needs of specific patient groups, special benefits of these formulas have not always been demonstrated in controlled trials, and their costs arc virtually always higher than those of standard formulas. Specialized formulas are therefore sometimes promoted for features that have little physiologic significance and no proven clinical superiority. For this reason, in selecting feeding formulas one must distinguish features that are major (important in all cases) from those that are minor (important only in selected cases) or inconsequential (virtually never important). Box 13–1 stratifies the compositional parameters of feeding formulas in this manner.

BOX 13–1   Criteria for Evaluating Enteral
Feeding Formulas

Major Criteria

Energy density (generally 1, 1.5, or 2 kcal/mL)
Protein content (less than or greater than 20% of total energy)
Route of administration (tube/oral vs. tube only)
Cost

Minor Criteria

Complexity (polymeric vs. oligomeric)
Osmolality
Protein source (e.g., casein, soy, peptides, amino acids)
Fat content
Fat source (long- vs. medium-chain triglycerides [MCTs])
Residue content
Electrolyte and mineral content
Form (liquid vs. powder; cans vs. ready-to-hang)
Vitamin content
Lactose content

Inconsequential Criteria

Carbohydrate source (e.g., corn starch or syrup, sucrose)
Method of preparation (compounded vs. blenderized)

Specialized or "Disease-specific" Formulas

Results of clinical studies needed to substantiate claims

Table 13–1 lists commercially available adult feeding formulas by categories, including specialized or "disease-specific" formulas.

Major Criteria

Appropriate choices can usually be made by considering only the major criteria. Energy density determines the amounts of most nutrients delivered per liter, including not only calories, but protein, water, and others as well. Higher energy-density formulas (1.5 to 2 kcal/mL) are very useful for delivering high-calorie loads or restricting fluid intake but can result in dehydration in patients who

Table 13-1	ENTERAL FEEDING FORMULAS						
Formula Category	Energy Density (kcal/mL)	Percent kcal			Macronutrient Sources	Formula Characteristics	Examples of Formulas*
		Protein	Carbohydrate	Fat			
Standard	1.0–1.2	14–18	50–57	29–37	Intact protein Glucose polymers Polysaccharides Canola oil MCT oil	Isotonic Lactose-free Some may be used as oral supplements	Boost Ensure Isocal Isosource Nutren 1.0 Osmolite
Fiber supplemented	1.0–1.5	15–25	50–57	29–33	Intact protein Maltodextrin Canola oil MCT oil	Fiber content 5–14 g/L Generally isotonic	Fibersource Jevity Nutren 1.0 with Fiber Probalance Ultracal
High-calorie (concentrated)	1.5–2.0	15–20	45–54	29–39	Intact protein Maltodextrin Canola oil MCT oil	Enable volume restriction	Deliver 2.0 Ensure Plus HN Isosource 1.5 Cal Nutren 1.5 Nutren 2.0 Two Cal HN
High-protein	1.0–1.5	18–25	38–53	25–40	Intact protein Maltodextrin	Some contain supplemental	Boost HP Fibersource HN

Table continued on following page

Table 13-1 ENTERAL FEEDING FORMULAS (Continued)

| Formula Category | Energy Density (kcal/mL) | Percent kcal | | | Macronutrient Sources | Formula Characteristics | Examples of Formulas* |
		Protein	Carbohydrate	Fat			
						vitamins and minerals to aid wound healing	Isosource VHN XL Replete Traumacal
Pulmonary (high-fat, low-carbohydrate)	1.5	17–20	27–38	42–55	Intact protein Maltodextrin Sucrose Canola oil MCT oil	One formula designed for patients with ARDS contains EPA, GLA, and antioxidants	Novasource Pulmonary Nutrivent Oxepa Pulmocare Respalor
Glucose intolerance	1.0–1.2	17–24	36–44	40–49	Intact protein Maltodextrin Hydrolyzed cornstarch Canola oil, MCT oil	Low carbohydrate content Often contain fiber	Resource Diabetic Boost Diabetic Diabetisource AC Glucerna Glytrol
Immune-enhancing	1.0–1.5	22–32	46–53	20–40	Sodium caseinate L-arginine Hydrolyzed cornstarch Maltodextrin Palm kernel oil Fish oil	For immuno-compromised patients Contain arginine, dietary nucleotides, fish oil	Crucial Impact Impact 1.5 Impact Glutamine

Category				Sources	Characteristics	Products
Renal	2.0	6–15	40–58	35–46	Intact protein Maltodextrin Corn syrup MCT oil Canola oil	Calorically dense for volume restriction Low in electrolytes Vary widely in protein	Magnacal Renal Nepro Novasource Renal NutriRenal Renalcal Suplena
Hepatic	1.2–1.5	11–15	57–77	12–28	Crystalline amino acids Monosaccharides MCT oil Polyunsaturated fatty acids	High in branched-chain amino acids, low in aromatic amino acids	Hepatic Aid II NutriHep
Oligomeric (small-peptide)	1.0–1.5	15–25	46–82	3–39	Maltodextrin Hydrolyzed proteins Free amino acids L-arginine MCT oil Soybean oil	Contain proteins hydrolyzed into small peptides, and/or free amino acids Sometimes called elemental or semielemental	Alitraq Crucial Optimental Peptamen Peptinex Subdue Vital High Nitrogen Vivonex T.E.N.

*Specific product information can be obtained by referring to package labels or visiting the companies' web sites. Manufacturers include Ross Products (http://www.ross.com), Novartis Medical Nutrition (http://www.novartisnutrition.com), Nestle Clinical Nutrition (http://www.nestleclinicalnutrition.com), and Hormel Health Labs (http://www.hormelhealthlabs.com)

MCT, medium-chain triglyceride.

are unable to consume additional water as needed or who have high water requirements. The fluid status of these patients should be carefully monitored.

Once the energy density has been selected, the formula of choice is usually determined by the protein content, route of administration (oral or tube), and cost. Protein content should be considered not only in absolute terms but also relative to total energy (as percent of calories). The term *high nitrogen* (HN) should be considered unreliable because some formulas designated as HN have protein contents as low as 16% of energy.

Minor Criteria

Among the minor criteria for formula selection, the issue of protein complexity received much attention in the 1990s. Oligomeric formulas that contain peptides (from hydrolyzed proteins) or free amino acids, often inappropriately referred to as "elemental formulas," had previously been thought to be more efficiently absorbed by patients with impaired gastrointestinal function. However, clinical trials have concluded that peptides confer minimal advantage, if any, over whole proteins (polymeric formulas) and that free amino acids are inferior to both. These formulas are also considerably more expensive than standard formulas.

Osmolality was once thought by many clinicians to have a major effect on the tolerance of enteral formulas, particularly with regard to diarrhea. However, several controlled clinical trials established that osmolality does not independently influence formula tolerance. Diluting formulas to half or quarter strength only delays adequate intake, and does not improve tolerance. Feedings should be started at full strength, and diluted only to provide supplemental water when other routes are not adequate.

Specialized Formulas

Many specialized or "disease-specific" enteral feeding formulas are available for patients with critical illness (e.g., trauma and sepsis), malabsorption, diabetes, pulmonary disease, hepatic encephalopathy, renal failure, or acquired immune deficiency syndrome (AIDS). Because these formulas are classified as foods by the U.S. Food and Drug Administration, they can be released on the market without the extensive clinical testing required for drugs. Although their compositions have most often been based on plausible ideas generated from basic or clinical research, these formulas still require clinical testing in order to substantiate special therapeutic properties and justify their inevitably higher costs. Such tests have not been conducted for all the specialized formulas, and when they have, the results have not always been positive. Therefore, it is important not to choose an enteral formula simply because a diagnosis is embedded in its name or it has an unusual compositional feature. Although certain formulas are listed as specialized in Table 13–1, this is not intended to suggest that they are truly disease-specific. Other formulas with disease-oriented names are listed among the general formulas because their features are not particularly unique, but this does not mean they are totally comparable to the others in the category. For more information, see the chapters devoted to the specific illnesses in question.

Hospital Formularies

Table 13–1 shows the characteristics of broad categories of enteral formulas. Stratification by categories aids clinicians in choosing appropriate formulas and in developing hospital enteral feeding formularies. The categories are developed by evaluating the formulas' nutrient contents, costs, vitamin and mineral contents, packaging, and in the case of specialized formulas, evidence of therapeutic efficacy. The categories are submitted to vendors for competitive bidding, and the lowest cost formulas in each category make up the hospital formula. Costs are often based on price per 1000 kcal, but labor costs should factored as well, because ready-to-hang formulas require less staff time to administer than do formulas delivered in cans that must be opened and poured into feeding containers.

Formularies are often developed for time frames stipulated by purchasing contracts, but they should be reviewed periodically.

As with hospital pharmaceutical formularies, when a clinician orders a nonformulary product, hospital policy can dictate that its formulary equivalent be substituted in order to contain costs. The use of specialized formulas can also be limited by hospital policy to specific clinical situations or hospital units, or require the approval of the hospital's nutrition support service. These measures help to confine the use of expensive formulas to situations in which they have proven therapeutic superiority.

Infusion Methods

The continuous-drip method with a closed, aseptic system delivered via a feeding pump is generally preferred. Continuous feeding assures more reliable nutrient delivery and may reduce the risks of gastric distention and pulmonary aspiration of feeding formula. The initial infusion rate and the rapidity of its increase should vary depending on the condition of the patient. A patient who has impaired mental status or has not used the gastrointestinal tract for more than 2 weeks should have feedings introduced and increased more slowly than alert patients whose intestines have been used recently.

The bolus method is most useful for long-term feeding in stable patients. It allows more mobility and reduces cost because a pump and infusion set are not required. The guidelines listed in Box 13–2 apply to adults.

Complications

Diarrhea

Diarrhea commonly complicates enteral feeding. Although it has been blamed on many factors, most factors have only been *associated* with diarrhea in tube-fed patients and there is little or no objective evidence for causal relationships. Factors that have been proposed but not proven include hypertonic feeding formulas,

---

BOX 13-2   Guidelines for Initiating and Discontinuing
Enteral Feeding

Continuous Feeding

Begin undiluted feeding at a rate between 10 and 50 mL/hr.
Greater doubts about gastrointestinal functions should prompt
  lower initial infusion rates.
Increase the rate in increments of 20–40 mL/hr every
  8–24 hours to attain the final rate (calculated to meet energy
  and protein requirements) in as little as 1 day or as many as
  5 days, depending on the state of the gastrointestinal tract.
  The final rate should generally not exceed 125–150 mL/hr;
  higher nutrient requirements should be met with 1.5–2 kcal/mL
  formulas.
Discontinue enteral feeding only when adequate oral intake
  has been achieved. When the likelihood of achieving
  adequate oral intake is uncertain, use weaning methods
  such as reducing the infusion rate, interrupting the infusion
  before meals, or infusing only at night to improve appetite
  and oral intake during the day.

Bolus Feeding

Place the patient in a sitting position, and limit feedings to
  waking hours whenever possible.
Begin with 50–100 mL boluses of undiluted feeding every
  2–4 hours. Increase the size of boluses every 8–24 hours,
  to 100 mL, 150 mL, 200 mL, etc. until requirements are met.
In alert patients it is often possible to begin with 250 mL
  (one can) boluses and increase the volume to as high as
  400 mL per feeding. If possible, avoid feeding during the night.
Flush the feeding tube with water after each infusion and cap
  the tube. If water requirements are not met by the
  formula, additional water should be given with the flush.
Rinse the infusion syringe after each bolus, and discard it daily
  if used in the hospital, or wash it well if used at home.
Do not allow opened formula to sit at room temperature for
  more than 4 hours.
Wean patients to oral intake by eliminating feedings that
  precede meals. Discontinue enteral feedings only when
  adequate oral intake has been achieved.

---

hypoalbuminemia, bacterial contamination of the feeding or dysentery, inadequate fiber in feeding formulas,
certain infusion methods (e.g., bolus infusions or rapid
increases in the infusion rate), fecal impaction, or lactose
or excessive fat in feeding formulas. The best-documented

> **BOX 13–3   Likely Causes of Diarrhea in Tube-Fed Patients**
>
> **Medications**
> Elixir medications containing sorbitol (acetaminophen, theophylline, cough preparations, codeine, vitamins, many others; see Chapter 15)
> Magnesium-containing antacids
> Oral antibiotics (definite); IV antibiotics (questionable)
> Phosphorus supplements, histamine-2 receptor blockers, metaclopramide, lactulose, other assorted medications
>
> **Pseudomembranous Colitis**
> **Gastrointestinal Disorders**

causal factors are medications, pseudomembranous colitis, and gastrointestinal dysfunction (Box 13–3), none of which are necessarily related to tube feeding. Tube feeding itself is rarely responsible for diarrhea and should not be identified as the cause until others have been ruled out.

Surprisingly, the medication that most commonly causes diarrhea in tube-fed patients is one that clinicians do not often request, so they are unaware that it is being administered. It is sorbitol, present in many liquid medications as a vehicle and sweetener. It is listed as an inactive ingredient and its quantity is not required on medication package inserts, so it was not suspected as a cause for diarrhea until a well-controlled study ruled out other causes.[1] Because they are easy to deliver, liquid medications are commonly administered to patients with feeding tubes. Medications previously administered orally or intravenously are often replaced by elixirs when a feeding tube is placed. Patients who receive more than one liquid medication or several doses of a single one may thus receive substantial amounts of sorbitol— commonly more than 20 g per day—which causes diarrhea in virtually all persons. Thus, there is a common scenario that is played out when a sorbitol-containing medication is started at the same time enteral nutrition begins—diarrhea develops, the tube feeding is unjustly identified as the cause, and tube feeding is stopped, resulting in inadequate intake.

Any form of magnesium given in sufficient quantities can cause diarrhea. Thus, when magnesium-containing antacids are used in tube-fed patients, diarrhea may result. Antacids based on aluminum alone or an aluminum-magnesium combination are practical alternatives. Some, but not all, oral antibiotics cause diarrhea by altering the intestinal flora. Although antibiotics administered intravenously have been implicated as well, confirmatory data are less firm, especially in critically ill patients who have multiple confounding factors. Additional medications that can have diarrhea as a direct side-effect are listed in Box 13-3. Many other medications may cause diarrhea, so product inserts and pharmaceutical references should be consulted whenever the cause for diarrhea is not obvious.

Box 13-4 lists measures to take and to avoid when a tube-fed patient develops diarrhea. The most important step is to consider all medications, particularly liquid ones, as possible causes. See Chapter 15 for a list of sorbitol contents of several common medications. These lists are not exhaustive, and because sorbitol concentrations are not listed on package inserts, pharmaceutical manufacturers may change them without notification. Therefore, all liquid medications should be suspected as causes of diarrhea and, if possible, discontinued or changed to other forms until the diarrhea has resolved.

When medications are clearly not responsible for the diarrhea, determine whether pseudomembranous colitis is the cause by measuring the stool *Clostridium difficile* titer. If this is negative, gastrointestinal dysfunction is a probable cause. The stool osmotic gap (see Box 13-4) can help establish a secretory cause if it is low or direct a further search for exogenous osmotic substances if it is high. The enteral feeding can be stopped temporarily to determine its role, but it should be resumed once a determination is made unless the diarrhea is compromising the patient. Changing to an isotonic feeding formula (much less diluting one) or to a

---

BOX 13-4 Managing Diarrhea in Tube-Fed Patients

Do's

Carefully review all medications.

Eliminate all elixirs containing sorbitol. If in doubt about the sorbitol content of any medication, discontinue it or change it to another form.

Eliminate magnesium-containing antacids.

Eliminate any other potential offenders.

Measure stool *Clostridium difficile* titer.

Consider measuring the stool osmotic gap to help distinguish between osmotic and secretory diarrhea by using the following equation:

Stool osmotic gap = stool osmolality − 2(stool sodium + stool potassium)

>140: osmotic diarrhea, likely a result of medications or (unlikely) tube feeding

<100: secretory diarrhea, possibly a result of pseudomembranous colitis or nonosmotic medications

Consider giving psyllium (e.g., Metamucil) or pectin (e.g., "banana flakes")

Dont's

Don't give antidiarrheal agents before a cause for the diarrhea is determined; use them only as a last report.

Don't infuse albumin IV with the assumption that it will remedy the diarrhea.

Don't stop the feeding any longer than is necessary to determine whether it is causing diarrhea.

Don't change the feeding formula with the assumption that doing so will relieve the diarrhea.

---

small-peptide or fiber-containing formula will *not* relieve the diarrhea. If there is still no clear cause, pectin may be administered to give substance to the stool. Antidiarrheal agents such as kaolin-pectin, loperamide, or diphenoxylate with atropine may be given, but only as a *last* resort.

Gastric Retention and Pulmonary Aspiration

Gastric retention has been defined as the presence of more than about 200 mL of tube feeding in the stomach.

The common practice of suctioning stomach contents has been shown to be an unreliable measure of gastric residual volumes; rather, it impedes adequate feeding and increases the risk of tube clogging.[2] Further, residual volumes obtained by suctioning do not correlate with tube-feeding tolerance and have not been shown to reduce the risk of pulmonary aspiration. Therefore, a combination of physical examination, questioning of the patient, and sometimes radiography should be used. If gastric suctioning is used, thresholds of 400 to 500 ml residual volume should be required before a pause in feeding is triggered.[2] Although ileus (the absence of bowel activity, usually because of sepsis, trauma, or surgery) is probably the most common cause of gastric retention, hypokalemia, drug side-effects, and obstruction must be ruled out.

The most serious and potentially lethal complication of tube feeding—pulmonary aspiration of gastric contents—is most common in patients with impaired mental status and intestinal ileus. In these patients, aspiration can usually be prevented by elevating the head during feeding (to avoid gastroesophageal reflux) and careful monitoring for distention. In patients at especially high risk, inserting the tube into the duodenum or jejunum is advisable.

Metabolic Complications

Enteral nutrition results in far fewer metabolic complications than does parenteral nutrition. The most common metabolic complication of enteral feeding is probably hyperglycemia, particularly in patients with pre-existing glucose intolerance. This can be handled through tighter diabetes control. Hyperglycemia rarely necessitates reduction of the feeding.

Tube-feeding formulas with high energy density or protein content do not contain enough water for some patients to handle the renal solute load. Patients receiving these formulas who are unable to regulate their fluid needs voluntarily and do not have adequate intravenous fluid intake may become dehydrated, hyperosmolar, and hyperglycemic. The osmolality of the formula is not related to these problems because carbohydrates (the major osmotic component) are metabolized and do not contribute to the renal solute load except when glycosuria occurs. The fluid status and blood glucose levels of patients at risk should be closely monitored.

REFERENCES

1. Edes TE, Walk BE, Austin JL: Diarrhea in tube-fed patients: Feeding formula not necessarily the cause. Am J Med 88:91–93, 1990.
2. McClave SA, Snider HL: Clinical use of residual volumes as a monitor for patients on enteral tube feeding. J Parent Ent Nutr 26:S43—S50, 2002.

SUGGESTED READINGS

American Society for Parenteral and Enteral Nutrition: ASPEN Nutrition Support Practice Manual, 2006. Available online at http://www.clinnutr.org/
American Society for Parenteral and Enteral Nutrition: The Science and Practice of Nutrition Support: A Case-based Core Curriculum. Dubuque, Iowa, Kendall/Hunt, 2001.
Rolandelli RH, Bankhead R, Boullata JI, Compher CW (eds): Clinical Nutrition: Enteral and Tube Feeding, 4th ed. Philadelphia, WB Saunders, 2005.

WEB SITES

American Society for Parenteral and Enteral Nutrition (ASPEN), http://www.clinnutr.org/
Enteral product manufacturer web sites, see Table 13–1.

14

Parenteral Nutrition

DOUGLAS C. HEIMBURGER, MD

Parenteral nutrition or intravenous feeding goes by many different names, the most common being total parenteral nutrition (TPN). More specific terms include central parenteral nutrition (CPN), central venous alimentation (CVA), peripheral parenteral nutrition (PPN), and peripheral venous alimentation (PVA). The term *hyperalimentation* (or hyperal) is not preferred because it implies that parenteral nutrition gives patients more than they require, which is inappropriate.

Parenteral nutrition can be used to satisfy all of a patient's nutritional requirements or to supplement an insufficient oral or enteral intake. In doing this, energy is supplied by dextrose and vegetable oil-derived lipid emulsions; protein by crystalline amino acids; and vitamins, minerals, and trace elements in pure forms. It is possible to add certain medications such as insulin.

Indications for Parenteral Nutrition

Parenteral nutrition is indicated when a patient's gastrointestinal tract is either unavailable for use or unreliable for more than 5 to 7 days or when extended bowel rest is desired for therapeutic reasons. Specific indications and contraindications are listed in Box 14-1.

Because there are no situations in which a person should absolutely not be fed, the contraindications are all relative. Surprisingly, some clinicians still tend to resort to TPN when enteral feeding can be used; this should be strongly discouraged. An aggressive commitment to obtaining access for enteral feeding often makes it possible to avoid using TPN.

> BOX 14-1   Indications and Contraindications for
> Parenteral Nutrition
>
> **Prolonged Unavailability or Unreliability of the
> Gastrointestinal Tract**
>
> Conditions obviating enteral access
>   Perioperative (bowel resection or other gastrointestinal
>   surgery; head and neck surgery)
>   Trauma to the abdomen or head and neck
> Intestinal obstruction not amenable to more distal feeding
> Intestinal ileus not amenable to duodenal or jejunal feeding
> Severe malabsorption (e.g., short bowel syndrome)
> Intractable intolerance of enteral feeding
>
> **Intentional Bowel Rest**
>
> Enteric fistulae
> Intractable diarrhea
> Unremitting pancreatitis
>
> **Relative Contraindications**
>
> Functional gastrointestinal tract
> Intended use for less than about 5 days
> Imminent death from underlying disease

As in any therapeutic feeding situation, before parenteral nutrition is begun, definitive objectives must be set. The patient's energy and protein requirements should be estimated or measured as described in Chapter 11, and a goal for weight maintenance or weight gain should be clear.

Methods of Administration

Central Parenteral Nutrition

To help patients attain sufficient energy intakes without giving them an excessive volume of fluid, the nonprotein energy must be given in a concentrated form. Using final concentrations of up to 35% dextrose results in a fluid osmolality of roughly 1800 mOsm/kg of water (before being admixed with lipids), which is very irritating to the venous endothelium. Therefore, these solutions must be infused into central veins where they are rapidly diluted by high blood-flow rates. The catheter tip is introduced into the superior vena cava or right atrium through the subclavian or internal jugular vein, or by using a peripherally inserted central catheter (PICC).

Peripheral Parenteral Nutrition

When central venous catheterization is undesirable or unavailable, more dilute solutions can be infused into peripheral veins. However, even with final dextrose concentrations of only 10 %, the osmolality of the dextrose/amino acid solution is 900 to 1100 mOsm/kg water, which causes phlebitis and venous occlusion after fairly short periods. To meet energy requirements and reduce osmolality, intravenous (IV) lipid emulsions must be admixed to create total nutrient admixtures (see "2-in-1 versus 3-in-1 Admixtures") or infused as a "piggyback." Total volumes of more than 3 L are often required, exceeding the tolerance of some patients. For these reasons, PPN is only feasible for very short periods of time, making its benefits questionable and requiring that careful consideration be given as to whether it is appropriate for each patient. PICCs provide a welcome alternative, allowing CPN to be infused through peripherally inserted catheters.

2-in-1 Versus 3-in-1 Admixtures

Parenteral nutrition may be administered as either 2-in-1 or 3-in-1 admixtures, also referred to as total nutrient admixtures (TNA). Two-in-one admixtures contain dextrose and amino acids with electrolytes, vitamins, minerals, and trace elements in one or more containers administered daily. Lipid is delivered as a piggyback infusion either daily or intermittently. TNAs contain all components, including lipids, in one daily container.

Each formulation method has advantages and disadvantages. Many institutions have chosen TNAs because they require only one large bag of parenteral nutrition per day, decreasing the pharmacy supplies and staff time required to compound and administer TPN. The use of one TPN container per day can also reduce physician error and inadequate nutrient delivery resulting from time gaps between TPN containers. Disadvantages of 3-in-1 formulations include difficulty visualizing precipitates or particulate material in the opaque solution and incompatibility of certain drugs with the lipid emulsion.

Macronutrients

Dextrose Monohydrate

The major source of nonprotein energy in TPN is dextrose (D-glucose). It is provided in the monohydrous form for IV use, which reduces its energy yield to 3.4 kcal/g rather than the 4 kcal/g of most carbohydrates. Dextrose contributes the majority of the osmolality of the TPN solution. It is supplied by manufacturers in concentrations ranging from 2.5% to 70%.

Lipid Emulsions

IV lipid emulsions, generally derived from safflower oil, soybean oil, or a combination of the two, are available in 10% (1.1 kcal/mL), 20% (2.0 kcal/mL), and 30% (3 kcal/mL) concentrations. The higher concentrations have the advantage of giving higher energy value in lower fluid volume. They can be admixed with dextrose and amino acids in 3-in-1 or TNAs in a variety of concentrations if certain guidelines are observed. The 30% lipid emulsion is only approved for compounding, not for direct administration. The lipids reduce the osmolality and hence the caustic nature of the high concentrations of dextrose used in parenteral nutrition.

In CPN, lipid emulsions must be used at least once or twice weekly to prevent essential fatty acid (EFA) deficiencies. The continuous infusion of concentrated dextrose and the consequent steady elevation of insulin levels can prevent mobilization of endogenous adipose tissue stores of EFAs, resulting in biochemical evidence of an EFA deficiency within 1 or 2 weeks. Lipid emulsions prevent this. When a clear contraindication to the use of lipid emulsions exists (which is extremely rare), a tablespoon of a vegetable oil, such as safflower oil, rubbed on the skin daily can prevent an EFA deficiency, but this may not be sufficient to correct a pre-existing deficiency.

Daily lipid intake is mandatory when PPN is used because it is virtually impossible to meet energy requirements with the more dilute glucose solutions required in PPN. Without adequate nonprotein calories, the infused amino acids will be oxidized to provide energy. This defeats one of the major purposes of parenteral nutrition, which is to meet all metabolic requirements. In addition, parenteral nutrition is more physiologic if lipids are provided daily as a source of nonprotein energy, as shown in Box 14–2.

In some patients, the inclusion of lipids as a daily energy source is particularly beneficial. Glucose-intolerant patients can achieve better glucose control and require less insulin when less dextrose is infused. Cachectic patients accrue lean body mass more efficiently and run less risk of developing glucose-induced complications of refeeding such as hypophosphatemia (see Chapter 11). Patients with ventilatory failure and CO_2 retention can benefit from the fact that less CO_2 production is associated with lipid oxidation than with glucose oxidation (see Chapter 24).

IV lipid emulsions have very few adverse effects, and documentation of adverse effects often consists of only one or two reports of single cases. Although potentially serious, hypersensitivity (reported as dyspnea, flushing,

---

BOX 14–2 **Advantages of Including Lipid as a Daily Energy Source in Total Parenteral Nutrition**

Improves glucose tolerance
Lowers insulin levels
Reduces the risk of refeeding complications
Facilitates nitrogen balance
Promotes synthesis of proteins such as albumin in the liver
Is readily used as an energy source by hypermetabolic, stressed patients
Lipid oxidation generates less CO_2 than does glucose oxidation

chest pain, back pain, and urticaria) is rare enough not to warrant the use of small test doses before lipid infusion. Hypoxemia can be aggravated by rapid infusion of lipids, if the clearance of circulating triglycerides is delayed. However, this complication can nearly always be prevented by infusing the lipids over 12 to 24 hours. Serum triglyceride levels greater than 500 mg/dL can cause pancreatitis, so it is prudent to document acceptable levels at least once during lipid infusion.

The common assumption that standard doses of lipid emulsions (e.g., 500 mL of 10 % lipids per day) cause or aggravate liver enzyme abnormalities or fatty deposits in the liver is not well founded. When associated with TPN, these abnormalities are generally a result of constant and sometimes excessive glucose delivery, which lipid emulsions can relieve. (See "Complications" later in this chapter).

Amino Acids

The crystalline amino acids used in TPN are available in concentrations between 3.5 % and 20 % (3.5 and 20 g/100 mL, respectively) and yield 4 kcal/g. Their energy content should be counted as part of the patient's total energy intake, despite the intent that they be used for protein synthesis. The reason for this is that most patients on TPN are at best in only a slightly positive protein balance, and the infused amino acids are used primarily to replace protein that is catabolized (and hence used as a fuel).

Among the specialized amino acid formulas designed for use in patients with specific diseases, efficacy has been documented only for those enriched with branched-chain amino acids for treating hepatic encephalopathy (see Chapter 22).

Micronutrients

Vitamins

The U.S. Recommended Dietary Allowances (RDAs) for micronutrients do not apply to parenteral nutrition because

TPN bypasses the absorptive process. The U.S. Food and Drug Administration developed requirements for maintenance parenteral vitamin intakes (Box 14–3), which are reflected in most of the commercial multivitamin preparations used in TPN.

These intake levels are appropriate for maintaining already normal circulating vitamin levels but cannot be assumed to be sufficient to correct pre-existing vitamin deficiencies or cover the needs of hypermetabolic, stressed patients. Consider whether the patient's vitamin intake has been adequate in the weeks preceding TPN and whether signs of a vitamin deficiency are present. If a deficiency is likely, parenteral vitamin intake should exceed maintenance levels for at least several days. This can be achieved by using single vitamin preparations such as vitamin C in added doses or by using multiple doses of multivitamin preparations, although the latter approach may still result in a low intake of some vitamins.

BOX 14–3   Parenteral Multivitamin Composition

Vitamin A: 3300 IU (990 μg)
Thiamin (vitamin B_1): 6 mg
Riboflavin (vitamin B_2): 3.6 mg
Niacin: 40 mg
Pyridoxine (vitamin B_6): 6 mg
Pantothenic acid: 15 mg
Vitamin B_{12}: 5 μg
Vitamin C: 200 mg
Vitamin D: 200 IU (5 μg)
Vitamin E: 10 mg (10 IU)
Folic acid: 600 μg
Biotin: 60 μg
Phylloquinone (vitamin K): 150 mcg

From Helphingstine CJ, Bistrian BR: New Food and Drug Administration requirements for inclusion of vitamin K in adult parenteral multivitamins. J Parent Ent Nutr 17:220, 2003.

BOX 14–4   Minerals Provided in Parenteral Nutrition

Cations and Associated Anions
Sodium: acetate, chloride, phosphate, bicarbonate
Potassium: acetate, chloride, phosphate
Calcium: gluconate, gluceptate, chloride
Magnesium: sulfate

Minerals

The major minerals provided in parenteral nutrition are shown in Box 14–4, paired with the salts most commonly used with each.

It is usually possible to make precise changes in the patient's mineral and acid-base status by altering levels of these except for calcium, which has levels that are tightly regulated by the parathyroid hormone. By substituting acetate for chloride with or without changes in sodium and potassium intake, it is usually possible to correct metabolic acidosis. Acetate is preferred over bicarbonate because buffering capacity can be lost if bicarbonate spontaneously converts to CO_2. Bicarbonate raises the pH of TPN and may precipitate with calcium or magnesium.

Although the amounts of minerals provided to patients in TPN must be individualized, there are suggested ranges for daily maintenance intake (Box 14–5).

When a patient needs more phosphorus, it can be provided in the sodium or potassium salt form. Because the co-solubility of admixtures of calcium, magnesium,

BOX 14–5   Daily Mineral Allowances in
Total Parenteral Nutrition

Phosphate: 20–40 mmol per day
Sodium: 60 or more mEq per day
Potassium: 60 or more mEq per day
Calcium: 10–15 mEq per day
Magnesium: 16–24 mEq per day

and phosphorus is limited, and varies according to the amino acid preparation used (particularly its pH), hospital pharmacies have strict guidelines governing admixtures based on the products they use. The relative amounts of phosphorus, sodium, and potassium patients receive from sodium phosphate and potassium phosphate depend on the pH of the solution and how it is ordered. Most commercial potassium phosphate preparations provide 4.4 mEq potassium and 3 mmol phosphorus per ml. Therefore, if an order is written for "20 mEq K^+ as K-Phos," the patient will receive 20 mEq of potassium and about 14 mmol of phosphorus; if the order is written as "20 mmol P as K-Phos," the patient will receive 20 mmol of phosphorus and about 29 mEq of potassium. The latter is preferred.

Trace Elements

As with vitamins, multiple-trace-element solutions that satisfy the maintenance requirements of most patients are available. The composition of a representative solution is shown in Box 14-6.

Patients who have losses of or increased requirements for zinc should be given additional doses—5 to 10 mg elemental zinc per day in patients who are stressed, postoperative, or have draining wounds, and up to 12 to 17 mg for each liter of upper intestinal fluid lost through diarrhea or fistulae.

Iron dextran can be added to non-lipid-containing parenteral nutrition solutions when needed to support iron status or correct deficiency. However, it is preferable to give iron dextran as a single IV total replacement dose separately from TPN. Because most patients are not on

---

BOX 14-6   Multiple-Trace-Element Solution for Total Parenteral Nutrition

Zinc (as sulfate): 4 mg
Copper (as sulfate): 0.8–1 mg
Chromium (as chloride): 10–12.5 μg
Manganese (as the sodium salt): 0.4–0.8 mg

TPN long enough for poor intake to deplete their body iron stores, this is usually necessary only in long-term TPN recipients. IV selenium and molybdenum are available but are generally reserved for patients on long-term home parenteral nutrition with no other source.

Drugs

Hyperglycemia is common in patients receiving TPN both because they receive a large dextrose load and because most patients who require TPN are in metabolic stress and some are diabetic. Regular human insulin is added to TPN when necessary to control hyperglycemia. A minimum dose of 15 units per bag of TPN should be provided to account for adsorption to the container and tubing, and the dose should be progressively increased to maintain blood glucose levels between 80 and 110 mg/dl. This level of glucose control was shown to decrease morbidity and mortality in critically ill patients on parenteral and enteral feeding.[1] This can be done by using a sliding scale of supplemental subcutaneous insulin based on frequent blood glucose monitoring, and increasing the TPN insulin dose each day by the total amount of subcutaneous insulin required on the previous day. If hypophosphatemia is present, phosphorus should be aggressively repleted, as it may be partly responsible for the hyperglycemia.

A number of other drugs such as cimetidine, ranitidine, heparin, octreotide, and hydrocortisone can be added to certain parenteral nutrition admixtures. However, drugs can disrupt the lipid emulsion in TNA formulations, so seek advice on the specific drug and TPN formulation to be admixed.

Management of Parenteral Nutrition

Inserting the Catheter

The method for inserting a subclavian central venous line is shown in Figure 14–1. For alternative methods using the internal jugular or PICC approach, see the

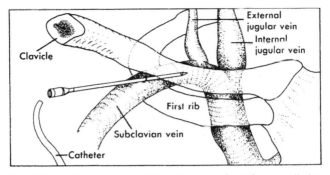

Figure 14–1. SUBCLAVIAN LINE INSERTION. To insert the catheter needle into the right subclavian vein, the index finger of the left hand should be placed in the sternal notch and the thumb along the clavicle. A point is selected just inside the middle third of the clavicle. The needle is inserted with the bevel pointed upward through the pectoralis major muscle. The needle should hug the undersurface of the clavicle and should be aimed toward the index finger.

Suggested Readings. Careful sterile technique is vital. Proper placement should be documented radiographically before TPN is infused. Appropriate standing orders for catheter care are shown in Box 14–7. The catheter port designated for TPN can be changed later

---

BOX 14–7 Nursing Guidelines for Total Parenteral Nutrition Patients

Obtain routine vital signs.

Record intake and output.

If a double- or triple-lumen catheter is used, label one lumen for total parenteral nutrition (TPN) use exclusively.

Use an IV pump to maintain a constant infusion rate. If the infusion falls behind schedule, the rate can be increased by up to 20% in order to achieve the energy goal.

If the infusion is interrupted for any reason, infuse $D_{10}W$ at the TPN infusion rate through a central or peripheral line. Notify the physician.

Change the IV administration set and tubing daily when a new bag or bottle is hung.

Maintain an aseptic, occlusive dressing, and change it according to hospital standards.

if necessary, but the TPN port should not be used simultaneously for anything else.

Ordering Solutions

Before parenteral nutrition is ordered, a few basic decisions must be made. First, energy and protein requirements should be calculated (see Chapter 11). Calculation of the relative protein requirement (percent of energy as protein; see Chapter 11) helps in choosing the relative amounts of amino acids and nonprotein calories to include in the TPN regimen.

A TNA order sheet resembling the electronic order entry screens at the University of Alabama Hospital is shown in Figure 14–2. The total calories desired must be

University of Alabama Hospital
ADULT PARENTERAL NUTRITION ORDER FORM

Date Due _____   Time Due _____   Bag # _____

The following information is required before the first bag of TPN will be formulated. See instructions on back of form.

Nutritional diagnosis *(circle any that apply):* kwashiorkor (260); marasmus (261)
Other protein-calorie malnutrition — severe (262), moderate (263.0), mild (263.1)

Problem requiring TPN use _____

Height _____   Weight _____ lb/kg   Age _____   Sex _____   BEE[1] _____

BEE x 1.1 to 1.4 [2] _____ Total calories per 24 hours (rounded to multiple of 200) _____

| Check one | Formula | Percent of calories from | | | Approximate volume per 1000 kcal |
		Dextrose	Amino acids[3]	Fat	
	15% protein	50	15	35	760
	20% protein (most often appropriate)	50	20	30	860
	25% protein	50	25	25	960
	Reduced carbohydrate	38	22	40	910
	Fat-free	75	25	0	940
	Peripheral vein	30	20	50	1632
	Special formula				

Additives	Quantity ordered	Suggested adult daily guidelines
Sodium acetate[4]	mEq	60+ mEq sodium
Sodium chloride	mEq	
Potassium acetate[4]	mEq	40-60 mEq potassium
Potassium chloride	mEq	
Phosphorus as potassium[5,6]	mmol	20 - 40 mmol phosphorus (*Note: max 15 mmol/L solution*)
Phosphorus as sodium[6]	mmol	
Calcium gluconate[6]	mEq	10 - 15 mEq (*Note: max 10 mEq/L solution*)
Magnesium sulfate[6]	mEq	16 - 24 mEq
Multivitamins[7]		Standard dose (check box)
Trace elements[8]		Standard dose (check box)
Optional additives		
Extra Ascorbic acid	mg	
Extra Zinc	mg	
Insulin, regular human	units	(*Note: approx. 10 units insulin is adsorbed to bag & tubing*)

Date ordered _____   Time ordered _____   M.D. signature _____

Figure 14–2. A, EXAMPLE OF A TOTAL NUTRIENT ADMIXTURE (TNA) ORDER FORM (FRONT).

Instructions

A. Use one of the listed formulas, if possible. Special formulas may require the approval of Pharmacy. For assistance, page the Unit Dietitian, Pharmacist, or Nutrition Support Service.
B. These mixtures may require up to 4 hours of preparation time; please allow for this. Orders received between 6:00 am and 4:00 pm will be filled the same day
C. All formulas utilize 70% dextrose, 10% amino acids, and 20% fat emulsion to provide maximally concentrated solutions. The peripheral vein formula includes sterile water to reduce concentrations and reduce the risk of phlebitis. Sterile water may be requested as an additive to any formula. In either case the total volume is determined by the formula, number of calories, and additives ordered. The approximate final volume and hourly infusion rate will be noted on each bag. The infusion rate may require adjustment so that the entire volume is infused in 24 hours.
D. If a cycled infusion is desired, use the following guidelines for calculating infusion rates. Consult the Nutrition Support Service for assistance.
Day 1: 20-hour cycle: Infuse for 19 hours at rate = (total volume − 50)/19 ml/hr
Day 2: 16-hour cycle: Infuse for 15 hours at rate = (total volume − 50)/15 ml/hr
Day 3: 12-hour cycle: Infuse for 11 hours at rate = (total volume − 50)/11 ml/hr
In all cases, infuse at 50 ml/hr during the final hour, then flush, heparinize, and cap the catheter.

Footnotes

1. Basal Energy Expenditure (BEE) is calculated as:

   Women $BEE = 655.1 + 9.56W + 1.85H - 4.68A$
   Men $BEE = 66.47 + 13.75W + 5H - 6.76A$

   where W = weight (kg), H = height (cm), and A = age (yrs). Use "dry" weights for edematous patients and adjusted weights for obese patients. Page the Unit Dietitian for assistance.

2. The BEE should be multiplied by 1.1 to 1.4 to estimate total calorie requirements. However, this amount should usually not be given on the first day of TPN. Rather, begin with about half the desired calories on the first day and increase to the desired calorie level as tolerated (usually on the second day) for stressed patients, but not before 4-6 days in severely cachectic patients)

3. Determine protein needs, preferably from a 24-hour urinary urea nitrogen (UUN) measurement, which can be used to calculate protein balance as long as the BUN and fluid status are stable:

   Protein loss (g/day) = (24-hour UUN [g] + 4) x 6.25
   Protein balance = protein intake − protein loss

4. Either acetate or chloride is acceptable for most patients; acetate assists in correcting metabolic acidosis but it may exacerbate metabolic alkalosis.

5. Use some phosphorus in each bag of TPN, *particularly in the first bag* unless specifically contraindicated. Each 3 mmol of phosphorus contains approximately 4 mEq of sodium or potassium.

6. Safe limits of compatible electrolyte concentrations *per 1000 ml final volume, in addition to the phosphorus present in the amino acid base solution*, are:

Formula	Central vein	Peripheral vein
Calcium, mEq	10	5
Magnesium, mEq	20	20
Phosphorus, mmol	15	10

7. The standard dose of multivitamins contains approximately the following: vitamin C 200 mg, vitamin A 990 mcg, cholecalciferol (vitamin D) 5 mcg, thiamine 6 mg, riboflavin 3.6 mg, pyridoxine 6 mg, niacin 40 mg, dexpanthenol (pantothenic acid) 15 mg, vitamin E 10 mg, vitamin K 150 mcg, folic acid 600 mcg, biotin 60 mcg, and vitamin B_{12} 5 mcg

8. The standard dose of trace elements contains approximately the following: zinc 4 mg, copper 1.6 mg, manganese 0.4 mg, chromium 16 mcg, and selenium 80 mcg. Some preparations also contain iodine. Concentrations vary by manufacturer.

Figure 14-2. *(Continued)* B, EXAMPLE OF A TNA ORDER FORM (BACK).

indicated and an admixture of carbohydrate, protein, and fat chosen. Ordering methods used in some institutions specify the volumes of base solutions (e.g., 500 mL D_{50} + 1000 mL 10% amino acids + 250 mL 20% lipid) or macronutrient amounts (e.g., total g or g/kg). Additional examples of TPN order sheets have been published.[2] In all cases the quantities of micronutrients must be specified and TPN orders must be renewed daily.

To facilitate ordering solutions the energy and protein content of a container of TPN can be calculated as follows:

Protein content = (mL aa)[aa conc (g/mL)]

Energy content = (protein content)(4 kcal/g) + (mL dex)[dex conc (g/mL)](3.4 kcal/g) + (mL lipid) (1.1 or 2.0 kcal/mL)

where

dex = dextrose
aa = amino acids
conc = concentration (e.g., 50% dextrose = 0.5 g/mL and 10% amino acids = 0.1 g/mL)
1.1 kcal/mL applies to 10% lipid and 2.0 kcal/mL to 20% lipid.

As an example, a solution containing 500 mL of 10% amino acids, 500 mL of 50% dextrose, and 500 mL of 10% lipid (either admixed or separately) has the following composition:

Protein content = (500 mL)(0.1 g/mL) = 50 g
Energy content = (50 g)(4 kcal/g) + (500 mL)(0.5 g/mL) (3.4 kcal/g) + (500 mL)(1.1 kcal/mL) = 200 kcal protein + 850 kcal dextrose + 550 kcal lipid
= 1600 kcal total

The relative contributions of carbohydrate, protein, and fat are calculated as:

850/1600 = 53% carbohydrate
200/1600 = 13% protein
550/1600 = 34% fat

The initial infusion rate varies among patients (see Chapter 11). Highly stressed patients who have been receiving IV dextrose infusions can begin at about 50 mL/hr and advance quickly (e.g., every 8 hours) to reach their full energy requirements within 24 to 48 hours. Severely cachectic, chronically starved patients should be fed more gradually (see Table 11–3). When TNAs are used, simply order gradually increasing calorie levels on the days preceding full feeding. With 1-L containers of 2-in-1 solutions, the pertinent number of containers should be ordered each day and the infusion rate set to achieve the appropriate energy intake. It is not necessary to start with low concentrations of dextrose (e.g., 20%

as opposed to 50% or 70%) when the initial rate of infusion is low.

Terminating the Infusion

Dextrose infusion stimulates insulin secretion, and insulin levels remain elevated for a short time after the dextrose infusion ceases. If the infusion is interrupted abruptly, hypoglycemia rarely ensues in hospitalized TPN patients because they generally have stress-induced insulin resistance. Nevertheless, it is prudent to infuse $D_{10}W$ in this event to prevent hypoglycemia. When TPN discontinuation is planned, it is wise to taper the infusion rate by 50% to 70% for 30 to 60 minutes before terminating it. Longer tapering periods are unnecessary, and no tapering is required if the patient is being fed enterally or orally.

Follow-up

Aside from proper general medical and nursing care, laboratory monitoring is the major requirement in following patients on TPN. Fluctuations in serum electrolytes often necessitate adjustment of the formula from day to day. However, additions should not be made to a container of TPN currently being infused, nor should TPN be used to correct major electrolyte abnormalities. In these situations, it more appropriate to use a separate IV line. A general outline for laboratory monitoring is given in Box 14-8.

Complications

Serious complications of parenteral nutrition can nearly always be avoided by careful patient management. Technical complications, which relate to central venous catheter placement and are therefore not unique to parenteral nutrition, are best prevented by careful, unhurried insertion of the central line by an experienced physician. The most common technical complications are pneumothorax and hemothorax.

**BOX 14–8   Laboratory Tests to Monitor in
Parenteral Nutrition**

Measure Daily Until Stable, then 2 to 3 times Weekly:

Electrolytes (sodium, potassium, chloride, bicarbonate)
Glucose
Phosphorus

Measure 1 to 2 times Weekly:

Calcium, magnesium
Liver function tests
Blood urea nitrogen (BUN), creatinine
Serum albumin

When sepsis occurs in a patient receiving TPN, it may indicate that a lapse in aseptic catheter-care technique has occurred. The organisms that cause TPN sepsis are usually skin contaminants such as *Staphylococcus aureus*, *Staphylococcus epidermidis*, and *Candida albicans*, but in hospitalized patients gram-negative bacteria such as *Pseudomonas* and *Klebsiella* are occasionally involved. Definite catheter sepsis usually requires removal of the catheter, but if the source of a fever is uncertain, the catheter can be cultured and replaced over a guidewire until the results of the catheter culture are available. If the catheter culture is positive, the replacement catheter should be removed and, if necessary, a new one placed in a different site. If the culture is negative, the replacement catheter need not be disturbed.

Infections involving tunneled silastic catheters can usually be treated with antibiotics while leaving the catheter in place. Treatment success may be enhanced by instilling a thrombolytic agent such as alteplase (TPA) or urokinase in the catheter to lyse an infected thrombus.

Metabolic complications of TPN are more common than technical and septic complications, because the metabolic requirements of individual patients cannot be fully reduced to standard guidelines. The most serious complication, as discussed in Chapter 11, is sudden, severe hypophosphatemia induced by dextrose infusion.

Although phosphorus levels drop in most patients after initiation of TPN, severely cachectic patients are the most susceptible to its potentially lethal effects. Normal phosphorus levels can be maintained by putting phosphorus in the *first* container of TPN in all patients, unless a specific contraindication exists (mainly hyperphosphatemia in renal failure). Because the risk of transient *hyper*phosphatemia is minimal except in hypercalcemic patients (whose risk of calcium-phosphate crystallization is greater), phosphorus should be included in all bags of TPN until the patient's requirements have been determined.

In patients receiving TPN, serum phosphorus levels below 2 mg/dL are potentially serious and should be corrected by infusing about 1 mmol/kg phosphorus over 24 hours. Levels below 1 mg/dL require immediate attention and should be treated by decreasing the rate of dextrose infusion and by giving about 1.5 mmol/kg phosphorus over 24 hours, preferably through another IV line. More rapid infusion rates (e.g., over 6 hours) can cause calcium-phosphate precipitation in the kidneys and muscles and should be avoided.

The most common metabolic abnormality in patients receiving TPN is hyperglycemia. After ruling out hypophosphatemia as a possible cause, it is treated by adding insulin to the TPN, ensuring that the total energy load is not excessive, or reducing the dextrose load by substituting lipid for dextrose. In intensive care units, hyperglycemia is often treated with insulin drips; when glucose control is achieved, insulin can be added to the TPN formula.

Hypokalemia and hyperkalemia are also common complications of TPN. They can be readily prevented and treated by using appropriate amounts of potassium in the TPN. Hypo- and hypernatremia require assessment of both sodium and water balance and should be treated by appropriate alterations in sodium and water intakes.

Mild to moderate elevations in liver enzymes and bilirubin occur frequently in patients receiving parenteral nutrition, in association with intrahepatic cholestasis and fatty deposition in the liver. Although the precise mechanisms of these abnormalities are not known, they are probably induced by constant dextrose infusion and perhaps by decreased levels of intestinal motility hormones when the intestine is not used for feeding. They are usually benign and self-limited, and require no intervention. If progressive increases are seen, causes other than the TPN should first be ruled out. If the TPN energy load is excessive, it should be reduced. If dextrose is the predominant energy source, it may help to substitute lipid for a portion of the dextrose calories.

If these are not the causes, cycling the TPN (i.e., infusing it in a shorter time and giving the liver a rest during part of each day) is often effective. This is done by increasing the infusion rate by 25% to 33% to deliver the TPN over 12 to 20 hours, then tapering at an intermediate rate for 1 hour and capping the infusion port or infusing non-glucose-containing IV fluids during the remaining 6 to 8 hours. As an alternative, the TPN infusion can be tapered and maintained at a "keep open" rate of about 10 ml/hr for 6 to 8 hours. For specific instructions for cycling, see Figure 14–2.

REFERENCES

1. Van den Berghe G, Wouters P, Weekers F, et al: Intensive insulin therapy in critically ill patients. N Engl J Med 345:1359–1367, 2001.
2. Task Force for the Revision of Safe Practices for Parenteral Nutrition: Safe practices for parenteral nutrition. J Parent Ent Nutr 28:S39–S70, 2004.

SUGGESTED READINGS

American Society for Parenteral and Enteral Nutrition Board of Directors and Clinical Guidelines Task Force: Guidelines for the use of parenteral and enteral nutrition in adult and pediatric patients. J Parent Ent Nutr 26(1 Suppl):1SA–138SA, 2002.
American Society for Parenteral and Enteral Nutrition: The Science and Practice of Nutrition Support: A Case-based Core Curriculum. Dubuque, Iowa, Kendall/Hunt, 2001.
Rombeau JL, Rolandelli RH (eds): Clinical Nutrition: Parenteral Nutrition, 3rd ed. Philadelphia, WB Saunders, 2000.

WEB SITES

American Society for Parenteral and Enteral Nutrition (ASPEN), http://www.clinnutr.org/

15

Drug-Nutrient Interactions

GLEN THOMPSON, PharmD

Drug-nutrient interactions can manifest in many ways. Foods can increase, decrease, or delay drug absorption. Foods can also influence the rate of drug metabolism by either increasing or decreasing the activity of drug-metabolizing enzymes (e.g., cytochrome P450) or by influencing splanchnic-hepatic blood flow. Varying the protein/carbohydrate ratio in a diet, consuming a diet high in charcoal-broiled beef or cruciferous vegetables, or consuming grapefruit juice or Seville orange juice with certain medications have all been found to influence the metabolism of some drugs. A drug loses efficacy when a food substance delays or prevents it from being absorbed or accelerates the rate of its metabolism or elimination. A toxic reaction from a drug is possible when a food increases its absorption or prevents its metabolism or elimination.

In general, drugs should be taken on an empty stomach unless doing so would cause significant gastrointestinal upset. Calcium supplements present some exceptions to this rule (see Chapter 28). Table 15–1 outlines the influence of foods on drugs when they are taken together and recommends optimal administration times. Drugs that inhibit monoamine oxidase can produce a hypertensive crisis when taken in conjunction with foods that have high tyramine contents. The severity of the response is related to the dosage of the drug and the level of tyramine in the particular food. The drugs and foods involved are listed in Table 15–1.

Grapefruit juice and Seville orange juice can inhibit drug-metabolizing intestinal cytochrome P450 enzymes, especially CYP3A4, for up to 72 hours. Because this significantly increases the bioavailability of many drugs

Table 15–1	**NUTRIENT EFFECTS ON DRUGS**

Decreased Absorption

Avoid taking these drugs with food. Take them at least 1 hour before or 2 hours after meals.

- Ampicillin
- Atenolol
- Biphosphonates
  - Alendronate
  - Etidronate
  - Risedronate
- Captopril
- Cefaclor
- Cephalexin
- Cholestyramine
- Cloxacillin
- Diltiazem
- Erythromycin stearate
- Furosemide
- Glipizide
- Hydralazine
- Iron
- Isoniazid
- Levodopa/carbidopa
- Midazolam
- Penicillin G
- Penicillin V
- Propantheline
- Proton Pump Inhibitors
  - Esomeprazole
  - Lansoprazole
  - Omeprazole
  - Pantoprazole
  - Rabeprazole
- Quinidine
- Quinolones
  - Ciprofloxacin
  - Norfloxacin
- Methotrexate
- Tetracycline
- Zafirlukast
- Zinc sulfate

Increased Absorption

Foods alter the amount of the drugs absorbed, therefore the drug should be taken at the same time(s) or way each day.

- Albenazole
- Atovaquone
- Carbamazepine
- Cefuroxime/Axetil
- Diazepam
- Fenofibrate
- Griseofulvin

Table 15–1	**NUTRIENT EFFECTS ON DRUGS** *(Continued)*

Increased Absorption *(Continued)*

Isotretinoin
Itraconazole capsule
Labetalol
Levothyroxine
Lithium
Mebendazole
Melphalan
Methoxsalen
Metoprolol
Metronidazole
Nitrofurantoin
Phenytoin
Propafenone
Propranolol
Saquinavir
Spironolactone
Sulfadiazine
Tamsulosin
Theophylline
Warfarin

Delayed Absorption
Foods delay the absorption of
these drugs but not the total
amount absorbed. Take them
at least 1 hour before or
2 hours after meals.

Acetaminophen
Aspirin
Cimetidine
Digoxin
Doxycycline
Hydrochlorthiazide
Hydrocortisone
Indomethacin
Ketoprofen
Misoprostol
Pentobarbital
Pentoxifylline
Sulfisoxazole
Tocainide

Monamine Oxidase Inhibitors
Foods to avoid or limit: Ale, beer,
Chianti and vermouth wines,
hard cheeses, breads, crackers
containing cheese, broad bean pods,
fava beans, sauerkraut, Brewer's yeast,
gravies, soups and sauces made from
meat extracts, sour cream, chocolate,
soy sauce, and yogurt.

Isocarboxazid
Pargyline
Phenelzine
Tranylcypromine

and can raise their blood levels into toxic ranges, these specific fruits and juices should be avoided by persons taking the medications listed in Table 15–2. Other citrus fruits do not have the same effects, and are safe to consume while taking the listed medications.

Drugs can induce nutritional deficiencies by decreasing nutrient intake, causing malabsorption or hyperexcretion

Table 15-2	DRUGS WHOSE BLOOD LEVELS ARE INCREASED BY GRAPEFRUIT JUICE

Anti-Infective Drugs
Albendazole
Erythromycin
Praziquantel
Saquinavir

Anti-Inflammatory Drugs
Methylprednisolone

Antilipemic Drugs
Atorvastatin
Lovastatin
Simvastatin

Cardiovascular Drugs
Amiodarone
Carvedilol
Felodipine
Nicardipine
Nifedipine
Nimodipine
Nisoldipine
Sildenafil
Vardenafil
Verapamil

Central Nervous System Drugs
Buspirone
Carbamazepine
Diazepam
Sertraline
Triazolam

Hormones
Estrogen

Immunosuppressive Drugs
Cyclosporine
Tacrolimus

of nutrients, increasing nutrient catabolism, or impairing nutrient utilization. The clinical significance of drug-induced deficiencies depends on the level of depletion reached, which is in turn influenced by the initial nutrient level and the presence of other risk factors such as poor intake, poverty, disability, alcohol abuse, etc. (see Chapter 10). The dose of the drug and the duration of its use are also very important. Table 15-3 lists drugs that can induce nutrient deficiencies and their clinical significance.

Table 15-3	DRUG EFFECTS ON NUTRIENTS
Drugs	**Nutrient Effects**
Anti-infective Agents	
Amikacin, gentamicin, and tobramycin	Hypokalemia, hypomagnesemia, and hypocalcemia; increased urinary potassium and magnesium loss
Amphotericin B	Increased urinary excretion of potassium and decreased serum potassium and magnesium levels
Isoniazid	Pyridoxine deficiency
Neomycin	Decreased absorption of iron, vitamin B_{12} and cholesterol
Rifampin	Decreased serum 25-hydroxyvitamin D
Sulfasalazine	Folate deficiency
Anticoagulants	
Warfarin and indanedione derivatives	Decreased vitamin K dependent coagulation factors
Cardiovascular Drugs	
Hydralazine	Pyridoxine deficiency
Sodium nitroprusside	Decreased total serum vitamin B_{12}
Central Nervous System Drugs	
Phenelzine and tranylcypromine	Pyridoxine deficiency
Phenobarbital	Decreased serum folate and vitamin K
Phenytoin	Decreased serum folate, calcium, and 25-hydroxyvitamin D
Propofol	Lipid emulsion vehicle provides 1.1 kcal/mL
Electrolyte Drugs	
Potassium chloride, slow release	Decreased vitamin B_{12} absorption

Table continued on following page

Table 15-3	DRUG EFFECTS ON NUTRIENTS *(Continued)*
Drugs	**Nutrient Effects**
Gastrointestinal Drugs	
Aluminum hydroxide antacids	Decreased absorption of iron, phosphate, and vitamin B_{12}
Cholestyramine	Decreased absorption of vitamins A, D, E, K, B_{12}, and folate along with decreased absorption of inorganic phosphate and fat
Cimetidine	Decreased absorption of protein-bound vitamin B_{12}
Mineral oil	Decreased absorption of vitamins A, D, E, K
Proton pump inhibitors	Decreased absorption of iron and vitamin B_{12}
Hormones	
Oral contraceptives	Decreased serum folate, pyridoxine deficiency, riboflavin deficiency
Other Agents	
Alcohol	Folic acid, thiamine, pyridoxine, vitamin A, magnesium, and zinc deficiencies; decreased serum phosphate; increased iron absorption
Aspirin	Decreased serum folate; decreased leukocyte and platelet ascorbic acid levels
Colchicine	Decreased absorption of vitamin B_{12}, sodium, potassium, fat, and nitrogen
Metformin	Decreased absorption of vitamin B_{12}
Penicillamine	Pyridoxine deficiency

The widespread use of complementary and alternative medicine (CAM) therapies introduces potential interactions with medications. Chapter 8 discusses ways to evaluate CAM therapies, and Table 8–3 lists a number of known interactions between dietary supplements and pharmaceutical agents.

The "active" ingredient in a drug is not always the agent involved in drug-nutrient interactions. A relevant example is sorbitol, which is used as a base in many liquid medicinal preparations because it enhances their palatability, improves solutions' stabilities, and does not crystallize like other syrup vehicles. It is not absorbed by the gastrointestinal tract and does not raise blood glucose levels. However, sorbitol is far from inactive.

Table 15-4 SORBITOL CONTENTS OF SELECTED LIQUID DRUG PREPARATIONS

Active Ingredient	Dosage Form	Brand Name	Manufacturer	Sorbitol Content (g/mL)	Sorbitol Content (g/common dose)
Acetaminophen	—	—	Roxane	0.35	7.1 g/650 mg
	Elixir	Tylenol	McNeil	0.2	4 g/650 mg
	Suspension	Tylenol	McNeil	0.2	4 g/650 mc
Acetaminophen with codeine	—	—	Carnick	0.06	0.9 g/15 mL
	—	Tylenol #3	McNeil	0	0 g/15 mL
Acyclovir	Suspension	Zovirax	GlaxoSmithKline	0.06	0.3 g/5 mL
Aluminum hydroxide	Suspension	Alternagel	Johnson & Johnson, Merck	0.12	1.8 g/15 mL
Aluminum hydroxide and magnesium carbonate	Suspension	Gaviscon	Marion Merrell Dow	0.073	1.1 g/1.5 mL
Aluminum hydroxide and magnesium hydroxide	Suspension	Maalox	Novartis	0.045	0.675 g/15 mL
		Maalox TC	Novartis	0.15	2.25 g/15 rL
		Maalox Plus Extra Strength	Novartis	0.1	1.5 g/15 mL
Amantadine	Solution	Symmetrel	DuPont	0.72	7.2 g/100 mg
Aminocaproic acid	Syrup	Amicar	Immunex	0.14	2.8 g/5 g
Aminophylline	—	—	Roxane	0.136	1.3 g/200 mg
Calcium carbonate	Suspension	—	Roxane	0.28	1.4 g/500 mg

Table continued on following page

Table 15-4 | **SORBITOL CONTENTS OF SELECTED LIQUID DRUG PREPARATIONS** *(Continued)*

Active Ingredient	Dosage Form	Brand Name	Manufacturer	Sorbitol Content (g/mL)	Sorbitol Content (g/common dose)
Carbamazepine	Suspension	Tegretol	Novartis	0.12	1.2 g/200 mg
Charcoal, activated	Syrup	—	Paddock	0.4	48 g/25 g
Chloral hydrate	Syrup	—	UDL	0.28	1.4 g/500 mg
			Roxane	0.14	0.7 g/500 mg
Chlorpromazine	—	—	Roxane	0.035	0.03 g/25 mg
Cimetidine	Solution	Tagamet	GlaxoSmithKline	0.56	2.8 g/300 mg
Codeine phosphate	—	—	Roxane	0.28	1.4 g/15 mg
Dexamethasone	—	Hexadrol	Organon Inc.	0.51	3.86 g/0.75 mg
			Roxane	0.24	1.8 g/0.75 mg
Diazepam	Solution	—	Roxane	0.21	1.05 g/5 mg
Diphenoxylate and atropine	Solution	Lomotil	Searle	0.21	1.05 g/5 mL
			Roxane	0.455	2.275 g/5 mL
Doxepin	—	—	Warner Chilcott	0.257	1.93 g/75 mg
Doxycycline	—	Vibramycin	Pfizer	0.7	7 g/100 mg
Felbamate	Suspension	Felbatol	Wallace Labs	0.3	2.25 g/900 mg
Furosemide	Solution	—	Roxane	0.49	049 g/40 mg
Guaifenesin	Syrup	—	Roxane	0.11	0.53 g/5 mL
Hydroxyzine	Suspension	Vistaril	Pfizer	1	5 g/25 mg
Hydromorphone	—	Dilaudid	Knoll	0.13	2.6 g/4 mg

Indomethacin	—	Indocin	Merck Sharp & Dohme	0.35	1.75 g/25 mg
Lithium	—	Cibalith-S	Ciba	0.77	3.86 g/300 mg
	Syrup	—	Roxane	0.54	2.7 g/300 mg
Methadone	Solution	—	Roxane	0.14	0.7 g/10 mg
Metoclopramide	Syrup	Reglan	Roxane	0.28	2.8 g/10 mg
			Wyeth-Ayerst	0.35	3.5 g/10 mg
			Warner Chilcott	0.42	4.2 g/10 mg
Milk of magnesia	—	—	Roxane	0.2	6.09 g/30 mL
Minocycline	—	Minocin	Lederle	0.1	1.03 g/100 mg
Molindone	Concentrate	Moban	DuPont	0.26	0.65 g/50 mg
Nalidixic acid	—	NegGram	Winthrop	0.7	7 g/500 mg
Naproxen	Suspension	Naprosyn	Roche	0.09	0.9 g/250 mg
Nitrofurantoin	Suspension	Furadantin	Dura	0.14	1.4 g/50 mg
Nortriptyline	—	Aventyl	Eli Lilly	0.64	8 g/25 mg
Oxybutynin	Syrup	Ditropan	Marion Merrell Dow	0.26	1.3 g/5 mg
Perphenazine	Solution	Trilafon	Schering	0.2	0.5 g/4 mg
Potassium chloride	Solution	—	UDL	0.18	0.45 g/10 mEq
Prednisolone	Liquid	Pediapred	Fisons	0.31	1.53 g/5 mg
Propranolol	—	—	Roxane	0.63	3.15 g/20 mg
Pseudoephedrine	Syrup	Sudafed	GlaxoSmithKline	0.35	1.75 g/30 mg
Pseudoephedrine and triprolidine	Syrup	Actifed	GlaxoSmithKline	0.49	2.45 g/5 mL
Pyridostigmine	Syrup	Mestinon	ICN	0.14	0.7 g/60 mg
Ranitidine	Syrup	Zantac	GlaxoSmithKline	0.1	1 g/150 mg

Table continued on following page

Table 15-4 SORBITOL CONTENTS OF SELECTED LIQUID DRUG PREPARATIONS *(Continued)*

Active Ingredient	Dosage Form	Brand Name	Manufacturer	Sorbitol Content (g/mL)	Sorbitol Content (g/common dose)
Sodium polystyrene sulfonate	Suspension	—	Roxane	0.235	14.7 g/15 g
Sucralfate	Suspension	Carafate	Hoechst Marion Roussell	0.14	1.4 g/1 g
Sulfamethoxazole	—	Gantanol	Roche	0.143	0.72 g/500 mg
Tetracycline	Suspension	Sumycin	Bristol-Myers Squibb	0.3	3 g/250 mg
Theophylline	—	Slo-Phyllin 80	Rorer	0.57	7.07 g/300 mg
			Roxane	0.455	25.6 g/300 mg
		Aerolate	Fleming	0.304	9.12 g/300 mg
Thiabendazole	—	Mintezol	Merck Sharp & Dohme	0.28	1.4 g/500 mg
Thiothixene	—	Navane	Roerig	0.6	0.6 g/5 mg
			Lemmon	0.5	0.5 g/5 mg
Trihexyphenidyl	—	Artane	Lederle	0.83	4.15 g/2 mg
Trimethoprim/ Sulfamethoxazole	Suspension	Septra	GlaxoSmithKline	0.45	2.25 g/5 mL
Valproate sodium	Syrup	Depakene	Abbott	0.15	1.5 g/250 mg
Vitamin E	Solution	Aquasol	Astra	0.2	0.04 g/10 IU

From Johnston KR, Govel LA, Andritz MH: Gastrointestinal effects of sorbitol as an additive in liquid medications. Am J Med 97:185, 1994; Feldstein TJ: Carbohydrate and alcohol content of 200 oral liquid medications for use in patients receiving ketogenic diets. Pediatrics 97:506–511, 1996.

Osmotic diarrhea almost always occurs in patients receiving 20 to 30 g per day of sorbitol, and some patients experience diarrhea with only 10 g per day. Because liquid drug preparations are very frequently given to patients receiving enteral feedings, sorbitol is a common but often unrecognized cause of diarrhea in these patients (see Chapter 13). Table 15–4 lists common liquid medications and their sorbitol contents. Note that drug manufacturers can change the amounts of sorbitol in their products at will because it is listed among the "inactive" ingredients, the contents of which are not disclosed on the label. If a patient has unexplained diarrhea, the current medications should be reviewed for any liquid dosage forms. If the drug manufacturer is contacted and will not divulge the content of sorbitol or other osmotic agent in the drug, administration of the the medication should be changed to crushed tablets or IV form to resolve the diarrhea.

SUGGESTED READINGS

Boullata JI, Armenti VT (eds): Handbook of Drug-Nutrient Interactions. Totowa, NJ, Humana Press, 2004.

American Society for Parenteral and Enteral Nutrition Board of Directors and Clinical Guidelines Task Force: Drug-nutrient interactions. In Guidelines for the Use of Parenteral and Enteral Nutrition in Adult and Pediatric Patients. J Parent Ent Nutr 26(1 Suppl):42SA–44SA, 2002.

Schmidt LE, Dalhoff K: Food-drug interactions. Drugs 62:1481–1502, 2002.

WEB SITES AND DIGITAL TOOLS

MD Consult (requires subscription), http://www.mdconsult.com

Martindale: The Complete Drug Reference (requires subscription), http://www.medicinescomplete.com

Medscape (requires registration), http://www.medscape.com/drugchecker

Personal Digital Assistant programs: Epocrates, Mobile PDR, and Tarascon Pharmacopoeia

PART III

*Nutrition in Specific
Clinical Situations*

16

Metabolic Syndrome

W. TIMOTHY GARVEY, MD • CRISTINA LARA-CASTRO, MD, PhD

Metabolic syndrome, also known as Insulin Resistance Syndrome (IRS) and Syndrome X, is a cluster of metabolic and anthropometric traits including glucose intolerance, upper body fat distribution (increased intra-abdominal fat mass), hypertension, dysfibrinolysis, and a dyslipidemia (characterized by high triglycerides, low high-density lipoprotein [HDL] cholesterol, and small dense low-density lipoprotein [LDL] particles).[1] Metabolic syndrome constitutes a powerful risk factor complex to identify individuals at increased risk for future Type 2 diabetes and cardiovascular disease (CVD). Insulin resistance and abdominal obesity are two central components of the syndrome and are integrally involved in its pathogenesis. Insulin resistance is a metabolic abnormality in which peripheral tissues exhibit a subnormal biologic response to the glucose-lowering action of insulin. Insulin resistance not only antedates the development of diabetes but is also a major metabolic defect (together with impaired insulin secretion and elevated hepatic glucose production) that maintains hyperglycemia in patients with overt disease. The central role of abdominal adiposity underscores the importance of body fat distribution regarding the metabolic consequences of obesity. Individuals with metabolic syndrome are also more prone to develop other pathologic conditions including polycystic ovary syndrome, non-alcoholic steatohepatitis (NASH), cholesterol gallstones, sleep disorders, and some types of cancer. Thus, metabolic syndrome is responsible for a tremendous burden of human disease and social costs, and nutritional therapy is key to both its prevention and limiting its progression to Type 2 diabetes and CVD.

Pathogenesis

Identifying the independent pathogenic role of insulin resistance is complicated by the fact that it is closely related to obesity. In general, insulin resistance increases as body fat increases. However, both lean and obese individuals can be either relatively insulin sensitive or resistant; only about 10% of individual differences in insulin sensitivity are explained by differences in body fat. Thus, while obesity is an important determinant of insulin resistance, individual variations in insulin sensitivity exist independent of the degree of total body fatness.

Other variables associated with insulin resistance include the accumulation of fat in the abdominal or omental compartment (i.e., upper body fat distribution) and intracellular lipid accumulation in muscle cells and hepatic cells, all of which can exist independent of the degree of general adiposity. Distribution of body fat in the omental compartment appears to have the greatest adverse effects, although increased subcutaneous fat also contributes to the association with insulin resistance. This observation is central to the hypothesis that increased omental fat helps promote the metabolic syndrome trait complex via the secretion of free fatty acids and adipocyte-derived proteins such as plasminogen activator inhibitor-1 (PAI-1), tumor necrosis factor alpha, leptin, adiponectin, resistin, cholesterol ester transfer protein, and multiple cytokines including interleukins 6, 8, and 10. Accumulating evidence suggests that several of these secreted factors can induce skeletal muscle and hepatic insulin resistance and constitute a mechanistic link between increased intra-abdominal fat, insulin resistance, and the full expression of the metabolic syndrome trait complex. In addition to insulin resistance and abdominal adiposity, genetic factors underlie susceptibility to metabolic syndrome, interacting with environmental variables including aging, physical inactivity, and low birth weight.

The involvement of insulin resistance and metabolic syndrome in the pathogenesis of atherosclerotic CVD is well established. One aspect of metabolic syndrome that is integrally involved in atherogenesis is the characteristic dyslipidemia that affects all lipoprotein classes. Hyperinsulinemia and elevated circulating free fatty acids may enhance the output of very-low density lipoprotein triglycerides and raise plasma triglycerides. A decrease in post-prandial lipoprotein lipase activity observed in insulin-resistant individuals, as well as other enzymatic changes, leads to a reduction in the number of large cardioprotective HDL particles and a shift toward increased numbers of small dense LDL particles, often without affecting the overall LDL-cholesterol level. In addition to effects on lipids and lipoproteins, insulin resistance and metabolic syndrome are associated with abnormalities in endothelial and vascular function. There is an increase in vascular reactivity that facilitates higher blood pressures and an increase in endothelial oxidative stress. Other potential manifestations of endothelial dysfunction include increased PAI-1 levels resulting in dysfibrinolysis, and elevated markers of systemic inflammation such as C-reactive protein (CRP). All of these factors are established risk factors for CVD and could adversely influence atherosclerotic plaque stability, plaque rupture, and the subsequent thrombosis that underlie acute clinical events.

Diagnosis

Diagnosing metabolic syndrome enables clinicians to identify patients at high risk for developing Type 2 diabetes and CVD and target them for more aggressive risk factor management and disease surveillance. Accordingly, several health organizations have devised diagnostic criteria for this syndrome, including the Adult Treatment Panel III (ATP III) of the National Cholesterol Education Program, the World Health Organization (WHO), and the International Diabetes Federation (Box 16–1).[2–4] The organizations' criteria are similar in many respects, although there is a relative emphasis on the presence of abnormal glucose tolerance in the WHO criteria and on waist circumference in the ATP III criteria. The criteria

NCEP Adult Treatment Panel III (ATP III)[3]

Three or More of the Following Risk Factors—

Risk Factor	Defining Level
Waist circumference	
Men	>102 cm (>40 in)
Women	>88 cm (>35 in)
Triglycerides	≥150 mg/dL
HDL Cholesterol	
Men	<40 mg/dL
Women	<50 mg/dL
Blood pressure	≥130/≥85 mm Hg
Fasting glucose	≥100 mg/dL

World Health Organization[2,3]

Insulin Resistance, Identified by One of the Following—
Type 2 diabetes
Impaired fasting glucose
Impaired glucose tolerance or, for those with normal fasting glucose levels (<110 mg/dL), glucose uptake below the lowest quartile for background population under hyperinsulinemic, euglycemic conditions

Plus Any Two of the Following—
Antihypertensive medication and/or high blood pressure (≥140 mm Hg systolic or ≥90 mm Hg diastolic)
Plasma triglycerides ≥150 mg/dl (≥1.7 mmol/L)
HDL cholesterol <35 mg/dl (<0.9 mmol/L) in men or <39 mg/dL (<1.0 mmol/L) in women
BMI >30 kg/m^2 and/or waist:hip ratio >0.9 in men and >0.85 in women
Urinary albumin excretion rate ≥20 μg/min or albumin:creatinine ratio ≥30 mg/g

International Diabetes Federation 2005[4]

Central Obesity, Defined as—
Waist circumference ≥94 cm for men of European descent and ≥80 cm for women of European descent, with ethnicity-specific values for other groups

Plus Any Two of the Following Four Factors—
Raised triglyceride level: ≥150 mg/dL (1.7 mmol/L), or specific treatment for this lipid abnormality
Reduced HDL cholesterol: <40 mg/dL (1.03 mmol/L) in males and <50 mg/dL (1.29 mmol/L) in females, or specific treatment for this lipid abnormality
Raised blood pressure: systolic BP ≥130 or diastolic BP ≥85 mm Hg, or treatment of previously diagnosed hypertension
Raised fasting plasma glucose ≥100 mg/dL (5.6 mmol/L), or previously diagnosed Type 2 diabetes

are based on limited empirical data regarding predictive value for future diabetes and CVD, and additional research is needed to refine them. The ATP III and WHO criteria exhibit low sensitivity for identifying patients with insulin resistance, dyslipidemia, and other risk factors, and do not take into account the impacts of age and race or ethnicity.[5] For example, the defining levels for elevated waist circumference and body mass index (BMI) should be lower to identify at-risk patients in relatively lean populations such as in India and East Asia. To address these issues, in 2005 the International Diabetes Federation recommended lower thresholds for waist circumference in people of European descent and even lower values for persons of East Asian ethnicity, and a lower threshold for abnormal fasting plasma glucose that matches the American Diabetes Association's definition of impaired fasting glucose (see Box 16-1). Because the formal diagnostic criteria are likely to change further, clinicians should take care to individualize patient evaluations and not overlook patients who may not strictly satisfy published criteria but could benefit from aggressive risk factor management.

Prevalence

The age-adjusted prevalence of metabolic syndrome in adults in the United States, using ATP III criteria, was 27% in the fourth National Health and Nutrition Examination Survey (NHANES IV, 1999–2000).[6] The prevalence increased with age, ranging from 6.7% among 20- to 29-year-olds to 43.5% among those 60 to 69 years old. The age-adjusted prevalence was similar for men (24%) and women (23.4%), and Mexican-Americans had the highest prevalence of the syndrome (31.9%) among major racial and ethnic groups. Although there is no standard pediatric definition of metabolic syndrome, its prevalence in children in the United States has been estimated to be about 1 in 10 for children aged 12 to 19 years, and 1 in 3 for overweight and obese children, suggesting that generalized obesity (as opposed to upper body fat distribution) is a more important determinant of the trait complex in children than in adults.

Nutritional Therapy

There is a consensus among advisory health organizations that first line therapy for metabolic syndrome is a lifestyle intervention consisting of diet and exercise. The dietary goals are twofold: (1) a moderate reduction in calories to achieve a 7% to 10% weight loss in the majority of patients, where weight loss is warranted, and (2) macronutrient composition that ameliorates insulin resistance and improves the cardiovascular risk factor profile. These components of therapy are best illustrated by the Diabetes Prevention Program (DPP) trial, which demonstrated that a lifestyle intervention resulting in a small degree of weight loss can dramatically prevent progression to Type 2 diabetes in high-risk individuals and improve the CVD risk profile.[7] The DPP was a multicenter prospective clinical trial that randomized 3234 adults with impaired glucose tolerance (at high risk for developing diabetes) to a control group, metformin treatment, or lifestyle intervention. The lifestyle intervention consisted of a moderately hypocaloric diet (1200 to1800 kcal/day) based on the U.S. Department of Agriculture Food Guide Pyramid and a National Cholesterol Education Program (NCEP) Step 1 diet plan that emphasized whole grains, fresh vegetables, and fruits with a goal of <25% calories from fat. This was combined with a program of moderate exercise (e.g., brisk walking) at a total duration of ~150 min/week. Subjects randomized to lifestyle intervention achieved and maintained a 5% to 7% weight loss over 4 years of observation. Results dramatically indicated that this degree of weight loss was associated with a 58% reduction in diabetes incidence over the 4-year period, and that this applied to white people, African Americans, Hispanic Americans, and Native Americans. Although the independent contributions of diet and exercise in the prevention of Type 2 diabetes were not rigorously assessed, the relative degree of diabetes prevention was correlated with the degree of chronic weight loss.

Weight Reduction

Sustained weight loss of as little as 5% to 10% of initial body weight can improve insulin sensitivity and cardio-vascular risk factors in metabolic syndrome, reduce cardiac events and related mortality in patients with previous myocardial infarction, and significantly decrease blood glucose, hemoglobin A1c concentrations, and medication requirements in obese patients with Type 2 diabetes.[8] Further weight loss does not lead to substantial further improvements in these parameters. It is important to note, however, that greater initial weight loss is associated with greater long-term weight-loss maintenance. Enhanced insulin sensitivity following moderate weight loss is partially related to the loss of total fat, and highly correlated with the loss of visceral and intramyocellular fat.

Negative energy balance produces weight loss regardless of the macronutrient composition of the diet. While various diet plans emphasize factors that affect hunger and satiety, caloric reduction is a *sine qua non* of weight loss. In recent years, a number of popular diets have advocated changes in macronutrient composition as a strategy for promoting weight loss without an emphasis on overall total energy intake. Diets such as the Atkins Diet, Zone Diet, and South Beach Diet reduce the amount and composition of carbohydrates to achieve a degree of unintentional calorie reduction through a blunting of the appetite. Many of these low-carbohydrate diets can also be termed high-fat diets since it is impractical to make up the carbohydrate caloric deficit with dietary protein. Randomized studies have shown that high-fat, low-carbohydrate diets are effective and safe for short-term weight loss, and after 12 months the amount of weight loss is comparable to that observed with low-fat diets. In fact, the major determinant of success is adherence to the diet, not the diet itself.[9] However, long-term safety has not been established for high-fat diets. This is of concern because high dietary fat content in subjects fed weight-neutral diets (i.e., isocaloric substitution of macronutrients with fat) worsens insulin resistance and cardiovascular risk factors. In the short-term, the beneficial effects of weight loss may predominate over the adverse effects of high fat content, but after weight equilibration, maintenance of high dietary fat could be harmful over the long-term. Many diets can be used to effectively and safely achieve weight loss; patient compliance is the chief determinant of success. The extent of weight loss is directly related to reductions in total energy intake. However, longer-term weight loss and weight maintenance should feature a dietary composition known to increase insulin sensitivity and improve the CVD risk profile.

An alternative approach that can be used effectively to promote weight loss is a diet consisting of high-fiber foods with low energy density. An example is the EatRight Weight Management Program employed at the University of Alabama at Birmingham (http://www.uab.edu/eatright), which emphasizes the ingestion of large quantities of high-bulk, low-energy-density foods (primarily vegetables, fruits, high-fiber grains, and cereals) and moderation in high-energy-density foods (meats, cheeses, sugars, and fats).[10] Details are provided in Chapter 17.

Dietary Composition

In addition to calorie reduction leading to moderate weight loss, nutritional therapy of metabolic syndrome should feature a nutrient profile designed to improve insulin sensitivity and lessen cardiovascular and metabolic disease risks. Alterations in the types of dietary fat and carbohydrate have been shown to affect these parameters.[11]

Dietary Fats

Epidemiologic studies have demonstrated that high intake of total fat (>40% of total calories) is associated with insulin resistance and higher rates of CVD.

In addition, the composition of dietary fatty acids, as opposed to total fat consumption, can independently modulate insulin sensitivity. Multiple cross-sectional studies have found that intake of both saturated and *trans* fatty acids are associated with hyperinsulinemia and with risk of Type 2 diabetes, independent of body adiposity. Isocaloric substitution of saturated fat with polyunsaturated fatty acids (PUFA) has resulted in both an increase in insulin sensitivity and a lowering of LDL cholesterol when compared with a diet rich in saturated fatty acids. However, it has not been determined whether the metabolic improvements observed were secondary to the increase in dietary PUFA or the decrease in saturated fat. Overall, because diets enriched in polyunsaturated fat have not consistently been shown to improve insulin sensitivity, and long-term intervention trials have not been conducted, intake of PUFA should be limited to ≤10 % of total energy. Compiled data further indicate that the intake of saturated fat should be limited to ≤10 %, and intake of *trans* fatty acids present in processed oils and foods should be minimized.

High relative intake of monounsaturated fatty acids (MUFA) as a component of overall dietary fat is felt to be critical for metabolic benefits of the Mediterranean diet. Dietary sources of MUFA include nuts and vegetable oils such as olive, canola, high oleic safflower, and sunflower oils that are liquid at room temperature. Short-term intervention studies in healthy volunteers have shown that the isocaloric substitution of MUFA for saturated fat, or even substituting MUFA for carbohydrates, can have positive effects on insulin sensitivity. In longer-term studies, beneficial effects of a high-MUFA diet on metabolic and cardiovascular risk factors in metabolic syndrome, and glycemic control in Type 2 diabetes have been demonstrated in randomized trials using isoenergetic high-MUFA diets. In the majority of diets employed in these studies, fat accounts for 30 % to 40 % of total calories, and largest component of total fat is MUFA, ranging from 12 % to 30 % of the total energy intake. In general, these effects are more evident when the total amount of fat is modest (<40 % of total calories).

Omega-6 and omega-3 fatty acids are the two major types of PUFA in the diet. Linoleic acid is the most abundant omega-6 fatty acid in the diet, found primarily in liquid vegetable oils including soybean oil, corn oil, and safflower oil. Vegetable sources of omega-3 fatty acid (linolenic acid) include soybean oil, canola oil, walnuts, and flaxseed. Eicosapentaenoic acid (EPA) and docosahcxacnoic acid (DIIA) are omega-3 fatty acids found predominantly in shellfish and fatty fish (e.g., salmon, trout, and herring). While evidence suggests that omega-3 fatty acids may help prevent heart disease, the effects of omega-3 and omega-6 fatty acids on glucose homeostasis are inconsistent. For example, fish oil supplementation (3 to 6 g/day), enriched in omega-3 fatty acids, has been reported to lower triglycerides, without any change in glucose control in diabetes and no change in insulin sensitivity.

Dietary Carbohydrates

As observed for fat, the composition of dietary carbohydrates can potentially influence insulin sensitivity and cardiovascular risk factors. Current carbohydrate recommendations range from 45% to 65% of total energy intake. The majority of those should come from whole grain, unrefined starches and fresh or frozen fruits and vegetables in order to guarantee an optimal fiber, mineral, and vitamin intake.

While avoidance of simple sugars and reliance on complex carbohydrates have been traditionally emphasized, the intake of fiber and whole grains may ultimately be responsible for beneficial effects of altered carbohydrate ingestion. Observational studies suggest that diets enriched in simple carbohydrates or fructose can be associated with low plasma HDL cholesterol and insulin resistance, whereas diets supplying higher amounts of complex carbohydrates and fiber are associated with increased insulin sensitivity. However, controlled intervention studies in humans indicate that high-sucrose or high-fructose diets do not have these same consequences, and do not worsen insulin sensitivity when assessed by hyperinsulinemic clamps. The dietary glycemic index has been established to physiologically classify carbohydrates based on post-meal glycemic responses, since this is not always predictable based on simple versus complex chemical structure. On balance, available data suggest that dietary fiber, rather than available carbohydrates or dietary glycemic index *per se*, is responsible for the effects of carbohydrates on insulin sensitivity in humans. A low glycemic index diet enriched in fiber and whole-grain products is associated with optimal glycemic and insulin responses and relatively low risk of Type 2 diabetes, indicating that the fiber content in low glycemic index foods may play a role in their metabolic effects. Studies on the effects of dietary intake of fiber, particularly whole-grain foods, have demonstrated an improvement in insulin sensitivity; the fiber and magnesium content of whole-grain foods account for a large proportion of this effect. Therefore, emphasis should be placed on achieving an optimal fiber intake of 14 g per 1000 calories consumed. To achieve metabolic benefits, intake of at least 3-ounce equivalents of whole grains per day should be recommended. Daily substitution of whole grains for refined grains will help achieve this goal. Whole grains that are consumed in the United States either as a single food or as an ingredient in a multi-ingredient food (i.e. multigrain breads) include whole wheat, whole oats or oatmeal, popcorn, brown rice, wild rice, and bulgur.

Exercise

Lifestyle intervention studies on insulin-resistant individuals have provided strong evidence for a direct role of physical activity in the prevention of metabolic syndrome and progression to Type 2 diabetes. Regular exercise was a key element of the lifestyle intervention in the Diabetes Prevention Program that resulted in a 58% reduction in Type 2 diabetes incidence. Physical activity increases energy expenditure and should be a component of all weight-loss programs. A weekly volume of low-to-moderate physical activity of about 150 min, equivalent to about 30 min on most days of the week, improves insulin sensitivity and associated traits independent of effects on body weight. Part of the metabolic benefit attained with exercise relates to preferential utilization of omental fat over subcutaneous fat. Moderate-intensity physical activity increases heart rate to about 70% of maximum (thc maximum can roughly be estimated in beats per minute as 220 minus the age in years). This can be achieved with brisk walking (about 3.5 miles/hr), bicycling (less than 10 mph), group aerobic exercise, hiking, or some types of yard work. It is possible to achieve greater health benefit through a more vigorous exercise training program. Under these circumstances, exercise intensity is the key variable leading to improvement in aerobic fitness (VO_2max), and may be achieved through high-intensity exercise (75% maximum heart rate and higher). In all instances, the exercise activity must be sustained over time in order to realize continued metabolic benefits.

Summary Recommendations

Lifestyle intervention consisting of diet and regular moderate exercise is key to both preventing the metabolic syndrome and preventing progression to Type 2 diabetes and cardiovascular disease. These recommendations are summarized in Box 16–2. The diet is hypocaloric to achieve and maintain a 7% to 10% weight loss in overweight and obese individuals, and it has a nutrient composition known to improve insulin sensitivity and reduce CVD risk. Weight loss can be achieved effectively and safely with many diet plans, and patient compliance is the main determinant of success. For longer-term weight maintenance, the nutrient composition becomes more important for risk factor reduction. The evidence supports diets low in total and saturated fat, relatively high in monounsaturated fat, and enriched in whole grains and dietary fiber. The EatRight plan achieves these goals for macronutrient composition and weight loss by emphasizing high-bulk,

BOX 16-2   Lifestyle Intervention for the Metabolic
Syndrome

Goal 1—Energy Intake

Limit energy intake to attain a weight loss of between 7% to
10% of initial body weight. Decreasing daily caloric intake by
500 to 1000 calories will induce an average weight loss of
1-2 pounds per week.

Goal 2—Macronutrient Composition of the Diet

Carbohydrates
    50%-60% of total daily calories
    Emphasis on whole grains, fiber-rich fruits,
        vegetables, and legumes
Fats
    Total fats <30% of total daily calories; additional amounts
        (up to 40% of calories) should be from MUFA,
        not saturated or *trans* fatty acids
    Saturated fat <10%
    MUFA ~ 15%
    PUFA <10%
    Minimal *trans* fatty acids
    Cholesterol <300 mg/day
Proteins 15%-20% of total calories

Goal 3—Physical Activity

~30 min per day of moderate-intensity physical activity on
most days of the week

MUFA, monounsaturated fatty acids; PUFA, polyunsaturated
    fatty acids.

low-energy-density, high-fiber foods. Mediterranean-
style diets with higher amounts of monounsaturated fat
can also be beneficial. It is important to individualize
the diet to account for personal and cultural dietary
preferences.

REFERENCES

1. Reaven GM: Pathophysiology of insulin resistance in human
    disease. Physiol Rev 75:473-486, 1995.

2. Alberti KG, Zimmet PZ: Definition, diagnosis and classification of diabetes mellitus and its complications. Part 1: Diagnosis and classification of diabetes mellitus provisional report of a WHO consultation. Diabetic Med 15:539–553, 1998.
3. Grundy SM, Cleeman JI, Daniels SR, et al: Diagnosis and management of the metabolic syndromes. Circulation 112:735–752, 2005.
4. International Diabetes Federation: The IDF consensus worldwide definition of the metabolic syndrome. Available at http://www.idf.org/webdata/docs/IDF_Metasyndrome_definition.pdf.
5. Liao Y, Kwon S, Shaughnessy S, et al: Critical evaluation of adult treatment panel III criteria in identifying insulin resistance with dyslipidemia. Diabetes Care 27:978–983, 2004.
6. Ford ES, Giles WH, Mokdad AH: Increasing prevalence of the metabolic syndrome among U.S. Adults. Diabetes Care 27:2444–2449, 2004.
7. Diabetes Prevention Program Research Group: Reduction in the incidence of type 2 diabetes with lifestyle intervention or metformin. N Engl J Med 346:393–403, 2002.
8. Wing RR, Koeske R, Epstein LH, et al: Long-term effects of modest weight loss in type II diabetic patients. Arch Intern Med 147:1749–1753, 1987.
9. Dansinger ML, Gleason JA, Griffith JL, et al: Comparison of the Atkins, Ornish, Weight Watchers, and Zone diets for weight loss and heart disease risk reduction: A randomized trial. JAMA 293:43–53, 2005.
10. Weinsier RL, Wilson NP, Morgan SL, et al: EatRight, Lose Weight: Seven Simple Steps. Birmingham, Ala, Oxmoor House, 1997.
11. Lara-Castro C, Garvey WT: Diet, insulin resistance, and obesity: Zoning in on data for Atkins dieters living in South Beach. J Clin Endocrinol Metab 89:4197–4205, 2004.

SUGGESTED READINGS

Grundy SM, Hansen B, Smith SC Jr, et al: Clinical management of metabolic syndrome: Report of the American Heart Association/National Heart, Lung, and Blood Institute/American Diabetes Association conference on scientific issues related to management. Circulation 109:551–556, 2004.

WEB SITES

Medline Plus, http://www.nlm.nih.gov/medlineplus/metabolicsyndromex.html
UAB EatRight Weight Management Program, http://www.uab.edu/eatright

17

Obesity

JAMY D. ARD, MD

Obesity is a public health problem of epidemic proportion and is one of the most significant nutritional problems in the United States today, as indicated by its designation as one of the 10 leading health indicators in the Healthy People 2010 initiative. Based on data from the National Health and Nutrition Examination Survey (NHANES), a majority (65.1%) of the U.S. adult population is overweight or obese, with 30.4% classified as obese.[1] Approximately 5% of adults in the United States are extremely obese. Some women of ethnic minority groups are disproportionately affected—nearly 50% of African-American women are obese compared to 30% of white women. These increases in the prevalence of obesity pose a direct risk to the health of the U.S. population by increasing the risk of other diseases, including coronary artery disease, diabetes, hypertension, and certain cancers. For example, reports from the 2001 Behavioral Risk Factor Surveillance Survey (BRFSS) indicated that the increased prevalence of obesity was associated with a seven times greater odds of being diagnosed with Type 2 diabetes mellitus and a six times greater odds of having hypertension.[2]

The increased prevalence of obesity also has a direct effect on health care expenditures. It is estimated that overweight employees cost businesses more than employees who have any other health risk, including smoking. Health insurance claims of overweight employees are about 37% higher than those of their slimmer counterparts, and the number of days spent in hospitals is 143% greater. Thus, in addition to direct adverse health effects, overweight employees represent a huge economic cost to employers and to collective productivity due to time lost from work. The overall economic cost of obesity is estimated to be approximately 6% of adult medical expenditures—well over $100 billion per year—including $75 billion in health care costs for obesity-related illness and $33 billion in expenditures on weight-loss products and services.[3]

Despite increasing attention to the health and economic effects of obesity, the prevalence continues to rise. This is particularly true for children, where 31% of children ages 6 to 19 are considered overweight or at risk of becoming overweight. Because overweight children are more likely to be obese in their adult years, this potentially signifies that the peak in obesity prevalence may be in the distant future.

Etiology

Obesity is a complex phenotype, resulting from the direct effects and interactions of genetic factors, the environment, and behavior. Although the mechanisms causing obesity are not completely understood, their net effect is an imbalance of energy intake and expenditure, creating an energy excess that is stored as fat.

Genetic Factors

It has been clearly established that genetic factors contribute to one's *predisposition to* or *protection from* obesity. Current estimates are that 25% to 40% of variation in body mass index (BMI) is likely due to genetically determined factors.[4] These factors include determinations of resting metabolic rate, where fat is stored (visceral vs. extremities), physiologic responses to overfeeding, and perhaps to some extent eating behaviors. What is unclear is how such genetic factors express themselves. To date there are no firm data to indicate that an individual who is lean but genetically predisposed to obesity will have certain characteristics, such as taste preferences, metabolically efficient muscle fiber types, or reduced maintenance energy requirements.

Discovery of the ob gene in the mouse model raised hopes that a gene or gene product that could directly benefit humans, such as leptin, might be found. This important discovery in inbred mice has important implications for our understanding of the etiology of obesity; however, clinical trials to increase leptin levels in obese patients have been disappointing. Despite these initial findings, significant research continues with other potential gene targets, including neuropeptide Y, β3-adrenergic receptor (ADRB3), peroxisome proliferator-activated receptor-γ (PPAR-γ), peroxisome proliferator-activated receptor-γ coactivator-1 (PGC-1), and adiponectin (APM1). These gene targets are likely to account for only a small degree of obesity susceptibility directly, but they may have significant interactions with other gene variants, amplifying this effect on obesity susceptibility.[5]

Having a genetic predisposition for or against obesity does not preclude an overriding environmental and behavioral influence. In fact, regardless of one's familial or genetic predisposition, environmental factors such as lack of access to or avoidance of energy-dense foods and behavioral factors such as regular physical activity can prevent the development of obesity.

Neuroendocrine Syndromes

Neuroendocrine abnormalities (Box 17–1) cause obesity in fewer than 1% of cases, and those that are more likely to cause obesity (e.g., hypothyroidism, Cushing's syndrome, and polycystic ovary syndrome) rarely cause severe degrees of obesity. Thus, markedly obese persons are *least* likely to have an underlying neuroendocrine disorder.

Metabolism

To predispose a person to weight gain, an abnormality in energy metabolism would have to cause a reduction in maintenance energy requirements. Thus, assuming that energy intake and voluntary physical activity remain the same, the metabolic disorder would have to reduce

---

BOX 17–1   Neuroendocrine Syndromes That (Rarely) Cause Obesity

Hypothyroidism and *hypopituitarism* may cause moderate obesity, but the main contributor to excess weight in these conditions is fluid, not adipose tissue.

Cushing's syndrome rarely causes gross obesity; typically, it has a truncal distribution.

Castration and *ovarian failure* predispose to obesity. They are usually accompanied by hot flashes and other symptoms of vasomotor instability plus elevated urinary gonadotropin levels.

Polycystic ovary (Stein-Leventhal) syndrome may cause a combination of hypothalamic and endocrine obesity. The syndrome is characterized by reduced or absent menses, moderate hirsutism, and weight gain. It usually develops in young women shortly after menarche.

Insulinoma may predispose to generalized obesity. Typical symptoms of hunger and hypoglycemia indicate the need for further evaluation.

Hypothalamic lesions caused by malignancy, trauma, or infection can, in rare instances, cause weight gain by affecting appetite control. Massive obesity may result.

Prader-Willi, Fröhlich's, and Laurence-Moon-Biedl syndromes are associated with childhood obesity, mental retardation, and failure of sexual development. Fröhlich's habitus (obesity and apparently delayed genital development) must be distinguished from true Fröhlich's syndrome.

---

daily energy expenditure. There are three major components of energy expenditure: resting energy expenditure (REE), thermic effect of food, and activity-related energy expenditure (Box 17–2).

Resting and total daily energy expenditure are somewhat variable among individuals, even those of the same size. REE is higher in men than in women, even after controlling for the higher lean mass and total weight. REE also decreases with age, primarily as a result of the loss of lean body mass. Furthermore, several studies have demonstrated that REE differs by ethnic background. Nevertheless, on average, energy requirements increase in proportion to the amount of weight gained, and heavier persons almost invariably have *higher* daily energy needs. Thus, at the present time there is

BOX 17-2   Major Components of Energy Expenditure

Resting energy expenditure (REE). Normally, REE accounts for more than 60% of the total energy expenditure and is related most directly to the amount of fat-free (lean) mass, which is more metabolically active than fat mass. Because obese persons tend to have increased amounts of fat-free mass (probably to support the increase in fat mass), they have increased REEs. Most studies have shown that REE adjusted for fat-free mass is normal in obese persons and in normal-weight persons who are predisposed to obesity.

Thermic effect of food (TEF). The contribution of TEF to total daily energy expenditure is small—approximately 10% of energy intake. Although a number of studies have found TEF to be blunted in obese persons, the potential energy "savings" from an abnormal TEF is probably less than 25 kcal per day, which is an insufficient amount to explain the development of obesity.

Activity-related energy expenditure (AEE). AEE normally represents 20%–30% of daily energy expenditure, depending on the amount of the person's physical activity. Although obese persons tend to be less physically active than lean persons, their AEEs are not necessarily lower because they require more energy to conduct the same amount of physical activity as lean persons. It is not known whether the reduced level of physical activity is secondary to their obese state or if it contributes to weight gain. There is no evidence that obesity-prone persons tend to perform identical physical activities more efficiently (using less energy) than normal persons.

no consistent, convincing evidence that reduced energy expenditure contributes meaningfully to the tendency of some individuals to gain weight.

Environmental Factors

Exogenous factors that may predispose to obesity include dietary excesses and physical inactivity. Without question, altered energy intake can cause weight gain or loss. Although the rate of the weight change may vary somewhat among individuals, one cannot avoid weight gain when energy intake continually exceeds requirements, or avoid weight loss when it fails to meet requirements. As noted above, obese persons must eat more calories to sustain their increased body mass. However, studies of eating behaviors of obese subjects have failed to identify any consistent patterns of calorie intake, eating frequency, or food preferences that account for their obese states.

Data supporting either increased energy intake or decreased physical activity as the sole etiology for the shift in the population weight in the United States are typically lacking, or at best conflicting. Depending on the study cohort and instruments used to assess food intake, one can find several reports that describe an increase in energy intake over the last 30 to 35 years, while other reports show no appreciable change. Changes in leisure time physical activity have demonstrated very little change in the same time frame. Despite increasing numbers of health clubs, fitness centers, and homes with exercise equipment, the amount of time spent in sedentary activities such as watching television, playing video games, or surfing the Internet has dramatically increased in the last 10 years.

While large secular-trend surveys may show little differences in general food intake or physical activity, there are significant trends occurring that have not been carefully measured to date. The availability of high-energy-density foods at low costs has increased, making these food items more accessible to a larger proportion of the population; soft drink and sugared beverage consumption has consistently increased, particularly in child and adolescent populations; work and neighborhood environments require less manual labor, and use of motorized transportation has increased, decreasing the energy expended during the course of a routine day; and fewer schools require physical education or allow time for physical activity during the school day while providing energy-dense foods with few healthy alternatives. Taken together, these trends affect everyone in the United States from childhood through the adult years, leading to consistent energy imbalance and an obesogenic environment that promotes weight gain.

Clinical Assessment of the Obese Patient

Medical History

The medical history should identify factors potentially contributing to the individual's obesity as well as possible comorbidities of obesity. As noted earlier, neuroendocrine causes are rare. Nevertheless, the symptoms listed in Table 17–1 should alert one to the possibility that a secondary cause may exist. The history-taking should also elicit signs of medical complications, which are discussed later.

Assessment of Degree of Obesity and Associated Risk

The primary objective in assessing obesity is to estimate the amount and distribution of body fat. While total body weight is a reliable clinical measure, it is not an accurate indicator of total body fatness because total body weight

Table 17–1	HISTORICAL FEATURES THAT SUGGEST SECONDARY CAUSES FOR OBESITY
History or Symptoms	**Consideration**
Cold intolerance, menstrual abnormalities, constipation, weakness (in adults); retarded mental and physical maturation (in children)	Hypothyroidism, hypopituitarism
Hypertension, glucose intolerance, menstrual dysfunction, weakness, back pain, compression fractures, easy bruising	Cushing's syndrome
Reduced or absent menses shortly after menarche, hirsutism	Polycystic ovary syndrome
Hypoglycemia	Insulinoma
Uncontrollable, ravenous appetite	Hypothalamic lesions
Childhood onset, mental retardation, failure of sexual development	Prader-Willi, Lawrence-Moon-Biedl, Fröhlich's syndromes
Medication use	Phenothiazines, corticosteroids

is a combination of fat mass and lean mass, including both bone and muscle. There are several imaging modalities for evaluating total and regional body fatness, including bioimpedance analysis (BIA), computed tomography (CT), magnetic resonance imaging (MRI), and dual energy x-ray absorptiometry (DEXA). However, the most efficient means of estimating total body and abdominal fatness are BMI and waist circumference, respectively.

In the general population, BMI is strongly correlated with total body fat, and therefore, BMI is a useful tool for classifying degrees of obesity. BMI is calculated by dividing weight (kg) by height squared (m²) (Table 17-2). BMIs between 18.5 and 24.9 kg/m² are considered normal; persons with BMIs between 25 and 29.9 kg/m² are considered overweight; and persons with BMIs greater than or equal to 30 kg/m² are classified as obese (Table 17-3). BMI is not gender specific, and unlike previous reference standards, it is not only associated with mortality, but with morbidity as well. However, BMI overestimates body fat in persons who are very muscular and underestimates body fat in those who have lost muscle mass without significant changes in weight, such as elderly persons.

Waist circumference is measured with the patient standing, at the end of expiration, one centimeter above the level of the umbilicus. This point typically corresponds to the smallest portion of the waist and is most reliably reproduced for follow-up measurements. Because intra-abdominal fat is associated with increased metabolic and cardiovascular disease risk (see section titled Complications later in this chapter), determining waist circumference is a particularly important part of the obesity assessment. Waist circumference holds the strongest association with higher disease risk at BMI levels below 35 kg/m².

The combination of BMI and waist circumference provides an adequate evaluation of body fatness for clinical purposes. Using this information, the clinician can classify the degree of obesity and associated risk for cardiovascular disease, hypertension, and dyslipidemia

Table 17-2 BODY MASS INDEX (BMI) CHART

Ft	5	5	5	5	5	5	5	5	5	5	5	5	6	6	6	6	6	6	KG
In	0	1	2	3	4	5	6	7	8	9	10	11	0	1	2	3	4	5	
Lb 100	19.5	18.9	18.3	17.7	17.2	16.6	16.1	15.7	15.2	14.8	14.3	13.9	13.6	13.2	12.8	12.5	12.2	11.9	44.6
105	20.5	19.8	19.2	18.6	18.0	17.5	16.9	16.4	16.0	15.5	15.1	14.6	14.2	13.9	13.5	13.1	12.8	12.5	46.9
110	21.5	20.8	20.1	19.5	18.9	18.3	17.8	17.2	16.7	16.2	15.8	15.3	14.9	14.5	14.1	13.7	13.4	13.0	49.1
115	22.5	21.7	21.0	20.4	19.7	19.1	18.6	18.0	17.5	17.0	16.5	16.0	15.6	15.2	14.8	14.4	14.0	13.6	51.3
120	23.4	22.7	21.9	21.3	20.6	20.0	19.4	18.8	18.2	17.7	17.2	16.7	16.3	15.8	15.4	15.0	14.6	14.2	53.6
125	24.4	23.6	22.9	22.1	21.5	20.8	20.2	19.6	19.0	18.5	17.9	17.4	17.0	16.5	16.0	15.6	15.2	14.8	55.8
130	25.4	24.6	23.8	23.0	22.3	21.6	21.0	20.4	19.8	19.2	18.7	18.1	17.6	17.2	16.7	16.2	15.8	15.4	58.0
135	26.4	25.5	24.7	23.9	23.2	22.5	21.8	21.1	20.5	19.9	19.4	18.8	18.3	17.8	17.3	16.9	16.4	16.0	60.3
140	27.3	26.5	25.6	24.8	24.0	23.3	22.6	21.9	21.3	20.7	20.1	19.5	19.0	18.5	18.0	17.5	17.0	16.6	62.5
145	28.3	27.4	26.5	25.7	24.9	24.1	23.4	22.7	22.0	21.4	20.8	20.2	19.7	19.1	18.6	18.1	17.6	17.2	64.7
150	29.3	28.3	27.4	26.6	25.7	25.0	24.2	23.5	22.8	22.2	21.5	20.9	20.3	19.8	19.3	18.7	18.3	17.8	66.9
155	30.3	29.3	28.3	27.5	26.6	25.8	25.0	24.3	23.6	22.9	22.2	21.6	21.0	20.4	19.9	19.4	18.9	18.4	69.2
160	31.2	30.2	29.3	28.3	27.5	26.6	25.8	25.1	24.3	23.6	23.0	22.3	21.7	21.1	20.5	20.0	19.5	19.0	71.4
165	32.2	31.2	30.2	29.2	28.3	27.5	26.6	25.8	25.1	24.4	23.7	23.0	22.4	21.8	21.2	20.6	20.1	19.6	73.6
170	33.2	32.1	31.1	30.1	29.2	28.3	27.4	26.6	25.8	25.1	24.4	23.7	23.1	22.4	21.8	21.2	20.7	20.2	75.9
175	34.2	33.1	32.0	31.0	30.0	29.1	28.2	27.4	26.6	25.8	25.1	24.4	23.7	23.1	22.5	21.9	21.3	20.8	78.1
180	35.2	34.0	32.9	31.9	30.9	30.0	29.1	28.1	27.4	26.6	25.8	25.1	24.4	23.7	23.1	22.5	21.9	21.3	80.3
185	36.1	35.0	33.8	32.8	31.8	30.8	30.0	29.0	28.1	27.3	26.5	25.8	25.1	24.4	23.8	23.1	22.5	21.9	82.6
190	37.1	35.9	34.8	33.7	32.6	31.6	30.7	29.8	28.9	28.1	27.3	26.5	25.8	25.1	24.4	23.7	23.1	22.5	84.8

Table continued on following page

Table 17-2 BODY MASS INDEX (BMI) CHART (Continued)

Ft / In / Lb	5 0	5 1	5 2	5 3	5 4	5 5	5 6	5 7	5 8	5 9	5 10	5 11	6 0	6 1	6 2	6 3	6 4	6 5	KG
195	38.1	36.8	35.7	34.5	33.5	32.4	31.5	30.5	29.6	28.8	28.0	27.2	26.4	25.7	25.0	24.4	23.7	23.1	87.0
200	39.1	37.8	36.6	35.4	34.3	33.3	32.3	31.3	30.4	29.5	28.7	27.9	27.1	26.4	25.7	25.0	24.3	23.7	89.3
205	40.0	38.7	37.5	36.3	35.2	34.1	33.1	32.1	31.2	30.3	29.4	28.6	27.8	27.0	26.3	25.6	25.0	24.3	91.5
210	41.0	39.7	38.4	37.2	36.0	34.9	33.9	32.9	31.9	31.0	30.1	29.3	28.5	27.7	27.0	26.2	25.6	24.9	93.7
215	42.0	40.6	39.3	38.1	36.9	35.8	34.7	33.7	32.7	31.7	30.8	30.0	29.2	28.4	27.6	26.9	26.2	25.5	96.0
220	43.0	41.6	40.2	39.0	37.8	36.6	35.5	34.5	33.5	32.5	31.6	30.7	29.8	29.0	28.2	27.5	26.8	26.1	98.2
225	43.9	42.5	41.2	39.9	38.6	37.4	36.3	35.2	34.2	33.2	32.3	31.4	30.5	29.7	28.9	28.1	27.4	26.7	100.4
230	44.9	43.5	42.1	40.7	39.5	38.3	37.1	36.0	35.0	34.0	33.0	32.1	31.2	30.3	29.5	28.7	28.0	27.3	102.7
235	45.9	44.4	43.0	41.6	40.3	39.1	37.9	36.8	35.7	34.7	33.7	32.8	31.9	31.0	30.2	29.4	28.6	27.9	104.9
240	46.9	45.3	43.9	42.5	41.2	39.9	38.7	37.6	36.5	35.4	34.4	33.5	32.5	31.7	30.8	30.0	29.2	28.5	107.1
245	47.8	46.3	44.8	43.4	42.1	40.8	39.5	38.4	37.3	36.2	35.2	34.2	33.2	32.3	31.5	30.6	29.8	29.1	109.3
250	48.8	47.2	45.7	44.3	42.9	41.6	40.4	39.2	38.0	36.9	35.9	34.9	33.9	33.0	32.1	31.2	30.4	29.6	111.6
255	49.8	48.2	46.6	45.2	43.8	42.4	41.2	39.9	38.8	37.7	36.6	35.6	34.6	33.6	32.7	31.9	31.0	30.2	113.8
260	50.8	49.1	47.6	46.1	44.6	43.3	42.0	40.7	39.5	38.4	37.3	36.3	35.3	34.3	33.4	32.5	31.6	30.8	116.0
265	51.8	50.1	48.5	46.9	45.5	44.1	42.8	41.5	40.3	39.1	38.0	37.0	35.9	35.0	34.0	33.1	32.3	31.4	118.3
270	52.7	51.0	49.4	47.8	46.3	44.9	43.6	42.3	41.1	39.9	38.7	37.7	36.6	35.6	34.7	33.7	32.9	32.0	120.5
275	53.7	52.0	50.3	48.7	47.2	45.8	44.4	43.1	41.8	40.6	39.5	38.4	37.3	36.3	35.3	34.4	33.5	32.6	122.7
280	54.7	52.9	51.2	49.6	48.1	46.6	45.2	43.9	42.6	41.3	40.2	39.1	38.0	36.9	35.9	35.0	34.1	33.2	125.0

Weight (lb / kg) versus height (cm); cell values are BMI.

lb	kg	152.4	154.9	157.5	160	163	165	168	170	173	175	178	180	183	185	188	191	193	196
285	127.2	55.7	53.9	52.1	50.5	48.9	47.4	46.0	44.6	43.3	42.1	40.9	39.7	38.7	37.6	36.6	35.6	34.7	33.8
290	129.4	56.6	54.8	53.0	51.4	49.8	48.3	46.8	45.4	44.1	42.8	41.6	40.4	39.3	38.3	37.2	36.2	35.3	34.4
295	131.7	57.6	55.7	54.0	52.3	50.6	49.1	47.6	46.2	44.9	43.6	42.3	41.1	40.0	38.9	37.9	36.9	35.9	35.0
300	133.9	58.6	56.7	54.9	53.1	51.5	49.9	48.4	47.0	45.6	44.3	43.0	41.8	40.7	39.6	38.5	37.5	36.5	35.6
305	136.1	59.6	57.6	55.8	54.0	52.4	50.8	49.2	47.8	46.4	45.0	43.8	42.5	41.4	40.2	39.2	38.1	37.1	36.2
310	138.4	60.5	58.6	56.7	54.9	53.2	51.6	50.0	48.6	47.1	45.8	44.5	43.2	42.0	40.9	39.8	38.7	37.7	36.8
315	140.6	61.5	59.5	57.6	55.8	54.1	52.4	50.8	49.3	47.9	46.5	45.2	43.9	42.7	41.6	40.4	39.4	38.3	37.4
320	142.8	62.5	60.5	58.5	56.7	54.9	53.3	51.6	50.1	48.7	47.3	45.9	44.6	43.4	42.2	41.1	40.0	39.0	37.9
325	145.1	63.5	61.4	59.4	57.6	55.8	54.1	52.5	50.9	49.4	48.0	46.6	45.3	44.1	42.9	41.7	40.6	39.6	38.5
330	147.3	64.4	62.4	60.4	58.5	56.6	54.9	53.3	51.7	50.2	48.7	47.3	46.0	44.8	43.5	42.4	41.2	40.2	39.1
335	149.5	65.4	63.3	61.3	59.3	57.5	55.7	54.1	52.5	50.9	49.5	48.1	46.7	45.4	44.2	43.0	41.9	40.8	39.7
340	151.7	66.4	64.2	62.2	60.2	58.4	56.6	54.9	53.3	51.7	50.2	48.8	47.4	46.1	44.9	43.7	42.5	41.4	40.3
345	154.0	67.4	65.2	63.1	61.1	59.2	57.4	55.7	54.0	52.5	50.9	49.5	48.1	46.8	45.5	44.3	43.1	42.0	40.9
350	156.2	68.4	66.1	64.0	62.0	60.1	58.2	56.5	54.8	53.2	51.7	50.2	48.8	47.5	46.2	44.9	43.7	42.6	41.5
355	158.4	69.3	67.1	64.9	62.9	60.9	59.1	57.3	55.6	54.0	52.4	50.9	49.5	48.1	46.8	45.6	44.4	43.2	42.1
360	160.7	70.3	68.0	65.8	63.8	61.8	59.9	58.1	56.4	54.7	53.2	51.7	50.2	48.8	47.5	46.2	45.0	43.8	42.7
cm		152.4	154.9	157.5	160	163	165	168	170	173	175	178	180	183	185	188	191	193	196

Table 17–3	**GUIDELINES FOR ASSESSING HEALTH RISK FROM OBESITY**			
			Disease Risk	
Weight Classification	**Body Mass Index (kg/m²)**	**Obesity Class**	**Normal Waist Circumference**	**Increased Waist Circumference**
Underweight	<18.5			
Normal	18.5–24.9			
Overweight	25–29.9		Increased	High
Obese	30–34.9	I	High	Very High
	35–39.9	II	Very High	Very High
Extremely obese	≥40	III	Extremely High	Extremely High

relative to individuals of normal weight and waist circumference (see Table 17–3).

Physical Examination

Precise physical examination can be difficult, depending on the degree of obesity. Accurate blood pressure measurement, auscultation of the heart and lungs, palpation of the abdomen, detection of breast masses, and other aspects of the exam require the use of proper technique and tools. Important aspects of the physical examination that are used to identify obesity-related comorbidities and to rule out endocrine abnormalities are listed in Box 17–3.

Laboratory Assessment

Although no particular laboratory test is indicated simply because a patient is obese, assessment of cardiovascular disease risk factors at the time of initial evaluation can be prudent, providing a more complete appraisal of the patient's global risk. Risk factors of note include low-density lipoprotein (LDL) and high-density lipoprotein (HDL) cholesterol, triglycerides, and fasting glucose. Testing to evaluate for secondary causes of obesity should be dictated by the patient's history and physical exam findings (Table 17–4).

BOX 17-3   Physical Examination of the Obese Patient

Blood pressure should be taken using a cuff size appropriate for the patient's arm circumference. Measure the mid-arm circumference to identify the appropriate cuff size. An arm circumference of 24-32 cm requires "Regular Adult"; 33-41 cm requires "Large Adult"; and 42-52 cm requires a "Thigh" cuff.

Skin. Red or purple depressed striae, hirsutism, acne, and moon facies with plethora suggest Cushing's syndrome; mild hirsutism is also seen in polycystic ovarian syndrome; dry, coarse, cool, and pale skin suggests hypothyroidism; dark-grey, velvety skin, prominent in flexural areas (neck, armpits) suggests acanthosis nigricans—an asymptomatic reactive skin lesion associated with insulin resistance and obesity.

Fat distribution. Android distribution pattern (central/trunk) associated with higher risk of cardiovascular disease, diabetes mellitus, and hypertension.

Abdomen. Right upper quadrant tenderness may be associated with gallstones; could also be associated with steatohepatitis, though typically asymptomatic.

Table 17-4	**LABORATORY TESTS FOR CAUSES OR COMPLICATIONS OF OBESITY**
Suspected Condition	**Diagnostic Tests**
Cushing's syndrome	Screening: 24-hr urinary free cortisol, or single low-dose dexamethasone suppression test (1 mg) plus Confirmation: 2-day low-dose dexamethasone suppression test (0.5 mg every 6 hours)
Diabetes	Fasting serum glucose
Gallstones	Ultrasonography
"Hypometabolism"*	Resting energy expenditure by indirect calorimetry
Hypothyroidism	Serum thyroid-stimulating hormone
Dyslipidemia	Fasting total cholesterol, triglycerides, high-density lipoprotein
Periodic/sleep apnea	Sleep studies for oxygen desaturation ENT exam for upper airway obstruction

*Some patients relate histories suggesting unusual energy efficiency, i.e., inability to lose weight despite energy intakes well below their estimated requirements. However, studies conducted in clinical research center conditions provide no conclusive evidence that significant variations in efficiency of energy expenditure exist. Nevertheless, the use of indirect calorimetry may be helpful in some patients to document normal energy expenditure relative to their body size.

Complications

Obesity is the second-leading modifiable cause of death in the United States, trailing only deaths related to smoking. It may surpass smoking as the principal modifiable cause of mortality in the near future. However, not all obese persons have medical complications, and the comorbidities of obesity are not evenly distributed among obese persons. Consequently, one cannot assume that an obese person will have a comorbid condition. Many other factors such as family history, levels of physical activity and fitness, and distribution of body fat contribute to the presence or absence of comorbid conditions. In particular, increased total body fatness is more likely to cause diseases associated with increased mechanical load on the joints or small muscle groups, whereas increased intra-abdominal fat is more strongly associated with cardiovascular and metabolic disease risk. In distinguishing the contribution of obesity *per se* to overall mortality, recent studies suggest that weight loss for the treatment of obesity is more likely to reduce mortality when comorbid conditions such as diabetes, hyperlipidemia, or hypertension are present. The following diseases and metabolic disorders have been associated with obesity.

Osteoarthritis

Osteoarthritis of the weight-bearing joints is more prevalent in obese persons. There is also increased likelihood of osteoarthritis in the non–weight-bearing joints, suggesting that the arthritis may not be simply a direct result of mechanical overload. Regardless of whether obesity is the direct cause of the joint disease, it aggravates joint symptoms, exacerbates postural faults, and complicates treatment.

Cancer

Obesity has been associated with increased risk for developing and dying from cancers of the colon and rectum, esophagus, liver, pancreas, kidney, gallbladder, uterus, postmenopausal breast, cervix, ovary, stomach, and prostate gland as well as non-Hodgkin's lymphoma and multiple myeloma. One potential mechanism relates to increased insulin resistance and resulting chronic hyperinsulinemia. As adiposity increases, adipocytes release more free fatty acids, tumor necrosis factor-alpha, and other adipokines that lead to increased circulating insulin and to increased bioavailability of insulin-like growth factor 1, which inhibits apoptosis and promotes cell proliferation in a number of tissues.

Coronary Artery Disease

In general, obese persons are at increased risk for developing coronary artery disease. However, it is unclear whether uncomplicated obesity is an independent risk factor for coronary artery disease in the absence of comorbid conditions such as diabetes, hyperlipidemia, and hypertension. Almost 4 decades of observation of the Framingham cohort suggest that body weight is a significant predictor of heart disease, independent of other standard risk factors, although not all studies support this conclusion. One important reason this finding is not consistent across all studies is that there may not be adequate control for the confounding effect of smoking. Typically, individuals who smoke have lower BMIs but higher rates of coronary artery disease.

Diabetes and Hyperinsulinemia

There is a positive association between degree and duration of obesity and risk for diabetes mellitus. The prevalence of diabetes is increased about 10-fold with moderate obesity and as much as 30-fold with extreme obesity. Elevated plasma insulin levels are uniformly found in obese individuals, in both the fasting and glucose-stimulated states, reflecting insulin resistance. Despite this, not all obese individuals become diabetic. It is likely that obesity only causes diabetes in individuals who are otherwise predisposed. The relationships between obesity and insulin resistance and diabetes are further detailed in Chapters 16 (Metabolic Syndrome) and 18 (Diabetes).

Hepatobiliary Disease

Obesity increases the risk of gallstone formation, probably by increasing fasting and residual gallbladder volumes with resultant bile stasis, and increasing cholesterol production and bile cholesterol saturation, which enhances cholesterol crystal nucleation. Women are approximately twice as likely as men to develop gallstones. On average, about 1% to 2% of obese women develop newly symptomatic stones each year. There is no threshold of body weight above which stones occur; i.e., even a moderate increase in weight can increase risk. From data collected among women, severe obesity increases risk of gallstone formation more than sixfold. Individuals who gradually reduce to a normal body weight normalize their risk for gallstones. By contrast, rapid weight loss increases the risk of stone formation during the period of active dieting by as much as 15- to 25-fold over that of the nondieting obese population. This problem is discussed further in a later section, Treatment.

Steatosis (fat accumulation within the liver) is reported to occur to some degree in as many as 88% of obese individuals. Of greater pathologic significance is steatohepatitis, which is fatty liver with the presence of a necroinflammatory component and possible fibrosis. This latter condition, known as nonalcoholic steatohepatitis (NASH), is a very common form of hepatitis, particularly in obese patients. NASH can progress to cirrhosis in up to 20% of patients and is now thought to be the leading cause of cryptogenic cirrhosis. The etiology of NASH is unclear; however, it is typically associated with obesity, hyperlipidemia, and diabetes mellitus. The diagnosis of NASH is made when a liver biopsy shows histologic features consistent with steatohepatitis, in the absence of a significant history of alcohol intake and negative serologies for hepatitis B and C. Serum aminotransferase levels are elevated in approximately 90 percent of patients with NASH. Although there are no proven therapies for NASH, lifestyle modification and weight loss are recommended and can result in normalization of liver enzymes and liver histology.

Hyperlipidemia

Serum triglyceride levels tend to be higher in obese individuals and HDL cholesterol levels tend to be lower. Total serum cholesterol levels are not consistently correlated with body fatness. Weight reduction generally improves serum cholesterol and triglyceride levels significantly during the active period of dieting, but the effect is largely due to energy restriction. During weight loss, increased intakes of polyunsaturated and monounsaturated fats and increased levels of physical activity act to increase HDL, while substitution of fat with refined grains and intake of *trans* fat lead to a decrease in HDL. Upon achieving a stable, reduced body weight, lipid levels partially rebound but tend to remain at an improved level as long as the weight loss is maintained.

Hypertension

In population studies there is a significant association between body weight and blood pressure. In the Framingham Heart Study, excess body weight accounted for 26% and 28% of the cases of hypertension in men and women, respectively. The relationship between increased body weight and blood pressure begins near a BMI of 25 kg/m^2. It is hypothesized that the physiologic link may be insulin resistance. As body weight increases, increased insulin levels promote sodium and water retention, expanding intravascular volume. The increase in intravascular volume and cardiac output without a concomitant decrease in systemic vascular resistance leads to elevated blood pressure. Weight reduction generally improves blood pressure levels, and its effects can be additive to other antihypertensive measures including sodium reduction and other dietary changes, physical activity, and medications. Maintenance of weight loss is associated with sustained blood pressure reduction.

Respiratory Problems

The obesity-hypoventilation or pickwickian syndrome is characterized by marked degrees of obesity, somnolence, periodic apnea (especially during sleep), chronic hypoxemia and hypercapnia (CO_2 retention), and secondary polycythemia. The explanations for the inadequate ventilation and reduced functional lung volume are not clear, although there appear to be decreased efficiency of respiratory muscles, reduced respiratory compliance, decreased ventilatory response to CO_2, and increased pulmonary dead space and atelectasis. Complications include pulmonary artery constriction resulting in pulmonary hypertension and right heart failure. Even a moderate weight reduction can reverse the hypoventilation syndrome. Periodic apnea can be caused by intermittent upper airway obstruction distinct from the alveolar hypoventilation syndrome. Such obstruction often responds to appropriate treatment, including surgical therapy, continuous positive airway pressure, and oral appliances designed to maintain airway patency during sleep.

Complications Associated with Increased Intra-abdominal Fat

Body fat distribution is a better predictor of the health hazards of obesity than is the absolute amount of body fat. Individuals with an upper body fat pattern, reflecting an excess of intra-abdominal or visceral fat, have significantly greater risk for diabetes, hypertension, hypertriglyceridemia, ischemic heart disease, some cancers, and death from all causes. The effect of intra-abdominal fat appears to be separate from that of total body fat *per se*. Waist circumference is a practical method for assessing body fat pattern (see section on Clinical Assessment of the Obese Patient earlier in this chapter).

Treatment

Overview

Not all persons desiring to lose weight should do so, and not all treatment programs can be equally endorsed. Table 17–5 offers several criteria to consider in selecting

Table 17–5	**CRITERIA FOR SELECTING WEIGHT CONTROL PROGRAMS**
Criteria	**Comments**
Patient selection	*Special attention if:* History of other eating disorders (anorexia nervosa, bulimia) *Avoid treatment:* Pregnant or lactating patients Patients with BMI <20 kg/m²
Weight loss claims	*Look for:* Prescribed rate of weight loss <1.5% or 1.5 kg/week Direct medical supervision for faster rates of weight loss Outcome data of ≥1 year post-treatment
Therapeutic approach	*Look for:* Team skilled in diet, exercise, and behavioral techniques Diet emphasizing self-selection of foods from conventional food supply for long-term weight maintenance Program of physical activity geared to individual needs Behavioral modification and psychosocial support
Medical supervision	*Recommended:* If obesity-related comorbidities exist If diet provides <800 kcal/day

a weight control program. For additional information, see the Suggested Readings for *Weighing the Options,* a report prepared by the National Academy of Sciences' Institute of Medicine.

Just as with other chronic conditions such as hypertension or diabetes, obesity must be treated with long-term goals and treatment plans. It cannot be corrected by short-term interventions, but requires ongoing effort and long-term support to help the individual establish and maintain control of the disorder. The goals are to establish permanent changes in eating habits and physical activity that become mutually supportive and self-reinforcing.

Safe Rate of Weight Loss

A safe rate of weight loss can be recommended on the basis of risk for gallstone formation because it is one of the few objective measures of morbidity associated with various rates of weight loss. Obese persons may transiently compound their risk during the period of active weight loss while attempting to achieve a lower-risk, nonobese state. Active weight loss results in the formation of new gallstones within just 4 weeks, and rapid rates of weight loss appear to enhance stone formation independently of the severity of obesity. Longer *periods* of weight loss increase risk in a linear fashion; however, faster *rates* of weight loss increase risk exponentially. On average, losing less than 1.5 kg/week is associated with gallstone development in fewer than 10% of dieters, but losing more than 2 kg/week results in stone formation in more than 25% of dieters. Therefore, it is recommended that weekly weight loss not exceed 1.5 kg, or about 1.5% of body weight.

Because resting energy expenditure varies significantly between individuals, accurate estimation of REE can have significant implications for prescribing appropriate calorie levels for weight loss. Total energy expenditure is the product of REE and a physical activity factor of 1.2 to 1.4. Using the estimated total energy expenditure, an energy deficit of 500 to 1000 kcal/d can be prescribed to achieve 1 to 2 lb of weight loss per week. REE is typically estimated using equations that include height, weight, age, and some adjustment for gender (see Chapter 11 for the Harris-Benedict equations). However, using the published equations, it is very difficult to predict the REE of free-living individuals within ±10% of measured REE. Several experts have recommended avoiding the use of equations to estimate REE given their lack of accuracy and the possibility of setting up false expectations for weight loss.[6] A simple approach for prescribing energy intake levels based on initial weight is suggested in Table 17–6.

Weight Cycling

Weight cycling or "yo-yo dieting" refers to repeated bouts of weight loss and regain without maintaining a

Table 17-6	SUGGESTED ENERGY INTAKE FOR A REDUCED–CALORIE DIET[6]
Initial Body Weight (lb)	**Energy Intake (kcal/d)**
150–199	1000
200–249	1200
250–299	1500
300–349	1800
≥350	2000

From Klein ST, Wadden T, Sugerman HJ, et al: AGA technical review on obesity. Gastroenterology 123(3):882–932, 2002.

lower weight. Unquestionably, weight cycling causes frustration on the parts of both the patient and therapist. However, it is less clear that repeated weight loss/regain cycles are hazardous to health or that they adversely affect parameters such as metabolic rate. A review by an NIH Obesity Task Force concluded that there is no convincing evidence that weight cycling has adverse effects on body composition, energy expenditure, risk factors for heart disease, or the effectiveness of future efforts at weight control. Obese individuals should not allow concerns about weight cycling to deter them from attempting to control their body weight.

Dietary Approach

The dietary approach used to achieve weight loss and long-term weight maintenance must satisfy three criteria: (1) it must be based on a sound scientific rationale, (2) it must be safe and nutritionally adequate, and (3) it must be practical and applicable to the patient's social and ethnic background so as to be conducive for long-term adherence.

Very-Low-Calorie Diets

These diets are designed to provide severe energy restrictions (less than 800 kcal/day) but sufficient protein to minimize loss of lean body mass. Protein losses tend to be less than losses associated with fasting but often continue to occur. The major concern about these diets is that they induce rapid weight loss that increases the risk of gallstone formation. They are sometimes useful for patients who are at substantial health risk from severe obesity (e.g., alveolar hypoventilation syndrome), where rapid weight loss is critical. When rapid weight loss is critical and a very low calorie diet is used, direct medical supervision is important.

Moderately-Low-Calorie, Balanced Diets

Most persons desiring weight loss may use these diets. Although they can have different characteristics, in general they should meet the three criteria outlined above, should provide at least 800 kcal/day (most often, 1000 to 1200 kcal), and should emphasize low-fat, high-complex-carbohydrate foods. One example is the *EatRight* Program developed at the University of Alabama at Birmingham (http://www.uab.edu/eatright).[7] Using the concept of time-calorie displacement, which involves ingestion of high-bulk, low-energy-density foods, displacing energy-dense foods, this dietary approach is based on the spectrum of energy densities of the food groups shown in Box 17–4. The low-energy-density, low-fat, high-bulk, slow-eating food groups to the right of the chart are emphasized.

Patients are given a list of foods in each category from which they can choose items according to their preferences. Most patients who are moderately overweight

---

BOX 17–4 *EatRight* Approach to Weight Control

High-calorie Low-bulk Fast-eating		[Eat "right"] ———————→		Low-Calorie High-bulk Slow-eating	
	Fat	*Meat/ Dairy*	*Starch*	*Fruit*	*Vegetables*
kcal/oz:	225	75	50	15	10
kcal/serving:	45	110	80–100	60	25
Servings/day:	Maximum 3–5	3–5	4–8	Minimum 3	Minimum 4

are instructed to eat the number of servings indicated under each food group. Fats are limited to a *maximum* of 3 to 5 servings per day, with no lower limit, whereas the fruit and vegetable prescriptions are a *minimum* of 3 and 4 servings per day, respectively, with no upper limit. By encouraging liberal amounts of complex carbohydrates, moderate amounts of low-fat meats and dairy products, and only small amounts of fat, satiety and nutritional adequacy are achieved with a low energy intake and without counting calories. Up to 200 kcal/week of sweets and snack foods are permitted as "special occasion" foods. Studies of the *EatRight* program indicate that it is nutritionally adequate, safe, and effective over the long-term. Participants lose an average of 6 to 8 kg by the end of the 12-week group program, and overall, half of participants maintain their reduced weight or continue to lose weight 2 years later, while only one quarter regain all their lost weight. It is also ideal for obesity prevention, and with very minor modifications it is appropriate for obese children and diabetic patients.

Any dietary approach to weight control must emphasize lifelong changes in eating patterns rather than short-term use of diets. The term *diet* implies temporary intervention, whereas the major challenge in treating obesity is not losing weight but maintaining weight loss.

Low-Carbohydrate Diets

As early as 1869 when William Banting published his "Letter on Corpulence," which described his successful weight loss of 46 pounds in 1 year by avoiding such items as "bread, butter, milk, sugar, beer, and potatoes," low-carbohydrate diets have been resurfacing in various forms. Most diets considered to be low-carbohydrate typically have less than 50 grams per day of carbohydrate intake with approximately 55% to 65% of calories from fat sources and 25% to 35% of calories from protein sources.

Public interest in low-carbohydrate diets stimulated a number of scientists to examine their effectiveness for weight loss. To date, we know that the initial weight loss with low-carbohydrate intake is more rapid than that seen with a calorically matched, low-fat, balanced diet. This difference persists through 6 months of intervention; however, at 1 year, there are no significant differences in weight loss between the two types of diets. Many of the improvements in cardiovascular risk factors seen with low-fat diets are also seen with low-carbohydrate diets; the latter produce even better improvements in serum triglycerides and HDL cholesterol. The risk factor improvements are primarily a function of the amount of weight lost, but are also due in part to energy restriction and decreased intake of refined grains and sugars. It is unclear whether maintenance of this type of dietary pattern has long-term detrimental effects on bone health, lipids, development of vascular disease, and cancer risk as a result of low-fiber, low-calcium, high-fat, and high-protein intake. More research is needed on the long-term effectiveness and safety of low-carbohydrate diets.

Physical Activity

Physical activity should be included in weight-management programs, with the objectives of promoting fat loss while maintaining lean body mass and engendering permanent changes in lifestyle without putting individuals at risk.

Increasing physical activity without controlling energy intake is generally an ineffective means of losing weight. However, multiple studies have demonstrated that a program of routine physical activity is critical to long-term maintenance of weight loss. As a complement to energy intake restriction, increased physical activity provides the advantages of improving cardiovascular conditioning and insulin sensitivity and, according to some studies, maintaining muscle mass and bone density while weight is lost. Increased physical activity may best be achieved with a combination of regular exercises several times weekly plus daily "step-losing" activities. When routinely established, step-losing behaviors such as walking or climbing stairs instead of driving or using the elevator may be even more effective than programmed exercise in maintaining weight loss.

For obese persons, aerobic exercises such as walking, swimming, bicycling, and low-impact dance and exercise classes are recommended to minimize damage to weight-bearing joints. The recommendation to "do a little more of what you are doing right now" and keep daily records is a reasonable way to begin increasing physical activity in overweight persons. For the untrained, sedentary person, initially aiming for a pulse rate of 60% to 65% of maximum (220 minus the person's age) sustained for about 20 minutes several times a week is reasonable. Another rough guide is to be able to maintain a conversation but not be able to sing during the exercise. Table 17–7 lists energy expenditures to expect from selected physical activities.

Behavioral Modification and Psychosocial Support

Behavioral modification and psychosocial support should be included in weight-control programs to (1) focus on methods of acquiring new behaviors, not merely on descriptions of desired behaviors; (2) incorporate standard therapeutic modalities including self-monitoring and cognitive restructuring; and (3) provide guidelines for maintaining weight loss, such as resuming record-keeping if weight is regained, practicing controlled intake of "fear" foods, and utilizing family and social support systems.

Patients attempting to modify their diets and physical activity patterns frequently require therapy for psychological and social problems. Keeping detailed records of dietary intake, exercise, and emotional factors is an important aspect of weight control and appropriately focuses attention on *patterns* and *problems* rather than on pounds. An important aspect of behavioral support is to help the patient maintain a positive outlook and emphasize even small, positive behavioral changes rather than setbacks. What patients perceive as major

Table 17-7	ENERGY EXPENDITURES OF VARIOUS PHYSICAL ACTIVITIES (KCAL PER 10 MIN OF ACTIVITY)								
		Body Weight (kg/lbs)							
Activity	Level	70 155	80 175	90 200	100 220	115 255	125 275	135 300
Inactivity	Sitting, riding in car, watching TV	12	13	15	17	19	21	23
Inactivity	Standing (little movement)	29	33	38	42	48	52	56
Bicycling, stationary	Very light effort (50 W)	35	40	45	50	58	63	68
Bicycling, stationary	Light effort (100 W)	64	73	83	92	105	115	124
Bicycling, stationary	Moderate effort (150 W)	82	93	105	117	134	146	158
Bicycling, stationary	Vigorous effort (200 W)	123	140	158	175	201	219	236
Bicycling	<10 mph, leisured pace	47	53	60	67	77	83	90
Bicycling	10–11.9 mph, slow, light effort	70	80	90	100	115	125	135
Bicycling	12–13.9 mph, moderate effort	93	107	120	133	153	167	180
Bicycling	14–15.9 mph, fast, vigorous effort	117	133	150	167	192	208	225
Bicycling	16–19 mph, very fast pace	140	160	180	200	230	250	270
Bicycling	>20 mph, racing, not drafting	187	213	240	267	307	333	360
Conditioning exercise	Calisthenics, light workout	53	60	68	75	86	94	101
Conditioning exercise	Circuit training, general	93	107	120	133	153	167	180
Conditioning exercise	Weight lifting, light workout	35	40	45	50	58	63	68
Conditioning exercise	Weight lifting, vigorous effort	70	80	90	100	115	125	135
Conditioning exercise	Stair-treadmill ergometer, general	70	80	90	100	115	125	135
Conditioning exercise	Rowing, stationary ergometer, light effort (50 W)	41	47	53	58	67	73	79
Conditioning exercise	Rowing, stationary ergometer, moderate effort (100 W)	82	93	105	117	134	146	158

Category	Activity							
Conditioning exercise	Rowing, stationary ergometer, vigorous effort (150 W)	99	113	128	142	163	177	191
Conditioning exercise	Rowing, stationary ergometer, very vigorous effort (200 W)	140	160	180	200	230	250	270
Conditioning exercise	Water aerobics, calisthenics	47	53	60	67	77	83	90
Dancing	Aerobic, low-impact	58	67	75	83	96	104	112
Dancing	Aerobic, high-impact	82	93	105	117	134	145	158
Home activities	Sweeping, vacuuming, playing with children	29	33	38	42	48	52	56
Home activities	Cleaning, vigorous effort	53	60	68	75	86	94	101
Home repair	Carpentry, painting, wall papering	53	60	68	75	86	94	101
Walking	<2 mph, very slow, strolling	23	27	30	33	38	42	45
Walking	3 mph, moderate pace	41	47	53	58	67	73	79
Walking	4 mph, very brisk pace	47	53	60	67	77	83	90
Running	5 mph (12 min mile)	93	107	120	133	153	167	180
Running	6 mph (10 min mile)	117	133	150	167	192	208	225
Running	8 mph (7.5 min mile)	158	180	203	225	259	281	304
Running	10 mph (6 min mile)	187	213	240	267	307	335	360
Skiing, snow	Downhill, moderate effort	70	80	90	100	115	125	135
Skiing, snow	Downhill, vigorous, racing	117	133	150	167	192	208	225
Swimming	Freestyle, slow	93	107	120	133	153	167	180
Swimming	Freestyle, fast	117	133	150	167	192	208	225
Sports, other	Basketball, nongame	70	80	90	100	115	125	135
Sports, other	Golf	53	60	68	75	86	94	101
Sports, other	Handball	140	160	180	200	230	250	270
Sports, other	Tennis	82	93	105	117	134	146	158
Yard work	Gardening, mowing	58	67	75	83	96	104	112

Derived from Ainsworth BE, Haskell WL, Whitt MC: Compendium of physical activities: an update of activity codes and MET intensities. *Med Sci Sports Exer* 32(9):S498-S516, 2000.

lapses are often no more than exaggerated responses to temporary indiscretions. Reminding patients that they can enjoy a limited amount of "special occasion" foods, such as desserts and snack items, helps to relieve the feeling of guilt from eating such foods and avoid relapsing into old habits. This is needed to prevent the all-or-none or on/off attitude toward dieting in which patients feel like failures if they eat prohibited foods. In addition, it is wise to encourage patients to practice controlled intake of highly desired foods that they fear they cannot eat in limited amounts, rather than to suggest total avoidance of the food. This may need to be done in a supervised clinic setting.

Drug Therapy

Drugs currently available for weight loss fall into two classes: those that both suppress appetite and stimulate energy expenditure, and those that promote malabsorption.[8] Stimulants increase the release of norepinephrine from synaptic granules. Appetite suppressants typically inhibit reuptake of neurotransmitters at synaptic clefts in the brain. As a group, their primary side effects include increases in heart rate and blood pressure, making them difficult to use in many obese patients. Sibutramine is the only drug in this class approved for long-term use in weight control. Stimulants such as phenteramine and benzphetamine are only approved for short-term use (less than 12 weeks), and patients can develop tolerance, or dependence, or both, to the medications. Orlistat, an inhibitor of pancreatic lipase that results in decreased digestion and absorption of fat, is the only other drug approved for long-term use by the FDA, at the time of writing. Decreased absorption of fat results in loose, fatty stools and flatulence, particularly if the diet consumed is not low in fat. Vitamin supplementation is often necessary due to reduced absorption of the fat-soluble vitamins (A, D, E, and K).

Pharmacotherapy is indicated for persons with a BMI 30 kg/m^2 or greater or those with a BMI of at least 27 kg/m^2 and associated comorbidities or risk factors.

The result of these medications on weight loss ranges from 2 to 10 kg. It is important to note that the successful implementation of any drug therapy is predicated on the implementation of a moderate-calorie, balanced diet that is low in fat, and consistent physical activity. Without these behaviors in place, the use of medications is futile, and in the case of orlistat, could result in negative side-effects.

Surgical Procedures

Bariatric surgery can be offered to individuals who have been extremely obese (BMI >40 kg/m^2) for at least 3 years, have serious medical conditions related to their obesity (with BMI >35 kg/m^2), have failed at attempts to lose weight through other means, and are judged able to tolerate the procedure.[9] Operations that have proven effective in producing sustained weight loss include: (1) those that restrict the volume of the stomach, such as banded gastroplasty; (2) those that restrict stomach volume and bypass some of the absorptive capacity of the small intestine, such as the Roux-en-Y gastric bypass; and (3) the biliopancreatic diversion with or without duodenal switch. Complications include vomiting, wound infections, marginal ulceration, and death. The amount of weight loss can be substantial; however, many patients do not reduce their BMIs to below 30 kg/m^2 because of their initial level of obesity. Despite changes in stomach volume and absorptive capacity, the long-term mainte-nance of weight loss is likely to depend on maintaining changes in eating behavior and physical activity. As more surgeries are completed, it is becoming apparent that weight regain is a significant concern for post-operative patients. Nevertheless, the improvements in obesity-related diseases and cardiovascular risk factors can be quite dramatic. Improvements in blood pressure, glucose control, and hyperlipidemia often precede the initiation of dramatic weight loss, leading to speculations that other neurohormonal mechanisms may be operative. Improvements in these risk factors have been shown to persist for up to 10 years following surgery.

REFERENCES

1. Hedley AA, Ogden CL, Johnson CL, et al: Prevalence of overweight and obesity among US children, adolescents, and adults, 1999–2002. JAMA 291(23):2847–2850, 2004.
2. Mokdad AH, Ford ES, Bowman BA, et al: Prevalence of obesity, diabetes, and obesity-related health risk factors, 2001. JAMA 289(1):76–79, 2003.
3. Finkelstein EA, Fiebelkorn IC, Wang G, et al: State-level estimates of annual medical expenditures attributable to obesity. Obes Res 12(1):18–24, 2004.
4. Wadden TA, Brownell KD, Foster GD: Obesity: Responding to the global epidemic. J Consult Clin Psychol 70(3):510–525, 2002.
5. Damcott CM, Sack P, Shuldiner AR: The genetics of obesity. Endocrinol Metab Clin North Am 32(4):761–786, 2003.
6. Klein S, Wadden T, Sugerman HJ: AGA technical review on obesity. Gastroenterology 123(3):882–932, 2002.
7. Weinsier RL, Wilson NP, Morgan SL, et al: EatRight, Lose Weight: Seven Simple Steps. Birmingham, Ala, Oxmoor House, 1997.
8. Li Z, Maglione M, Tu W, et al: Meta-analysis: Pharmacologic treatment of obesity. Ann Intern Med 42:532–546, 2005.
9. Maggard MA, Shugarman LR, Suttorp M, et al: Meta-analysis: Surgical treatment of obesity. Ann Intern Med 42:547–559, 2005.

SUGGESTED READINGS

Bray GA: Medical consequences of obesity. J Clin Endocrinol Metab 89(6):2583–2589, 2004.

Klein S, Burke LE, Bray GA, et al: Clinical implications of obesity with specific focus on cardiovascular disease: A statement for professionals from the American Heart Association Council on Nutrition, Physical Activity, and Metabolism: Endorsed by the American College of Cardiology Foundation. Circulation 110(18):2952–2967, 2004.

McTigue KM, Harris R, Hemphill B, et al: Screening and interventions for obesity in adults: Summary of the evidence for the U.S. Preventive Services Task Force. Ann Intern Med 139:933–949, 2003.

National Heart, Lung, Blood Institute Obesity Education Initiative and the North American Association for the Study of Obesity: Practical Guide to the Identification, Evaluation, and Treatment of Overweight and Obesity in Adults. NIH Publication Number 00-4084, 2000.

Thomas PR (ed): Weighing the options: Criteria for evaluating weight-management programs, Food and Nutrition Board, Institute of Medicine. Washington, DC, National Academy Press, 1995.

WEB SITES

American Obesity Association, http://www.obesity.org/
American Society for Bariatric Surgery, http://www.asbs.org/
NAASO, The Obesity Society, http://naaso.org/
NIH Obesity Research, http://obesityresearch.nih.gov/
NIH Weight Control Information Network, http://win.niddk.nih.gov/
UAB *EatRight* Weight Management Program, http://www.uab.edu/eatright

18

Diabetes

JAMES M. SHIKANY, DRPH, PA

Diabetes mellitus affects approximately 17 million persons in the United States, although up to one third of those may be undiagnosed. Diabetes comprises a group of disorders of glucose metabolism with a common phenotype of hyperglycemia. The pathogenesis of diabetes involves a deficiency of insulin secretion, defects in insulin action, or both. Type 1 diabetes, which accounts for 5% to 10% of diabetes cases, is caused by predominantly immune-mediated pancreatic islet β-cell destruction and is characterized by absolute insulin deficiency. Type 2 diabetes, which accounts for 90% to 95% of cases, is characterized by insulin resistance and a defect in compensatory insulin secretion, resulting in relative rather than absolute insulin deficiency.

Diabetes is the leading cause of blindness, amputations, and end-stage renal disease in the United States. Coronary heart disease (CHD) is the main cause of death in persons with diabetes. Careful dietary management can improve quality of life and lessen the risk of complications in these patients. Regarding nutritional management of diabetes, multiple misconceptions and recommendations with little supporting evidence abound. An example is the endorsement of specially formulated "diabetic" or "dietetic" foods for which there are is no evidence of significant clinical benefit for important diabetic outcomes. This chapter will focus on evidence-based recommendations for the nutritional management of diabetes.

Medical Nutrition Therapy for Persons with Diabetes

Nutrition therapy is essential for successful diabetes management. The American Diabetes Association (ADA) is the main advisory body that develops guidelines for the treatment of diabetes. The ADA has promulgated the goals of medical nutrition therapy shown in Box 18-1 for all persons with diabetes.

The advent of home blood glucose monitoring has made it possible for persons with diabetes to directly observe the effects of changes in their diets and physical activity on blood glucose control. As such, regular home glucose monitoring is an important adjunct to diet and exercise in the treatment of this disease.

Carbohydrates

Perhaps no other dietary component in the nutritional management of diabetes is as misunderstood

---

BOX 18-1   Goals of Medical Nutrition Therapy for Persons with Diabetes[1]

Attain and maintain optimal metabolic outcomes, including:
   Blood glucose levels in the normal range or as close to
      normal as is safely possible, to prevent or reduce the risk
      for complications of diabetes
   A lipid and lipoprotein profile that reduces the risk for
      macrovascular disease
   Blood pressure levels that reduce the risk for vascular disease
Prevent and treat the chronic complications of diabetes.
   Modify nutrient intake and lifestyle as appropriate for the
   prevention and treatment of obesity, dyslipidemia,
   cardiovascular disease, hypertension, and nephropathy.
Improve health through healthy food choices and physical activity.
Address individual nutritional needs, taking into consideration
   personal and cultural preferences and lifestyle while respecting
   the individual's wishes and willingness to change.

From American Diabetes Association: Nutrition principles and
   recommendations in diabetes. Diabetes Care 27(Suppl 1):
   S36–S46, 2004.

as carbohydrate. Severe restriction of dietary carbohydrates in diabetes is not indicated. To the contrary, moderate intake of carbohydrates should be permitted in most persons with diabetes. Within the total caloric recommendation based on a person's optimal weight and physical activity level, carbohydrates should be 45% to 60% of total energy intake.

The classification of carbohydrates as "simple sugars" and "complex carbohydrates" is imprecise and should be discarded in favor of the more meaningful terms, sugars (monosaccharides and disaccharides), starch (glucose polymers), and fiber (nondigestible carbohydrate). There is little, if any, evidence supporting the long held belief that the intake of sugars causes adverse metabolic effects compared to the consumption of starches in persons with diabetes. In fact, there is evidence that sugars raise blood glucose and insulin concentrations less than isocaloric amounts of starches (i.e., have lower *glycemic index* values; the glycemic index is a ranking of carbohydrate-containing foods based on their postprandial blood glucose responses). As such, sucrose and sucrose-containing foods need not be overly restricted in diabetes, as previously believed. However, although it is clear that carbohydrates produce differing glycemic responses, there is currently no convincing evidence that substituting low- for high-glycemic index carbohydrates will affect long-term glycemic control. Until such evidence becomes available, the total amount of digestible carbohydrate is considered more important than the source or type of carbohydrate in this respect.

Dietary fiber intake has been shown to be beneficial in the management of diabetes. Soluble fibers such as pectins, gums, mucilages, and β-glucan found in such foods as apples, oranges, legumes, and oats, may be particularly useful. Viscous soluble fiber tends to blunt postprandial glycemic and insulinemic responses primarily by inhibiting starch hydrolysis and glucose absorption, and to a lesser extent by delaying gastric emptying. Soluble fiber may also reduce fasting glucose levels by improving insulin sensitivity. A high fiber intake also has indirect benefits such as promoting satiety and is associated with small reductions in serum cholesterol and blood pressure. High-fiber foods also provide vitamins, minerals, and other substances that promote good health. A total fiber intake of 14 g/1000 kcal from foods is recommended, of which a significant portion should be soluble fiber.

While nutritive sweetener alternatives to sucrose have been promoted as beneficial in persons with diabetes, their value has not been proven. Although fructose produces a lower glycemic response when substituted for sucrose or starch in the diet, its use as a sweetening agent should be avoided because of possible adverse effects on blood lipids. Naturally occurring fructose in foods such as fruits does not need to be restricted. Corn syrup, fruit juice, honey, molasses, dextrose, and maltose offer no clear benefits over sucrose. Sugar alcohols, such as sorbitol and mannitol, produce a lower glycemic response than sucrose, but are not non-caloric, and osmotic diarrhea may occur with high intakes. Non-nutritive sweeteners including saccharin, aspartame, acesulfame potassium, and sucralose may play a role as weight-loss adjuncts in persons with diabetes, especially when used in frequently consumed beverages.

In summary, the primary sources of carbohydrate in the diet should be whole grains, fruits, vegetables, and low-fat dairy products. Sucrose does not need to be overly restricted as a sweetener because of concerns over aggravating hyperglycemia, although its contribution to energy intake should not be ignored. The recommendation to the general population to limit intake of added sugars is particularly relevant for persons with diabetes who are trying to meet other carbohydrate intake goals (i.e., fiber) while staying within a calorie range that promotes weight maintenance or weight loss. The use of other sweeteners by persons with diabetes is of dubious value, with the possible exception of non-nutritive sweeteners in weight-loss efforts.

Fats

Diabetes is a major risk factor for cardiovascular disease. Lipid abnormalities are twice as common in persons with Type 2 diabetes compared to those without diabetes, due in part to a greater prevalence of obesity and insulin resistance/hyperinsulinemia. Elevated triglycerides and, to a lesser extent, low-density lipoprotein (LDL)-cholesterol, as well as depressed high-density lipoprotein (HDL)-cholesterol are common in persons with diabetes, especially when glycemic control is poor. Serum lipid and lipoprotein goals for persons with diabetes are: LDL-cholesterol <100 mg/dL (<70 mg/dL with established CHD); HDL-cholesterol >40 mg/dL (>50 mg/dL may be appropriate in women); and triglycerides < 150 mg/dL.

Clinical trial data on recommended levels of fat intake specific to persons with diabetes are lacking. Therefore, recommendations are the same as for the general population, or 20% to 35% of total energy. Overly fat-restricted diets have no proven benefit for persons with diabetes, and the concomitant high-carbohydrate intake may lead to an increase in triglycerides and a reduction in HDL-cholesterol. Instead, more attention should be given to the types of fat consumed. It should be remembered, however, that fat is more energy-dense than other macronutrients, and this can impair weight-loss efforts.

Saturated fats are the primary serum cholesterol-raising fats in the diet, and should be limited to <10% of total energy intake (<7% if LDL-cholesterol is ≥100 mg/dL). The most important dietary sources of saturated fats are meats, full-fat dairy products, and tropical oils. Lean meats, low- or non-fat dairy products, and non-tropical cooking oils should be substituted. Dietary cholesterol intake should be <300 mg/day (<200 mg/d if LDL-cholesterol is ≥100 mg/dL). The major sources of dietary cholesterol are eggs, meats, and full-fat dairy products.

Polyunsaturated fats (supplied primarily by plant oils) tend to reduce total and LDL-cholesterol levels when substituted for saturated fat. N-3 polyunsaturated fatty acids in particular (found in fatty fish, soybean and canola oils, and flax seed), reduce triglyceride levels and have been shown to have cardiopreventive effects in the general population (including antiplatelet aggregation, anti-inflammatory, antiarrythmic, and antihypertensive effects). They can therefore be recommended to persons with diabetes. Intake of polyunsaturated fat should be in the range of 7 % to 10 % of total energy intake, with an emphasis on n-3 fatty acids. While n-3 fatty acid supplements and concentrated fish oils have been shown to lower triglycerides in persons with diabetes, their potential deleterious effects on LDL-cholesterol and glycemic control limit their usefulness. However, the beneficial effects of n-3 fatty acids on triglycerides can be attained without adverse effects on hyperglycemia if intake does not exceed 3 g per day.

Cis monounsaturated fatty acids (MUFAs) found in olive oil, canola oil, and nuts have several properties that may be beneficial in persons with diabetes. When substituted for saturated fatty acids, MUFAs lower serum total and LDL-cholesterol to an even greater degree than polyunsaturated fatty acids. In addition, high-MUFA diets result in improved insulin sensitivity and glycemic control, lower triglycerides, and higher levels of HDL-cholesterol compared to low-saturated-fat, high-carbohydrate diets. MUFAs may also reduce LDL oxidation, as well as intra-arterial inflammation. Overall, replacement of saturated fats with MUFAs is associated with a greater reduction in CHD risk than that obtained by replacement of saturated fats with carbohydrates. Accordingly, MUFAs should compose 15 % to 20 % of total energy intake, with carbohydrates and MUFAs together composing 60 % to 70 % of total energy intake.

Trans fatty acids are created primarily through the hydrogenation of polyunsaturated fatty acids. They are found mainly in processed foods such as shortening, margarines, and baked and deep-fried foods. *Trans* fats not only increase LDL-cholesterol, but also decrease HDL-cholesterol levels. Some studies suggest adverse effects of *trans* fats on insulin sensitivity. Accordingly, the intake of *trans* fats should be limited as much as possible. Many food companies are currently reducing or eliminating the use of hydrogenated oils in their products.

Protein

In Type 1 diabetes, severe insulin deficiency may result in a loss of body protein, increasing the dietary protein requirement. In most persons with Type 2 diabetes, however, severe insulin deficiency does not occur, and the protein requirement is generally similar to persons without diabetes. However, a chronic hyperglycemic state can contribute to increased protein turnover, increasing the protein requirement. Because most adults in the United States consume at least 50% more protein than the Recommended Dietary Allowance, persons with diabetes are generally protected against protein malnutrition. In well-controlled Type 2 diabetes, ingested protein does not increase plasma glucose concentrations.

There is no evidence that protein intake in the recommended range is associated with the development of diabetic nephropathy, or that restricting protein in persons with diabetes will prevent or delay the onset of renal insufficiency. The recommendation for protein intake in the absence of renal insufficiency is 0.8 g/kg of body weight/day. In most persons this amounts to 10% to 20% of total enery intake. The risk of nephropathy associated with long-term protein intakes of >20% of total energy is not known; consequently, intakes above this level should be avoided.

Even with overt nephropathy, the benefits of decreasing protein intake are questionable. However, once the glomerular filtration rate (GFR) begins to decline (heralding the onset of renal insufficiency), decreasing protein intake may slow further decline in GFR in some patients. Therefore, protein intake should be reduced to 0.6 g/kg of body weight/day in the setting of renal insufficiency. More severe restrictions should be avoided because they may lead to protein deficiency with loss of lean body mass and symptoms including muscle weakness.

Energy and Body Weight

A minority of persons with Type 2 diabetes have normal body weights (body mass index [BMI] <25 kg/m^2). For these patients, efforts should be directed at maintaining weight and preventing weight gain. Unfortunately, the majority of persons with Type 2 diabetes are overweight

(BMI ≥25 kg/m^2) or obese (BMI ≥30 kg/m^2). A high proportion of excess body fat in these persons is intra-abdominal (visceral), which has been associated with multiple adverse metabolic and physiologic outcomes, including insulin resistance, impaired glucose tolerance, dyslipidemia, and hypertension. Therefore, weight loss is imperative in most persons with diabetes.

Even modest weight loss, as little as 5% to 10% of body weight, has beneficial effects on many of the adverse metabolic and physiologic effects listed above, including improved insulin sensitivity and measures of glycemia and dyslipidemia, and reduced blood pressure. In addition, modest weight loss can restore the efficacy of oral hypoglycemic agents that have lost their effectiveness (secondary failure), and may obviate the need for initiating or increasing doses of insulin. Weight loss has been associated with increased life expectancy in persons with Type 2 diabetes. Energy restriction *per se* improves glycemic control within days of initiation, independent of weight loss.

While the benefits of weight loss in persons with diabetes have been demonstrated in clinical trials, the long-term effectiveness of weight-loss interventions outside of research settings has yet to be documented. As in the general population, many persons with diabetes regain lost weight. There are several reasons for failure of weight loss programs: long-term adherence to the strict dietary requirements of many programs is challenging; not all obese persons with diabetes respond as expected to a hypocaloric diet; and maintenance of weight is difficult once the weight-loss goal is achieved and the program, with its associated support structure, is terminated.

Nevertheless, these challenges should not deter clinicians from recommending weight loss when indicated in persons with diabetes because it offers significant benefits. The selection of a weight-loss program is critical. Programs and plans that result in gradual weight loss should be promoted over those that promise rapid, unrealistic reductions. Individualized or group dietary counseling (behavioral modification) should be included in weight-loss programs, as well as regular physical activity. Generally, a gradual decrease in body weight (i.e., 1 to 2 kg/month) is more likely to result in sustained weight loss. This translates into a reduction from usual intake of 250 to 500 kcal/day. Fat is probably the most important nutrient to restrict in weight-loss efforts because of the increased energy intake associated with diets high in fat. Consuming a low-energy-density diet promotes increased satiety, decreased energy intake, and weight loss in healthy persons. Currently, the multicenter study Look AHEAD (Action for Health in Diabetes), sponsored by the National Institutes of Health, is underway to evaluate the long-term effectiveness of weight loss using a low-fat diet and physical activity in obese persons with diabetes. Very-low-calorie diets (400 to 800 kcal/day) are an option for severe obesity. However, although these diets are safe when medically supervised and effective in the short-term, long-term efficacy is questionable due to their highly restrictive nature. Because weight loss and maintenance of weight loss can be difficult, the clinician should intervene with most patients to prevent further weight gain and impress upon them the important role that body weight plays in managing diabetes.

Sodium

Clinical trials of sodium restriction have not been conducted exclusively in persons with diabetes. Accordingly, the recommended Upper Limit (UL) for sodium intake in persons with diabetes is generally the same as for the general population, less than 2300 mg, or about 6 g (1 teaspoon) of table salt per day. Intake should be below 2000 mg per day in persons with diabetes with concomitant hypertension or nephropathy. Because 1600 mg per day of sodium meets the sodium requirement in most persons, intakes of 2000 to 2300 mg protect against sodium deficiency. The sodium/potassium ratio may be a critical factor in the development of hypertension. In order to promote adequate intake of potassium while minimizing sodium intake, the consumption of foods with a low sodium/potassium ratio, such as fresh fruits and vegetables, should be encouraged. Unprescribed potassium supplements should not be recommended, particularly in patients with chronic renal insufficiency, because of the possibility of excessive intake with potentially lethal effects.

Micronutrients

Several micronutrients have been reported to be deficient in persons with diabetes, including chromium, magnesium, zinc, and the antioxidant nutrients vitamin C, vitamin E, β-carotene, and selenium. However, clinical trial data demonstrating benefits of supplementing with these nutrients in persons with diabetes are lacking. As a result, vitamin and mineral supplementation is of dubious benefit except in cases of documented deficiency. An exception to this is calcium, for which the daily recommended intake of 1000 to 1500 mg per day is difficult to meet through diet alone. In all persons with diabetes, the intake of vitamins and minerals should be encouraged through natural food sources, most notably vegetables and fruits.

Alcohol

While alcohol intake can pose some problems in persons with diabetes, moderate intake can be allowed, provided some precautions are taken. Because alcohol is not metabolized to glucose in the body and inhibits gluconeogenesis, if it is consumed without food by persons on insulin or oral hypoglycemic therapy, hypoglycemia may result. However, if alcohol is consumed in moderation and with food, blood glucose levels are minimally affected when diabetes is well controlled. Moderate alcohol intake has been associated with a reduced incidence of CHD in observational studies of persons with diabetes. However, alcohol contributes 7 kcal/g and may impair weight-control efforts. Excessive intake also aggravates hypertriglyceridemia, and should be avoided in persons with pancreatitis, liver disease, advanced neuropathy, or history of abuse. If alcohol consumption is permitted, intake should be limited to two drinks per day for men and one drink per day for women. A drink is usually defined as 12 oz of beer, 5 oz of wine, or 1.5 oz of distilled spirits.

Exercise

Exercise should be encouraged in persons with Type 2 diabetes because of the potential substantial benefits to the metabolic derangements associated with the disease and lowered risk of cardiovascular disease. Regular physical activity improves insulin sensitivity and acutely reduces blood glucose levels, which may reduce the need for oral hypoglycemic medications and insulin. Because insulin resistance has been linked with dyslipidemia, hypertension, inflammation, and impaired fibrinolytic activity (see Chapter 16), regular exercise has the potential to positively impact these cardiovascular disease risk factors. Several studies have demonstrated a consistent beneficial effect of regular physical activity on carbohydrate metabolism and insulin sensitivity when the activity is performed at 50% to 80% VO_2max (the maximum amount of oxygen, in ml, one can use per kg of body weight per minute), 3 to 4 times a week for 30 to 60 minutes per session. Although physical activity has only modest effects on weight loss when not accompanied by a reduction in energy intake, it is an important adjunct for maintenance of weight loss.

Persons with Type 1 diabetes who do not have complications and have adequate blood glucose control can safely participate in all levels of physical activity. The hypoglycemia that can occur during or after physical activity can be avoided by knowledge of the previously measured glycemic response to the activity, careful self-monitoring of blood glucose levels, and the use of intensive insulin therapy, which allows for flexibility to make insulin dose adjustments for various activities.

Dietary and exercise recommendations for persons with diabetes are summarized in Box 18-2. See also Table 12-1 (Dietary Therapies for Specific Diagnoses) and Table 12-2 (Diabetic Exchanges).

BOX 18-2   Dietary and Exercise Recommendations
for Persons with Diabetes

Carbohydrate	45%–60% of total energy intake
Dietary fiber	14 g/1000 kcal
Total fat	20%–35% of total energy intake
Saturated fat	<10% of total energy intake
Polyunsaturated fat (emphasizing n-3)	7%–10% of total energy intake
Monounsaturated fat	15%–20% of total energy intake
Trans fat	As low as possible
Cholesterol	<300 mg/day
Protein	10%–20% of total energy intake
Absence of renal insufficiency	0.8 g/kg of body weight/day
Presence of renal insufficiency	0.6 g/kg of body weight/day
Energy	Maintain body mass index <25 kg/m^2
Sodium	<2300 mg/day
Calcium	1000–1300 mg/day
Alcohol	
Men	≤2 drinks/day
Women	≤1 drink/day
Exercise	30–60 minutes, 3–4 times/week

SUGGESTED READINGS

American Diabetes Association: Physical activity/exercise and diabetes. Diabetes Care 27 (Suppl 1):S58–S62, 2004.
Sheard NF, Clark NG, Brand-Miller JC, et al: Dietary carbohydrate (amount and type) in the prevention and management of diabetes. A statement by the American Diabetes Association. Diabetes Care 27:2266–2271, 2004.

WEB SITES

American Diabetes Association, http://www.diabetes.org
NIH-sponsored Look AHEAD clinical trial, http://www.niddk.nih.gov/patient/SHOW/lookahead.htm

19

Hypertension

JAMY D. ARD, MD

Approximately 50 million adults in the United States have hypertension (systolic blood pressure ≥140 mmHg or diastolic blood pressure ≥90 mmHg), a known risk factor for premature death from cardiovascular disease (CVD). Further, most adults in the United States are at increased risk for heart disease because their blood pressure (BP) is above the optimal level (120/80 mmHg), even if they do not have frank hypertension. The range between optimal BP and hypertension is termed pre-hypertension (systolic BP 121 to 139 mmHg or diastolic BP 81 to 89 mmHg). The complete classification of blood pressure levels is shown in Table 19–1.

The relationship between diet and BP has been well established. Populations with vegetarian or low-salt diets have lower BPs. Lower BP has also been correlated to higher intakes of potassium, calcium, magnesium, protein, and fiber, along with lower intakes of alcohol and fat. The typical American diet does not mirror these dietary patterns. The average daily American diet contains 33% calories from fat, 3100 to 3600 mg of sodium, 4.8 servings of fruits and vegetables (with significant portions provided by fried potatoes), and 5.1 servings of meat.[1,2]

Table 19–1	BLOOD PRESSURE CLASSIFICATION		
Classification	**Systolic (mmHg)**		**Diastolic (mmHg)**
Optimal	≤120	and	≤80
Prehypertension	121–139	or	81–89
Stage I Hypertension	140–159	or	90–99
Stage II Hypertension	≥160	or	≥100

In addition to adverse dietary patterns, overweight and obesity, major risk factors for hypertension, are increasing at dramatic rates in all segments of the population. In the United States, both dietary patterns and the prevalence of overweight or obese individuals are significant contributors to the high incidence of hypertension. Fortunately, if dietary changes are implemented, the effects of these factors on BP can be reversed. Implementation of dietary changes can produce significant benefits on BP levels within 2 weeks and can persist over time if the changes are maintained.

Behavior modification is important not only for treating high BP but also for preventing it. Several interventions including the Dietary Approaches to Stop Hypertension (DASH) diet,[3] sodium reduction,[4] weight reduction,[5] and moderation of alcohol intake,[6] have been shown to lower BP in patients with hypertension as well as in those with prehypertension. Therefore, these interventions are included in the guidelines of the Seventh Report of the Joint National Committee on Prevention, Detection, Evaluation and Treatment of High Blood Pressure (JNC-7, Box 19–1) for treating all stages of

---

BOX 19–1   JNC-7 Lifestyle Recommendations for Preventing and Treating Hypertension

Maintain a normal body weight or lose weight if body mass index/24.9 kg/m[2].
Reduce sodium intake to 2.4 g (6 g salt) or less per day.
Limit alcohol intake to 2 drinks or less per day for men and 1 drink for women (1 drink = 14 g of ethanol, contained in 12 oz beer, 5 oz wine, or 1.5 oz distilled spirits).
Eat a dietary pattern that is high in fruits, vegetables, and low-fat dairy and lower in fat, saturated fat, and cholesterol (DASH dietary pattern).
Engage in moderate level aerobic physical activity, 30 min/day, most days of the week.

DASH, Dietary Approaches to Stop Hypertension
From Chobanian AV, Bakris GL, Black HR, et al: The Seventh Report of the Joint National Committee on Prevention, Detection, Evaluation, and Treatment of High Blood Pressure: The JNC-7 report. JAMA 289(19) 2560–2572, 2003.

hypertension, with or without concomitant antihypertensive medication.[7] Lowering BP in persons with prehypertension can reduce risk in two ways: It can prevent the rise in BP associated with aging and therefore prevent the development of hypertension; and it can move nonhypertensive individuals to more optimal BP levels. Framingham Heart Study data showed that compared to those with optimal BP, persons with BP in the prehypertension range had a higher 10-year incidence of CVD. Effective use of dietary interventions in patients with prehypertension could lead to more optimal pressure, thereby reducing their risk of CVD.

Weight Reduction

As a group, hypertensives tend to be overweight, and there is a strong positive association between blood pressure and body weight that is independent of other factors. The risk of hypertension is twofold to sixfold higher in obese individuals compared to lean individuals. Because obesity is very prevalent in the U.S. population, it is estimated that a significant percentage of hypertension is attributable to this risk factor, accounting for up to 78% of hypertension cases in some cohort studies. Deposition of adipose tissue in the abdomen is particularly detrimental (see Chapter 17).

Weight reduction in obese hypertensives generally reduces systolic and diastolic BP levels, and is an important therapeutic maneuver in conjunction with pharmacologic therapy. In fact, blood pressure is usually reduced with as little as 10 lb of weight loss. A systematic review of over 18 randomized controlled trials concluded that weight loss of 3% to 9% leads to an average decrease in both systolic and diastolic BP of 3 mmHg.[5] Others have estimated that BP declines 1.2/1.0 mmHg for every kg of weight lost. In addition to direct effects on BP, weight loss may lead to a decrease in the dosages of medications required to control BP.

Weight reduction is also important for prevention of hypertension, as demonstrated in the Trials of Hypertension Prevention, Phases I and II.[8,9] In phase I, individuals with higher than optimal blood pressures (diastolic BP 80 to 89 mmHg) were assigned to a weight-loss intervention or control and followed for 18 months. The intervention group lost an average of 5.6 kg at 6 months, and 3.9 kg by 18 months. This modest amount of weight loss decreased the risk of developing hypertension. When compared to the usual care control group, the weight-loss intervention reduced the risk of developing hypertension during the study period by 34%. In phase II, with an average weight loss of only 1.9 kg at 36 months, the weight-loss group had a relative risk reduction for hypertension of 14.8%. There was a linear relationship between maintenance of weight loss and prolonged BP reduction; patients with the greatest weight loss had the greatest decline in mean BP at 36 months (systolic BP 5 mmHg, diastolic BP 7 mmHg).

Sodium Restriction

Sodium is found in almost all foods and is a common additive to many prepared and processed foods. Sodium requirements for both children and adults are on the order of less than 200 mg per day, although most societies consume many times that amount, ranging from 6 to 12 g of salt per day (2.4 to 5 g of sodium).

Populations such as the United States that have high sodium intakes tend to have a higher prevalence of hypertension and a rise in blood pressure with age. The effects of salt restriction on blood pressure are likely to increase with age and with the severity of hypertension, and are greater in African Americans. However, individuals vary in their responses to salt restriction. Controlled studies of moderate sodium restriction in hypertensives have shown modest reductions of 5 and 3 mmHg in systolic and diastolic blood pressure, respectively. The mechanism of action is thought to involve reducing intravascular volume, vessel wall sodium content, or vascular reactivity. In studies of hypertension prevention, a reduction of approximately 50 mmol (1.1 g) of sodium resulted in an 18% decreased risk of developing hypertension over 4 years of follow-up. Sodium reduction was equally effective at preventing hypertension in African-American and non–African-American subjects. Reducing sodium intake can be a particularly effective method of preventing hypertension in elderly populations as well. Sodium reduction of 50 mmol in elderly populations has been demonstrated to reduce the need for antihypertensive therapy or an adverse cardiovascular event by 32% over approximately 28 months of follow-up. A meta-analysis of clinical trials reported a dose-response relationship between sodium reduction and BP, such that for every 100 mmol/day (2.3 g) decrease in sodium, BP decreased 5.8/2.5 mmHg in patients with hypertension and 2.3/1.4 mmHg in those without hypertension.[4] Critics of the efficacy of reducing BP through sodium reduction point to the difficulty of implementation and the lack of a significant response in certain subsets of the population. They also cite concerns for possible adverse effects of reduced sodium intake, including increased lipids. However, the weight of evidence currently supports the JNC-7 recommendation to lower sodium intake.

Because there is no known benefit from consuming more sodium than is needed to meet daily losses, moderate reductions in healthy persons' salt intake to less than 6 g (2.4 g of sodium) per day is recommended. This level is achievable and palatable after a brief period of adaptation, and it may adequately control BP in some patients with stage 1 hypertension. In those who still need drug therapy, medication requirements may be decreased by sodium reduction.

Alcohol Moderation

Population studies consistently show a higher prevalence of hypertension as alcohol consumption rises. Studies have identified a linear relationship between population alcohol intake and BP, and a cause-effect relationship has been confirmed in intervention studies. Possible mechanisms for the relationship include a direct effect of alcohol on the vessel wall, sensitization of resistance vessels to pressor substances, stimulation of the sympathetic nervous system, and increased production of adrenocorticoid hormones. Excessive alcohol intake can also cause resistance to antihypertensive therapy, and reductions in alcohol intake may prevent hypertension.

The JNC-7 guidelines recommend limiting alcohol intake to less than 2 drinks per day for men and less than 1 drink per day for women. This recommendation is primarily supported by evidence from a meta-analysis of 15 clinical trials that studied the effects of alcohol reduction on BP in individuals who typically drank 3 or more drinks per day. Following a median self-reported reduction in alcohol intake of 76%, systolic BP (SBP) decreased by 3.31 mmHg and diastolic BP (DBP) decreased 2.04 mmHg.[6] Many expert panels and clinicians endorse this recommendation due to the additional health benefits and safety of limiting alcohol intake in nondependent drinkers.

Dietary Patterns

Observational studies demonstrate that blood pressure is inversely related to the intake of several nutrients (potassium, calcium, protein, magnesium, and fiber). However, intervention studies of individual nutrient supplements have led to small and inconsistent BP changes. The sum of the parts, i.e., the dietary pattern, may be more important than the intake of individual nutrients. Indeed, part of the epidemiologic link between diet and BP was established by observations of the dietary intake of vegetarians. Vegetarian diets are high in several nutrients including potassium, magnesium, and fiber, while being low in fat, and are associated with lower blood pressure. Moreover, when vegetarians switch to a more typical American diet (including meat), their blood pressures tend to increase, and when meat-eaters adopt a vegetarian diet, their blood pressures tend to decrease. These data suggest that the effects of individual nutrients on BP are only apparent when they are consumed as part of a dietary pattern.

DASH combines the aforementioned individual nutrients using various food groups to create a dietary pattern that lowers blood pressure. The DASH dietary pattern emphasizes fruits, vegetables, and low-fat dairy products and contains reduced amounts of red meat, sugar-containing beverages, and sweets. As a result, it is high in potassium, magnesium, calcium, total protein, and dietary fiber while being low in saturated fat, total fat, and cholesterol. The mean BP reduction achieved with the DASH diet compared to a diet typical of American intake was 5.5/3.0 mmHg.[3] For patients with hypertension, the mean BP reduction was even greater, 11.4/5.5 mmHg. The DASH diet was more effective for African Americans, especially for African Americans with hypertension, who had a mean BP reduction of 13.2/6.1 mmHg.[10] Even nonhypertensive participants who followed the DASH diet had a BP reduction of 3.5/2.2 mmHg. This clinical trial evidence of significant BP reductions as a result of following the DASH diet led to its inclusion in the JNC-7 guidelines.

Combined Interventions

In addition to dietary modifications, regular aerobic exercise, even of low to moderate intensity, appears to help prevent and control high blood pressure, independent of its effect on body weight. Also, combinations of any of the dietary approaches discussed should be attempted whenever feasible. This strategy is recommended because several studies have demonstrated that the combination of two approaches (e.g., weight loss or DASH combined with sodium reduction) was more effective at reducing BP than any one alone. Other multiple lifestyle interventions for BP reduction that included at least three interventions (dietary modifications, weight reduction, and physical activity) similarly demonstrated success in lowering BP. For the highly motivated patient, implementing multiple lifestyle changes can be an effective way to reduce BP.

Beyond the impact on individual patients, widespread implementation of lifestyle modifications could result in a small decrease in mean BP levels across the population, which could have a highly significant impact on CVD outcomes. For example, it is estimated that a population-wide decrease in systolic BP of 5 mmHg would result in a 14% reduction in mortality due to stroke, a 9% reduction in mortality due to coronary heart disease, and a 7% decline in all-cause mortality.[11] At least three facts underscore the importance of population-wide lifestyle changes in the United States to minimize the risk for developing hypertension: (1) in most cases hypertension is permanent, (2) many U.S. adults are unaware that they have prehypertension, and (3) the increase in blood pressure that occurs in the United States as people age appears to be lifestyle-related. Especially given their consistency with lifestyle recommendations to prevent and treat other chronic conditions, the JNC-7 recommendations are worthy of universal adoption for preventing and treating hypertension.

REFERENCES

1. US Department of Agriculture: Data Tables: Results from USDA's 1994–96 Continuing Survey Of Food Intakes By Individuals and 1994–96 Diet And Health Knowledge Survey. 1997.
2. Karanja NM, McCullough ML, Kumanyika SK, et al: Pre-enrollment diets of dietary approaches to stop hypertension trial participants. Dash Collaborative Research Group. J Am Diet Assoc 99(8 Suppl): S28–S34, 1999.
3. Appel LJ, Moore TJ, Obarzanek E, et al: A clinical trial of the effects of dietary patterns on blood pressure. Dash Collaborative Research Group. N Engl J Med 336(16):1117–1124, 1997.
4. Cutler JA, Follmann D, Allender PS: Randomized trials of sodium reduction: An overview. Am J Clin Nutr 65(2 Suppl):643S–651S, 1997.
5. Mulrow CD, Chiquette E, Angel L, et al: Dieting to reduce body weight for controlling hypertension in adults. Cochrane Database Syst Rev 2000(2):CD000484.
6. Xin X, He J, Frontini MG, et al: Effects of alcohol reduction on blood pressure: A meta-analysis of randomized controlled trials. Hypertension 38(5):1112–1117, 2001.
7. Chobanian AV, Bakris GL, Black HR, et al: The seventh report of the Joint National Committee on Prevention, Detection, Evaluation, and Treatment of High Blood Pressure: The JNC-7 report. JAMA 289(19):2560–2572, 2003.

8. Stevens VJ, Corrigan SA, Obarzanek E, et al: Weight loss intervention in phase 1 of the trials of hypertension prevention. The Tohp Collaborative Research Group. Arch Intern Med 153(7):849–858, 1993.

9. Stevens VJ, Obarzanek E, Cook NR, et al: Long-term weight loss and changes in blood pressure: Results of the trials of hypertension prevention, phase II. Ann Intern Med 134(1):1–11, 2001.

10. Svetkey LP, Simons-Morton D, Vollmer WM, et al: Effects of dietary patterns on blood pressure: Subgroup analysis of the dietary approaches to stop hypertension (DASH) randomized clinical trial. Arch Intern Med 159(3):285–293, 1999.

11. Whelton PK, He J, Appel LJ, et al: Primary prevention of hypertension: Clinical and public health advisory from the National High Blood Pressure Education Program. JAMA 288(15):1882–1888, 2002.

WEB SITES

American Society of Hypertension, http://www.ash-us.org/

Facts about the DASH eating plan (downloadable material to assist patients), http://www.nhlbi.nih.gov/health/public/heart/hbp/dash/index.htm

National Heart, Lung, Blood Institute (NIH) hypertension website, http://www.nhlbi.nih.gov/hbp/index.html

National High Blood Pressure Education Program, http://www.nhlbi.nih.gov/guidelines/hypertension/

20

Cardiovascular Disease

JAMY D. ARD, MD, • FRANK A. FRANKLIN, JR, MD

When aggregated across all age groups, cardiovascular disease (CVD) is the leading cause of death in the United States; it was responsible for 38% of deaths in 2002. CVD primarily includes ischemic (coronary) heart disease and other forms of heart disease; pulmonary heart disease and diseases of pulmonary circulation; cerebrovascular disease (stroke); and atherosclerosis and other diseases of arteries, arterioles, and capillaries. Despite declines in the prevalence of coronary heart disease (CHD) over the past 2 decades, it still affects more than 70 million people in the United States, or 34% of the population. Even though CVD seems almost ubiquitous, it is largely preventable, with many of the major risk factors, including physical activity, diet, body weight, and smoking, being modifiable. It is estimated that 15% of deaths in 2000 were related to poor diet and physical inactivity.

Atherogenesis

The atherosclerotic process begins in childhood with fatty streaks, lesions that are composed of cholesteryl ester-filled macrophages but do not compromise the arterial lumen. Low-density lipoprotein (LDL) particles that are chemically altered by oxidation, acetylation, or glycosylation, are particularly atherogenic, and these altered LDL particles are taken up by activated macrophages. These cells, laden with cholesterol, remain in the arterial wall as the foam cell component of atherosclerotic plaques and stimulate inflammatory responses. Oxidized LDL may promote several additional steps in the atherogenic process, including endothelial cell damage, foam cell accumulation and growth, and synthesis of auto-antibodies. Some fatty streaks develop into fibrous plaques, which are raised lesions with a collagen cap and smooth muscle cell proliferation. These plaques enlarge and rupture and, if they stimulate thrombosis, can precipitate an acute CVD event such as a myocardial infarction. This major component in the pathogenesis of atherosclerosis is recognized as an inflammatory process, mediated by activated macrophages that secrete chemotactic and cytokine factors that facilitate the inflammatory response. Markers of inflammation such as C-reactive protein are strongly correlated with risk for vascular disease and may become useful clinical tools for identifying high-risk populations for preventive intervention.

Cardiovascular Risk Factors

A consensus method for assessing cardiovascular risk and recommendations for its prevention and treatment have been promulgated by the National Cholesterol Education Program's (NCEP) Adult Treatment Panel III (ATP III).[1] Modifiable and non-modifiable risk factors for cardiovascular disease identified by the ATP III and other groups are shown in Box 20–1. Because many of them are modifiable, a significant proportion of cardiovascular events is preventable. The lipoprotein and metabolic syndrome risk factors comprise the emphasis in risk assessment and therapeutic approaches for CVD risk reduction.

The relationship between serum total cholesterol (TC) levels and CHD deaths is curvilinear, so that the mortality risk from a TC level of 250 mg/dL is twice that of 200 mg/dL, and at 300 mg/dL the risk is fourfold higher (Fig. 20–1). In addition, the risk declines with TC levels below 200 mg/dL, suggesting that even 200 mg/dL is not optimal. Although TC is an important identifier of risk, its subfractions have differential effects on risk. Both epidemiologic studies and controlled clinical trials have indicated that each 1 mg/dL increment in LDL causes an increase in CHD risk of 1 %. Similarly, a 1 mg/dL decrease in high-density lipoprotein cholesterol (HDL-C) increases

---

BOX 20–1   Risk Factors for Cardiovascular Disease

Non-modifiable

Age (males ≥45; females ≥55 years)*
Male sex
Family history of premature coronary heart disease
  (definite myocardial infarction or sudden death in male first
  degree relative <55 years, or in female first degree relative
  <65 years)*

Modifiable (direct)

High low-density lipoprotein cholesterol (LDL-C) level
Low high-density lipoprotein cholesterol (HDL-C) level
  (males ≤40 mg/dL; females ≤50 mg/dL)*
High total cholesterol/HDL-C or LDL-C/HDL-C ratio
Hypertriglyceridemia
Current cigarette smoking*
Hypertension (≥140/90 mmHg confirmed on several
  occasions, or on antihypertensive medication)*
Metabolic syndrome
Diabetes mellitus (considered a CHD equivalent)

Modifiable (indirect)

Obesity (may act mainly through hypertension, high LDL-C,
  low HDL-C, and diabetes)
Physical inactivity

---

*Considered major independent risk factors by the ATP III and
  included in its algorithm for calculating CHD risk.

CHD risk by 2% to 3%. At any LDL level, the concentration of HDL-C has an inverse association with CVD risk. Therefore, the ATP III has identified LDL as the primary target for cholesterol-lowering therapy to reduce CVD risk. Recommended serum lipid levels are shown in Table 20–1.

Lowering LDL is effective and safe for primary and secondary prevention of CHD. Nutrition modifications can have a significant impact on LDL levels. In two randomized trials, a low-fat diet combined with smoking cessation or medication in persons with CHD resulted in less progression and more regression of coronary

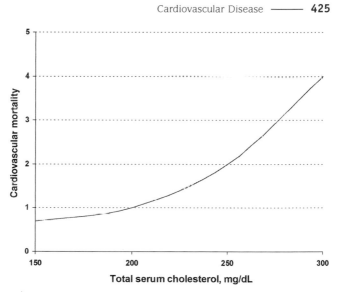

Figure 20–1. Relationship of serum cholesterol to cardiovascular risk.

artery lesions than did the control regimen. The improvement in artery luminal diameter correlated with the extent of LDL lowering. In the Lifestyle Heart Trial, a diet with less than 10% of energy from fat and no dietary

Table 20-1	ATP III CLASSIFICATION OF SERUM LIPID LEVELS[1]			
Classification	Total Cholesterol (mg/dL)	LDL-C (mg/dL)	HDL-C (mg/dL)	Triglycerides (mg/dL)
Optimal	<200	<100	≥60	<150
Near optimal		100–129		
Borderline high	200–239	130–159		150–199
High	≥240	160–189		200–499
Very high		≥190		≥500
Low			<40	

HDL-C, high-density lipoprotein cholesterol; LDL-C, low-density lipoprotein cholesterol.
From Third Report of the National Cholesterol Education Program (NCEP) Expert Panel on Detection, Evaluation, and Treatment of High Blood Cholesterol in Adults (Adult Treatment panel III). Executive Summary; available at http://www.nhlbi.nih.gov/guidelines/cholesterol/atp_iii.htm.

cholesterol reduced angina symptoms in only 1 month, suggesting an impact on vascular relaxation, while later angiograms showed net regression of CHD.

Elevated serum triglycerides (TG) appear to be an independent CVD risk factor as well. High serum TG levels are often associated with a pattern of dyslipidemia characterized by reduced HDL-C levels and raised levels of chylomicron remnants, very-low-density lipoprotein (VLDL) remnants, intermediate-density lipoprotein (IDL), and small, dense, cholesterol-depleted, apolipoprotein (Apo) B-rich LDL. This phenotype is often part of metabolic syndrome (discussed later).

At any given serum TC level, there is synergy with other CVD risk factors that greatly increases CVD risk. This has led the NCEP to propose a clinical strategy of diet and medications for individuals in the highest quintile of CVD risk, and a public health approach involving lifestyle modification for the general population.[1] Dietary modification is an important part of both strategies.

The diagnosis of metabolic syndrome, as defined by the ATP III (see Chapter 16), is appropriate for persons with at least three of the following five criteria: elevated fasting plasma glucose levels ($\geq$110 mg/dL); abdominal obesity (waist circumference >35 inches in women or >40 inches in men); hypertension ($\geq$130/$\geq$85 mmHg); hypertriglyceridemia ($\geq$150 mg/dL); and low HDL-C (<50 in women, <40 in men). Up to 40% of the U.S. population older than 50 has metabolic syndrome. Compared to persons without metabolic syndrome, those who have it are twice as likely to have CHD.

Nutrient Effects on Serum Lipids and Cardiovascular Disease

Fatty Acids and Cholesterol

The recommended diet for dyslipidemia is based on the major nutrients that affect serum total cholesterol. The Keys equation (Box 20–2) demonstrates that saturated fatty acids (SFAs) raise total cholesterol levels twice as much as polyunsaturated fatty acids (PUFAs) lower it,

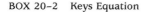

BOX 20-2   Keys Equation

$$\Delta C = 1.35 (2S - P) + 1.5Z$$

where
ΔC = Change in serum TC (mg/dL)
  S = Change in percent energy intake from SFAs
  P = Change in percent energy intake from PUFAs
  Z = Difference in square roots of old and new cholesterol
      intakes (mg/1000 kcal)

and more than dietary cholesterol raises it. However, the relationship is curvilinear so that higher dietary intakes have progressively smaller effects on serum TC.

SFAs raise TC predominantly by raising LDL. However, SFAs of different chain lengths have variable influences on TC and LDL: palmitic (16:0), lauric (12:0), and myristic (14:0) acids raise both serum TC and LDL, whereas stearic acid (18:0) has no effect on them. Reductions in SFA intake are generally associated with decreased intake of cholesterol; therefore, reducing saturated fat provides the benefits of lowering serum total cholesterol and LDL.

An important and controversial issue is what should replace SFAs in the diet. Four major possibilities are stearic acid, PUFAs, carbohydrates, and monounsaturated fatty acids (MUFAs). The data on stearic acid are too limited to make a population recommendation, and the potential for promotion of thrombogenesis indicates that caution is warranted. Regarding PUFAs, no population has ever consumed high amounts for long periods with proven safety. Because of concerns about suppressing the immune response and promoting tumor development in laboratory animals, it has been suggested that intakes of PUFAs be limited to less than 10% of total energy. On the other hand, high-carbohydrate diets are consumed by many populations that have low rates of CVD, and appear to be safe. If consumed in the form of fruits and vegetables, the intake of vitamins that function as antioxidants or promote homocysteine metabolism will likely increase, providing additional benefit. If consumed as whole grains and legumes, the increased carbohydrate will increase soluble and insoluble fiber. Further, high-carbohydrate diets usually have lower energy density than do high-fat diets, which should lower the prevalence of obesity in the population. However, the drawback to this strategy is that refined grains are often used to replace calories from saturated fat, resulting in little net increase in fiber, continued levels of high energy intake, and adverse effects on serum triglycerides and HDL-C.

MUFAs, which are rich in the olive oil based Mediterranean diet, have been suggested as other potential replacements for SFAs. Although MUFAs were initially thought to be neutral with respect to cholesterol levels, they have now been shown to lower LDL levels without lowering HDL-C levels as do carbohydrates. Low rates of CHD in Mediterranean cohorts of the Seven Countries Study support the efficacy and safety of MUFAs. However, because they are energy-dense, MUFAs could make weight management more difficult. Key plant sources of MUFAs include high-oleic acid vegetable oils such as olive, canola, or high-oleic safflower or sunflower oils, and nuts and avocados. Overall, both carbohydrates and MUFAs are valid options for replacing SFAs, but carbohydrates are preferred in obesity-prone individuals.

Trans Fatty Acids

Trans fatty acids are isomers of the normal *cis* fatty acids, produced when PUFAs are hydrogenated, such as in the production of margarine and vegetable shortening. Hydrogenated vegetable oils were developed mainly as an alternative to animal fats and tropical oils used in frying, baking, and spreads. The effects of *trans* fatty acids on serum lipoproteins markedly differ from those of the natural *cis* isomer. *Trans* fatty acids uniformly raise LDL concentrations and lower HDL-C concentrations. In addition, *trans* fatty acids raise serum LP(a), an atherogenic LP.

There is evidence that intake of *trans* fatty acids increases the risk of CHD. Results from the Nurses' Health Study suggest that for every 2% increase in energy from *trans* fat there is a 1.93 relative risk of CHD.

There appears to be no benefit from consuming *trans* fat, and it appears prudent to limit intake as much as possible. These concerns have prompted new nutrition labeling guidelines that include identification of the percent of energy from *trans* fat in food products and the manufacturing of food items with lower levels of *trans* fat.

Fish and Fish Oil

Two types of PUFAs occur in the diet: (1) those with the terminal double bond 6 carbons from the methyl end are designated n-6; (2) those with the terminal double bond 3 carbons from the methyl end are designated n-3. Linoleic acid (18:2), the major n-6 fatty acid in the diet, is found mainly in plant oils. N-3 fatty acids such as eicosapentaenoic (EPA) and docosahexaenoic (DHA) are found primarily in fish. Observational studies of low CHD mortality rates in populations with high consumption of fish (200 to 400 g per day) have contributed to the hypothesis that n-3 fatty acids may have antiatherogenic and antithrombotic properties. The rarity of CHD in Greenland Eskimos and their low plasma TG were linked to their diet of seafood. Similar associations were observed in Japan, where CHD mortality and platelet aggregability were found to be lower in areas where fish intake was higher. The favorable disease pattern in Eskimos and Japanese may also be partially a result of a diet low in SFAs and high in n-3 PUFA intake.

Several prospective studies found statistically significant inverse trends between fish intake and CHD mortality. In the Zutphen (the Dutch cohort of the Seven Countries Study) and the Chicago Western Electric studies, which involved almost 2800 men free of CHD at entry, CHD mortality after 20 and 25 years was inversely related to fish intake. In Zutphen, consumption of as little as 30 to 44 g per day (about 1 or 2 fish meals per week) was associated with 64% fewer deaths compared to those with no fish intake. In the Western Electric study there was a 25% reduction in CHD mortality with fish intake of 18 to 34 g per day. There was some evidence of dose-response, with the highest mortality being among those who ate no fish. In a controlled clinical study, the Diet and Reinfarction Trial (DART), 2033 men who had recently recovered from myocardial infarction (MI) were randomly allocated to two groups; one group was advised to eat two fatty fish meals per week and the other group was not. Two years later the fish group had a significant reduction in mortality of 29%, although there was no reduction in new myocardial infarctions. Additionally, other studies have shown a risk reduction in sudden cardiac death in persons who consumed fish more than once per week. This effect is thought to be related to the effect of n-3 fatty acids on cardiac membrane stability and suppression of arrhythmias. Thus, patients with CVD as well as healthy persons can be encouraged to consume fish, including fatty ones such as salmon and mackerel, in the place of other fatty meats to lower their intake of SFAs and increase n-3 PUFA levels.

Soluble Fiber

Water-soluble fibers including pectin, gums, mucilages, algal polysaccharides, some hemicelluloses, and some storage polysaccharides can reduce serum lipid levels more effectively than insoluble fibers. The reduction in serum total cholesterol levels attributable to soluble fiber may range from 0.5% to 2% per g of dietary fiber intake, and the reduction is greater in patients with initially higher serum total cholesterol levels. Serum TC can be lowered approximately 5% by daily consumption of any of the following: 6 to 40 g pectin, 8 to 36 g gums (e.g., guar gum), 100 to 150 g (0.5 to 0.75 cups) dried bean or leguminous seeds, 25 to 100g (0.3 to 1.2 cups) dry oat bran, 57 to 140 g (0.7 to 1.7 cups) dry oatmeal, or 10 to 30 g (3 to 9 tbsp) psyllium.

Soluble fiber acts directly by increasing fecal bile acid excretion and slowing absorption of dietary sugars; they act indirectly by displacing fat from the diet. Data from the Health Professionals Follow-Up Study suggest that an increase in dietary fiber of 10 g per day decreases the risk of fatal coronary heart disease by 19%. Fiber may have effects on atherosclerosis independent of serum total cholesterol level; supplemental pectin caused atherosclerotic lesions to regress in swine maintained on a high-fat diet without lowering serum total cholesterol concentrations.

Dietary Guidelines for adults recommend total dietary fiber intake of about 20 to 30 g per day, with about 25% as soluble fiber from whole fruits and vegetables and whole-grain products. Average dietary fiber intake in U.S. adults is well below this. Supplemental soluble fiber (e.g. oat bran, gums, or psyllium) may produce additional modest lowering of LDL cholesterol and may be useful in treating hypercholesterolemic patients.

Soy Protein

Dietary proteins of plant origin can lower cholesterol levels. In a meta-analysis, replacement of animal protein with soy protein (averaging 47 g per day), without changing dietary saturated fat or cholesterol, resulted in 10% to 12% reductions in serum total and LDL cholesterol levels without adverse effects on HDL-C. Those with higher initial total cholesterol levels experienced greater effects. Consuming 25 g soy protein per day could decrease serum total cholesterol by 9 mg/dL, with linear dose-related effects through 75 g per day. The effect may be from the protein itself (e.g., the amino acid pattern or peptide structure) or from phytochemicals such as isoflavones or saponins. Intakes of 30 g soy protein per day can be achieved by consuming 2 to 3 servings of soy protein daily from sources such as soy milk, tofu, or soy powders.

Alcohol

The relationship between alcohol and total mortality is depicted by a J-shaped curve, with the lowest risk among persons who take 1 to 2 drinks per day, due almost entirely to lower CHD death rates. Epidemiologic studies have consistently shown that moderate alcohol drinkers have approximately 30% to 40% lower CHD mortality risk and 10% lower total mortality risk than nondrinkers. This relationship is independent of numerous potential confounders including age, sex, ethnicity, cigarette smoking, education, adiposity, and dietary habits. The mechanism apparently involves higher HDL-C levels and an antithrombotic effect of alcohol.

Because it is dangerous to consume high levels of alcohol, advice about the health benefits and risks of alcohol must be individually based on age, sex, and personal or family history of problem drinking, CHD, certain cancers, or liver disease. Nondrinkers and established light or moderate drinkers should not be advised to begin or increase alcohol consumption in order to reduce their CHD risk. Recommendations call for no more than 2 drinks per day for men and no more than 1 drink per day for women. A drink is defined as 5 oz wine, 12 oz beer, or 1.5 oz 80-proof liquor.

Homocysteine, Folic Acid, and Vitamins B_6 and B_{12}

Homocysteine is a sulfhydryl-containing amino acid produced by the demethylation of methionine, an amino acid derived primarily from animal protein. To conserve methionine, homocysteine is recycled using a pathway that requires folic acid and vitamins B_6 and B_{12}. Marginal deficiencies of these vitamins, in addition to genetic defects and polymorphisms in the key enzymes of homocysteine metabolism, can elevate homocysteine levels. High levels of homocysteine adversely affect endothelial cells and produce abnormal clotting, thus increasing CVD risk. Persons with CHD or peripheral atherosclerosis have significantly higher mean plasma homocysteine levels than do controls. The reliable and reproducible association between high homocysteine levels and vascular disease in disparate groups and from different study designs suggests that homocysteine is an independent CVD risk factor. A 25% lower homocysteine level is associated with an 11% reduction in ischemic heart disease.

Folic acid is the vitamin with the most potent influence on homocysteine levels. Doses of 0.4 to 1 mg of folic acid, especially when combined with vitamins B_{12} and B_6, reduce serum homocysteine levels. Randomized trials are underway to test the ultimate effect of this treatment on the natural history of CHD. Dietary changes that are reasonable for other reasons as well, such as reducing intake of meat and increasing that of vegetables and legumes (for folic acid), can most often reduce plasma homocysteine concentrations.

Antioxidants

The oxidative modification of LDL and other lipoproteins is important, and possibly obligatory, in atherogenesis. Thus, it is possible that inhibiting the oxidation of LDL will decrease or prevent atherosclerosis. Vitamin E, β-carotene, and vitamin C, all antioxidant vitamins, delay and reduce the oxidation of LDL when it is subjected to an oxidative challenge *in vitro*.

In the oxidation hypothesis, the susceptibility of LDL oxidation is determined by the balance between the pro-oxidant challenge and the capacity of antioxidant defenses. Epidemiologic evidence suggests an inverse relation between the intake of antioxidant vitamins, particularly vitamin E, and CHD. Several large observational studies have suggested that antioxidant supplementation reduces CHD risk, after adjusting for risk factors and for use of multivitamins, β-carotene, or vitamin C. However, at least two randomized prospective trials of vitamin E supplementation have not shown benefit for primary or secondary prevention of CHD, and there is evidence of an adverse effect on mortality from vitamin E supplementation in excess of 200 IU per day (see Chapter 3). Therefore, antioxidant supplements are not recommended for prevention of heart disease.

Phytochemicals

Dietary substances from plants can lower serum total cholesterol levels and reduce CHD risk. Examples of these phytochemicals are phytosterols, tocotrienols, and flavonoids. Phytosterols are plant sterols that inhibit absorption of both endogenous and exogenous cholesterol and lower serum total cholesterol levels. Food sources of sterols include barley seedlings, almonds, cashews, peanuts, sesame seeds, sunflower seeds, whole wheat, corn, soybeans, and many vegetable oils. Commercial spreads enriched with plant sterols and stanols such as Benecol and Take Control can be incorporated into the treatment of patients with dyslipidemia. The ATP III recommends the daily intake of 2 to 3 g of plant sterols, which can reduce LDL cholesterol levels by 6% to 15%.

Tocotrienols are related chemically to tocopherol (vitamin E). In animals and humans these substances inhibit HMG CoA reductase activity and reduce serum total cholesterol levels. Tocotrienols are found in cereal seeds and palm oil. Flavonoids are antioxidant polyphenolic compounds that are ubiquitously present in vegetables, fruits, and beverages of vegetable origin including tea and red wine. Flavonoid intake has been inversely associated with CHD mortality and explains a significant proportion of the variance in CHD rates regardless of its dietary source. This suggests that flavonoids have an impact on CHD risk that is independent of associated dietary factors.

Evaluation and Management of Cardiovascular Disease Risk

The third report of the NCEP, published in 2002 and updated in 2004, provides a concise clinical approach to the evaluation and management of CHD risk, focusing on serum lipids as the key intervention target. This portion of the chapter will provide an overview of the approach suggested by the ATP III, with additional focus on the dietary intervention for CHD risk reduction. The full report is referenced in the Suggested Readings.

Step 1: Determine Serum Lipid Levels

The recommendations begin with obtaining a fasting lipid profile on all adults age 20 years and older at least once every 5 years. Screening for lipid abnormalities and other CVD risk factors such as smoking and hypertension is recommended at an early age to allow interventions to be initiated early to prevent the progression of athero-sclerotic disease. Although atherosclerotic lesions can be reduced later in life with aggressive dietary and medical therapy, the remaining risk is unacceptably high when compared to those who never had such disease progression. Patients should ideally be in a fasted state (nothing to eat for at least 9 hours) to ensure accurate assessment of the triglyceride level, which is most acutely altered by eating. However, if the inconvenience of fasting hinders successful screening, the initial measurement may be done without fasting, and abnormal levels confirmed after fasting. In laboratories where LDL cholesterol is not measured directly, fasting measurements allow reasonable estimation of LDL from the following equation:

LDL = Total cholesterol – HDL-C – Triglycerides/5.

This estimate is only useful when triglyceride levels are less than 400 mg/dL. Screening should be done more frequently than once in 5 years for those with multiple risk factors or if there is a history of elevated LDL cholesterol (LDL-C).

Step 2: Identify CHD/CHD Equivalents and Major Risk Factors Other Than Elevated LDL-C

While the major consideration is atherosclerotic disease that affects the vessels supplying the heart, the athero-sclerotic process is paralleled in other vessels of the body and can have associated signs and symptoms. When evidence of other vascular disease is present, it can be associated with the same degree of risk for a major CHD event, such as myocardial infarction or cardiac death, as having known CHD. This is referred to as a CHD risk equivalent. Patients with CHD risk equivalents have a greater than 20% risk per 10 years of suffering a major CHD event. The forms of clinical atherosclerotic disease that are considered CHD risk equivalents include peripheral artery disease, symptomatic carotid artery disease, and abdominal aortic aneurysm. Patients with diabetes mellitus (Types 1 or 2) are also at increased risk for CHD and considered to have the same risk for a major event as those diagnosed with CHD.

The major risk factors for CHD are highlighted in Box 20–1. When patients have known CHD or a CHD risk equivalent, knowledge of risk factors is helpful primarily to target modifiable behaviors that can improve global disease risk (e.g., smoking cessation, optimal control of blood pressure, or increasing HDL). This is true because therapeutic goals for those with greater than 20% 10-year risk is typically uniform (with one exception, see Step 3) and should be pursued aggressively. However, for those without CHD or risk equivalents, the number of major risk factors is a key aspect of determining CHD risk and subsequent therapeutic goals for LDL-C.

Step 3: Determine 10-year Coronary Heart Disease Risk

Persons who have no risk or one risk factor typically have less than 10% risk of suffering a CHD event in 10 years, and therefore, calculation of the 10-year CHD risk is not necessary. For those with two or more major risk factors, 10-year CHD risk is determined using Tables 20–2 and 20–3 for men and women, respectively. The algorithms are derived from results of the Framingham Heart Study and provide an easy method to estimate 10-year risk of myocardial infarction or death from CHD. Risk factors included in the calculation encompass most major ones, including age, total cholesterol, HDL-C, systolic blood pressure levels and treatment status, and smoking status. For each risk factor, a point value is given; however, in some instances, such as when total cholesterol is optimal, no additional points are added to the score. Optimal levels of HDL-C (≥60 mg/dL) result in subtraction of 1 point. Systolic blood pressure should be the average of several measurements. Because of residual risk even with pharmacologic treatment of hypertension, 1 point is added to the score for those on therapy. This is not to imply, however, that risk reduction should occur by allowing patients to have less than optimal blood pressure without medication.

| Table 20-2 | CARDIOVASCULAR DISEASE 10-YEAR RISK CALCULATOR FOR MEN |

Framingham Point Scores

Age	Points
20–34	−9
35–39	−4
40–44	0
45–49	3
50–54	6
55–59	8
60–64	10
65–69	11
70–74	12
75–79	13

	Points				
Total Cholesterol	Age 20–39	Age 40–49	Age 50–59	Age 60–69	Age 70–79
<160	0	0	0	0	0
160–199	4	3	2	1	0
200–239	7	5	3	1	0
240–279	9	6	4	2	1
≥280	11	8	5	3	1

	Points				
	Age 20–39	Age 40–49	Age 50–59	Age 60–69	Age 70–79
Nonsmoker	0	0	0	0	0
Smoker	8	5	3	1	1

HDL (mg/dL)	Points
≥60	−1
50–59	0
40–49	1
<40	2

Systolic BP (mmHg)	If Untreated	If Treated
<120	0	0
120–129	0	1
130–139	1	2
140–159	1	2
≥160	2	3

Table continued on following page

Table 20–2	CARDIOVASCULAR DISEASE 10-YEAR RISK CALCULATOR FOR MEN *(Continued)*

Point Total	10-year Risk%
<0	<1
0	1
1	1
2	1
3	1
4	1
5	2
6	2
7	3
8	4
9	5
10	6
11	8
12	10
13	12
14	16
15	20
16	25
≥17	≥30

Third Report of the Expert Panel on Detection, Evaluation, and Treatment of High Blood Cholesterol in Adults (Adult Treatment Panel III); available at http://www.nhlbi.nih.gov/guidelines/cholesterol/atp3_rpt.htm.
Reproduced as material in the public domain. Originally published by the National Heart, Lung, and Blood Institute (NHLBI), part of the National Institute of Health; see http://www.emall.nhlbihin.net/reuse.asp.

Smoking is defined as any cigarette usage in the past month. The points from each risk factor are summed and matched to the corresponding risk percentage to provide an estimate of the 10-year CHD risk.

Step 4: Determine Risk Category

The underlying principle for the ATP III guidelines is that therapy for CHD risk reduction, primarily through LDL reduction, should be dictated by the level of risk for CHD. Each risk category modifies the LDL goal, with increasing risk resulting in lower LDL goals. In the previous three steps, all of the information needed to determine the 10-year risk category for CHD has been obtained.

Table 20–3	**CARDIOVASCULAR DISEASE 10-YEAR RISK CALCULATOR FOR WOMEN**

Framingham Point Scores

Age	Points
20–34	−7
35–39	−3
40–44	0
45–49	3
50–54	6
55–59	8
60–64	10
65–69	12
70–74	14
75–79	16

			Points		
Total Cholesterol	Age 20–39	Age 40–49	Age 50–59	Age 60–69	Age 70–79
<160	0	0	0	0	0
160–199	4	3	2	1	1
200–239	8	6	4	2	1
240–279	11	8	5	3	2
≥280	13	10	7	4	2

			Points		
	Age 20–39	Age 40–49	Age 50–59	Age 60–69	Age 70–79
Nonsmoker	0	0	0	0	0
Smoker	9	7	4	2	1

HDL (mg/dL)	Points
≥60	−1
50–59	0
40–49	1
<40	2

Systolic BP (mmHg)	If Untreated	If Treated
<120	0	0
120–129	1	3
130–139	2	4
140–159	3	5
≥160	4	6

Table continued on following page

Table 20–3	CARDIOVASCULAR DISEASE 10-YEAR RISK CALCULATOR FOR WOMEN *(Continued)*
Point Total	**10-year Risk%**
<9	<1
9	1
10	1
11	1
12	1
13	2
14	2
15	3
16	4
17	5
18	6
19	8
20	11
21	14
22	17
23	22
24	27
≥25	≥30

Third Report of the Expert Panel on Detection, Evaluation, and Treatment of High Blood Cholesterol in Adults (Adult Treatment Panel III); available at http://www.nhlbi.nih.gov/guidelines/cholesterol/atp3_rpt.htm.
Reproduced as material in the public domain. Originally published by the National Heart, Lung, and Blood Institute (NHLBI), part of the National Institute of Health; see http://www.emall.nhlbihin.net/reuse.asp.

The levels of risk are less than 10%, 10% to 20%, and greater than 20%. As stated before, those with 0 to 1 risk factor will typically fall into the less than 10% range. On the opposite end of the spectrum, those with CHD equivalents or CHD, by definition, have greater than 20% risk of a major CHD event in 10 years. Patients with two or more risk factors may fall into the 10% to 20% risk category or the greater than 20% category. Because those with a risk greater than 20% are considered high-risk or CHD-equivalent, the major therapeutic distinction is for those with 2 or more risk factors and a 10-year risk of 20% or less.

The ATP III therapeutic goals for LDL-C are shown in Table 20–4. In general, the trend for LDL-C reduction

Table 20-4 LOW-DENSITY LIPOPROTEIN CHOLESTEROL (LDL-C) GOALS BY RISK CATEGORY[1]

Risk Factors	Risk Category (10-year CHD risk)	LDL-C goal	Initiate Therapeutic Lifestyle Changes (TLC)	Consider Drug Therapy
0–1	Not necessary to calculate	<160 mg/dL	≥160 mg/dL	≥190 mg/dL
≥2	<10%	<130 mg/dL	≥130 mg/dL	≥160 mg/dL
	10–20%	<130 mg/dL (Therapeutic option: <100 mg/dL)	≥130 mg/dL	≥130 mg/dL
	>20%	Same as CHD Risk Equivalent		
CHD or CHC Risk-Equivalent	>20%	<100 mg/dL (Therapeutic option for very high-risk: <70 mg/dL)	≥ 100 mg/dL	≥ 100 mg/dL

CHD, coronary heart disease.

From Third Report of the National Cholesterol Education Program (NCEP) Expert Panel on Detection, Evaluation, and Treatment of High Blood Cholesterol in Adults (Adult Treatment Panel III). Executive Summary; available at http://www.nhlbi.nih.gov/guidelines/cholesterol/atp_iii.htm.

has been to push levels lower, with a therapeutic option to set a goal of less than 70 mg/dL for very high-risk patients—those with a recent myocardial infarction, or those with a combination of CHD and either diabetes or severe, poorly controlled risk factors or metabolic syndrome. There is also now a therapeutic option to reduce LDL-C levels below 100 mg/dL for moderately high-risk patients (those with two or more risk factors and 10-year CHD risk of 10% to 20%). This trend has been fueled largely by results of large clinical trials involving treatment with HMG Co-A reductase inhibitors (statins) that showed benefits of progressively lower levels of LDL-C in both very high and moderately high risk patients.

Step 5: Initiate Therapy

Dietary saturated fat and cholesterol are both major LDL-raising components and are the focus of the therapeutic lifestyle changes (TLC) diet recommendations. The ATP III recommends that persons with LDL-C levels above goal reduce their saturated fat intake to less than 7% of energy intake and maintain a cholesterol intake of less than 200 mg per day. Additional dietary strategies for lowering LDL-C levels include increasing intake of plant sterols or stanols and soluble dietary fiber. The basic premise of the dietary intervention is to identify frequently consumed foods that are high in saturated fat and cholesterol and replace them with better alternatives (Table 20–5). This often results in reduced energy intake, particularly when energy-dense items are replaced with lower-energy-density items. The initial changes should be made in the context of a diet that has a composition of macronutrients shown in Table 20–6.

The lifestyle changes recommended by the ATP III are not limited to dietary modification, but include weight reduction and increased physical activity. For overweight or obese persons, a 10% decrease in body weight is recommended along with achieving regular physical activity while decreasing sedentary activities (e.g., driving or watching television). These lifestyle modifications have

Table 20-5	MAJOR SOURCES OF AND ALTERNATIVES FOR SATURATED FAT AND CHOLESTEROL IN THE AMERICAN DIET (MEDICS MNEMONIC)	
Food Group	**Major Sources**	**Preferred Foods**
Meat	Hamburgers, beefsteaks, roasts, hot dogs, ham, luncheon meats, pork, bacon, sausage	Fish, shellfish, poultry without skin, lean red meats (if used at all), beans, peas, other meat substitutes
Eggs	Egg yolks	Egg whites, egg substitutes
Dairy Products	Whole milk, whole-milk beverages, cheeses, butter, ice cream, frozen desserts	Skim or 1% milk or buttermilk; low-fat varieties of cheese, cottage cheese, yogurt, and frozen desserts (e.g., sherbet, sorbet)
Invisible Fats	Processed, packaged foods; bread, rolls crackers	Home-baked whole-grain breads, low-fat rolls and crackers
Cooking Fats	Margarine, oils, dips, sauces, mayonnaise, lard; breaded/fried foods, mixed dishes (pizza, soups, casseroles, chili, pot pies)	Unsaturated, unhydrogenated oils (olive, canola, safflower) and margarines, low-fat mayonnaise
Sweets and Snacks	Doughnuts, cookies, cakes, nuts, peanut butter	Angel food cake, low-fat sweets, fruit

been included because a large proportion of individuals with increased CHD risk are overweight and sedentary. In addition, the ATP III specifically targets persons with metabolic syndrome to provide therapeutic interventions to remedy elevated triglycerides, low HDL-C, higher than optimal blood pressure, or abdominal obesity. As described in the guidelines, it is expected that the interventions for weight loss and increased physical activity be implemented after addressing the initial two dietary strategies (dietary SFAs and cholesterol), particularly if metabolic syndrome is present. However, synergy among all components of the TLC plan is readily apparent: reducing intake of foods high in SFAs and cholesterol will likely result in decreased total energy intake and assist in weight control efforts; increasing fiber intake can increase satiety and reduce total energy intake, leading to weight reduction; increasing physical activity

Table 20-6	NUTRIENT COMPOSITION OF THE THERAPEUTIC LIFESTYLE CHANGE (TLC) DIET TO REDUCE SERUM CHOLESTEROL LEVELS[1]	
Nutrient	**Recommended Intake**	**Average American Diet***
Fat, % energy	25–35+	33
SFAs, % energy	<7	11
MUFAs, % energy	Up to 20	13
PUFAs, % energy	Up to 10	6
Cholesterol, mg	≤200	331 (men)
		213 (women)
		228 (children, 6–11 yrs)
Carbohydrate, % energy	50–60+	52
Protein, % energy	~15	15

*Data Tables: Results from USDA's 1994–1996 Continuing Survey of Food Intakes by Individuals and 1994–1996 Diet and Health Knowledge Survey, 1997.

+For persons with metabolic syndrome, up to 35% of calories can come from fat. In this instance, carbohydrates should be reduced to ~50% of energy and the increase in fat calories should be from MUFAs and PUFAs.

MUFAs, monounsaturated fatty acids; PUFAs, polyunsaturated fatty acids; SFAs, saturated fatty acids.

From Third Report of the National Cholesterol Education Program (NCEP) Expert Panel on Detection, Evaluation, and Treatment of High Blood Cholesterol in Adults (Adult Treatment Panel III). Executive Summary; available at http://www.nhlbi.nih.gov/guidelines/cholesterol/atp_iii.htm.

is a key component of successful weight loss and weight maintenance strategies; and weight loss can result directly in lowering of LDL-C. Therefore, in the proper clinical situation (i.e., motivated patient with multiple risk factors), it can be advantageous to implement the TLC components broadly rather than stepwise, to enhance effectiveness in achieving CHD risk reduction. The motivated patient can be counseled to lose weight by decreasing total fat intake, with a focus on SFAs, increasing fiber intake, and establishing a moderate physical activity regimen.

Responses to the TLC interventions should be evaluated at approximately 6-week intervals. If the LDL-C goal is achieved at the first assessment, the patient should be encouraged to continue the dietary changes, as resumption of prior dietary intake will result in a return to previous LDL-C levels. If the LDL-C goal has not been achieved, intensification of the dietary intervention and additional education may be necessary. Referral to a nutrition professional is recommended for more formal counseling and instruction. Following a second assessment of LDL-C levels, the addition of medication may be considered if goal levels have not been achieved. If the patient is nearing the LDL-C goal, consideration should be given to continuing dietary therapy before adding medication.

The Polymeal Approach

Significant interest exists for developing broad population-based strategies to reduce cardiovascular risk. One interesting concept is known as the Polypill—a daily pharmacologic intervention that combines six different medications shown independently to reduce risk of a major CVD event. It is proposed that these medications, when combined, could potentially produce multiplicative effects on CVD risk reduction—perhaps totaling more than 80%. This provocative assertion resulted in debate about associated costs and potential adverse events. As a result, a group of researchers proposed an alternative known as the Polymeal—a dietary pattern that consists of food items individually shown to reduce CVD risk.[2]

The ingredients of the Polymeal include wine (150 mL/day), fish (114 g 4 times/week), dark chocolate (100 g/day), fruit and vegetables (400 g/day), garlic (2.7 g/day), and almonds (68 g/day). Another proposed dietary portfolio including plant sterols, soy protein, soluble fiber, and almonds proved as effective as a low-dose statin for reducing LDL-C and C-reactive protein.[3]

Assuming that the benefits of consuming these items in a dietary pattern are additive, Polymeal proponents estimate that they could total approximately 76% CVD risk reduction. While no randomized, controlled trial has yet tested this specific claim, the idea of using a dietary pattern rather than individual food items or supplements as the basis for intervention strategies directed at CVD risk reduction is supported by epidemiologic data and randomized, controlled trials such as the Dietary Approaches to Stop Hypertension (DASH) trial (high fruit, vegetable, low-fat dairy intake) and the Lyon Heart Study (Mediterranean diet). This strategy is gaining popularity because of potential benefits on multiple levels, including quality of life and risks of other chronic diseases such as cancer, whereas use of its components in isolation may not produce the same broad impact on multiple disease risk factors. Few lifestyles involve consuming food items in isolation anyway, and optimal cardiovascular health will most likely be achieved in the context of a balanced diet that may include specific items to address a given CVD risk (e.g., plant sterols or stanols for LDL reduction).

REFERENCES

1. Third Report of the National Cholesterol Education Program (NCEP) Expert Panel on Detection, Evaluation, and Treatment of High Blood Cholesterol in Adults (Adult Treatment Panel III). Executive Summary; available at http://www.nhlbi.nih.gov/guidelines/cholesterol/atp_iii.htm

2. Franco OH, Bonneux L, de Laet C, et al: The Polymeal: A more natural, safer, and probably tastier (than the Polypill) strategy to reduce cardiovascular disease by more than 75%. BMJ 329:1447–1450, 2004.

3. Jenkins DJA, Kendall CWC, Marchie A, et al: Effects of a dietary portfolio of cholesterol-lowering foods vs lovastatin on serum lipids and C-reactive protein. JAMA 290:502–510, 2003.

SUGGESTED READINGS

American Heart Association: Heart Disease and Stroke Statistics—2005 Update. Dallas, Tex, American Heart Association, 2005.

Grundy SM, Cleeman JI, Merz CN, et al: Implications of recent clinical trials for the National Cholesterol Education Program Adult Treatment Panel III Guidelines. Circulation 110:227–239, 2004.

Hu FB, Willett WC: Optimal diets for prevention of coronary heart disease. JAMA 288:2569–2578, 2002.

Mokdad AH, Marks JS, Stroup DF, et al: Actual causes of death in the United States, 2000. JAMA 291:1238–1245, 2004.

WEB SITES

American Heart Association, http://www.americanheart.org

Cardiovascular Health Branch of the Centers for Disease Control and Prevention, http://www.cdc.gov/cvh/

National Cholesterol Education Program, http://www.nhlbi.nih.gov/about/ncep/index.htm

21

Cancer

DOUGLAS C. HEIMBURGER, MD

Cancer Prevention

Cancer is the leading cause of death in the United States for persons under the age of 85.[1] Although survival rates after diagnosis of the major lethal cancers (those of the lung, colon, and breast) have increased in recent years, prevention remains a key component of the war on cancer.

The risk for cancer is related to nutrients, non-nutritive dietary constituents, and nutritional status in a variety of ways. Part of the complexity stems from the fact that the development of cancer is a multistage process that usually begins with exposure to an environmental substance called a precarcinogen that must be activated *in vivo*. Once active, the carcinogen effects tumor initiation by producing a mutation that activates an oncogene or inactivates a tumor suppressor gene. Although this is a necessary step, it is not sufficient, as many mutant cells are probably destroyed before they form clones. Tumor promotion and progression, which require additional mutations and growth factors and often take many years, must occur before a tumor that is large enough to produce symptoms develops. Nutrition interacts with each of the stages of carcinogenesis, making the relationship complex.

To complicate matters further, the evidence linking nutritional variables to cancer is of many different types and strengths. Evidence for the involvement of particular nutrients in carcinogenesis often begins with epidemiologic observations in human populations. Prospective epidemiologic studies of cohorts, without intervention, have become quite valuable in confirming cross-sectional observations. Yet the diets of individuals are extremely complex, making it virtually impossible to distinguish the effects of single nutrients from those of groups of nutrients and other environmental and lifestyle variables on cancer risk. Animal carcinogenesis studies are often next, and perhaps thousands of them have been conducted. Carefully controlled to isolate single variables of interest, these studies allow causal inferences to be drawn, but extrapolation to the conditions and metabolism of free-living humans can be fraught with uncertainty. *In vitro* investigations, such as studies of factors that regulate oncogenes in cell cultures, provide important insights into the mechanisms of nutrient-cell interactions, but it is often unclear how each observation fits into the overall scheme of cancer development. Randomized, controlled human trials can provide the most definitive causal links in humans but are often quite expensive and lengthy, and sometimes use doses of single nutrients or synthetic analogues that are unavailable from food sources.

Nevertheless, taken together, there is compelling evidence of causal links between diet and cancer. It is estimated that nutritional factors account for about one third of the cancer deaths in the United States, with tobacco accounting for another one third and all other causes sharing the final one third. Nutritional risk factors for cancer include both dietary patterns and obesity and physical inactivity. Together they comprise the most important lifestyle choices that persons who do not use tobacco products can make to reduce their cancer risk. Evidence regarding them, distilled and updated every 5 years by the American Cancer Society, is summarized in the recommendations shown in Box 21–1. These recommendations will be used as an outline for consideration of the topic in this chapter.

Eat a Variety of Healthful Foods, with an Emphasis on Plant Sources

Eat Five or More Servings of a Variety of Vegetables and Fruits Each Day

Evidence suggests that consuming a generous quantity of fruits and vegetables reduces risk for several cancers,

---

BOX 21–1   Recommendations for Nutrition
and Physical Activity for Cancer Prevention*

Recommendations for Individual Choices

*Eat a Variety of Healthful Foods, with an Emphasis
on Plant Sources.*
Eat five or more servings of a variety of vegetables and
  fruits each day.
Choose whole grains in preference to processed (refined)
  grains and sugars.
Limit consumption of red meats, especially those high in fat
  and processed.
Choose foods that maintain a healthful weight.

Adopt a Physically Active Lifestyle.
Adults: Engage in at least moderate activity for 30 minutes or
  more on 5 or more days of the week; 45 minutes or more of
  moderate to vigorous activity on 5 or more days per week may
  further enhance reductions in the risk of breast and colon cancer.
Children and adolescents: Engage in at least 60 minutes per day of
  moderate to vigorous physical activity at least 5 days per week.

Maintain a Healthful Weight Throughout Life.
Balance caloric intake with physical activity.
Lose weight if currently overweight or obese.

If You Drink Alcoholic Beverages, Limit Consumption.

ACS Recommendation for Community Action

Public, private, and community organizations should work
  to create social and physical environments that support the
  adoption and maintenance of healthful nutrition and
  physical activity behaviors.
Increase access to healthful foods in schools, worksites, and
  communities.
Provide safe, enjoyable, and accessible environments for physical
  activity in schools and for transportation and recreation in
  communities.

---

*From American Cancer Society, http://www.cancer.org.

---

including those of the lung, stomach, esophagus, and
oral cavity, and the overall cancer death rate. Studies
suggest that the low energy density and high fiber content of these foods, plus folic acid, vitamin E, selenium,
and perhaps other nutrients as well as non-nutritive

phytochemicals naturally present in them, may be collectively responsible for this effect.

Epidemiologic studies show that both smokers and nonsmokers who have lower intakes or plasma levels of carotenes are at increased risk for lung cancer. A number of human intervention studies testing β-carotene or synthetic retinoids as cancer chemopreventive agents have been completed. Some of these have confirmed the expected protective effects, but two large trials showed small but significant *increases* in lung cancer in smokers who were supplemented with β-carotene; a third trial showed no effect. This unexpected result may have occurred because carcinogenesis had already progressed in the subjects, who had smoked for an average of 36 years, beyond the point where β-carotene could exert a beneficial effect. It also likely indicates that other constituents of fruits and vegetables may be responsible for some of the protective effect previously attributed to β-carotene.

Because folic acid is required for nucleic acid synthesis and repair and for DNA methylation, folic acid may offer protection against cancer. It is inactivated by certain environmental substances, particularly cigarette smoke, and it is marginally sufficient in the diets of many Americans (although this has improved since mandatory fortification of grains and cereals with folic acid took effect in 1998). There is evidence for a protective effect of folic acid against cancers of the colon, cervix, and lung.

Vitamin C, also present in fruits and vegetables, has been investigated, but its cancer-protective role has been difficult to isolate because of the presence of other protective nutrients and phytochemicals in the same foods. Its most direct role is probably as a water-soluble antioxidant that blocks the formation of nitrosamines in the stomach after the ingestion of foods containing nitrates and nitrites. In this way it may reduce the risk of stomach cancer.

The ability of vitamin E to protect lipid membranes against oxidation suggests that it could inhibit the actions of carcinogens. Another antioxidant, selenium, may have a protective role against several cancers, particularly those of the gastrointestinal tract. Results from large supplementation trials in the United States, China, and Finland have suggested that vitamin E and selenium may reduce risk for prostate cancer. Additional trials are underway to confirm these effects.

Non-nutritive substances in fruits and vegetables are probably responsible for some of their benefits. Many of these, including sulforafanes, indoles, sterols, phenols, terpenes, protease inhibitors, flavonoids, isoflavones, allylic sulfides, and capsaicin, have demonstrated anti-cancer actions *in vitro*. Lycopene, a carotenoid present in tomatoes, may reduce risk for prostate cancer. Because many of these substances can be obtained only from foods, it is inadvisable to use dietary supplements to prevent cancer instead of changing dietary habits. Vitamin A and selenium supplements, except in multivitamin/ multimineral preparations, should be particularly discouraged, as they can cause toxicity. Although it is not clear which nutrients or substances are most responsible, there are clear benefits from consuming substantial quantities of fruits and vegetables as part of a predominantly plant-based diet. Including a wide variety of them in the diet is likely to increase exposure to a broad range of beneficial phytonutrients.

There is little evidence that the food additives commonly used in the United States are responsible for any human cancers. A number of pesticides are carcinogenic *in vitro*, but whether they cause cancer in humans is the subject of continuing debate. It has been estimated that humans ingest at least 10,000 times as many naturally occurring carcinogens as they do synthetic ones.

Choose Whole Grains in Preference to Processed (Refined) Grains and Sugars

Since the inverse association of dietary fiber and whole-grain foods with colon cancer rates was first described in the 1970s, it has been investigated extensively. The mechanisms proposed to explain the association include dilution of carcinogens by increased stool bulk, direct binding of carcinogens by fiber, and alterations in colonic bacterial metabolism, which decreases the luminal pH and inhibits the formation of fecal mutagens such as secondary bile acids. The short-chain fatty acid metabolites of fiber also exert a trophic effect on the colonic mucosa, which may help to maintain a better defense against carcinogens.

Whole-grain foods, including legumes (e.g., dried beans, pinto beans, lentils, soybeans, and many others) are good sources of other nutrients including folate, vitamin E, and selenium. In human populations, dietary fiber intake varies inversely with dietary fat, and directly with the intake of other potentially beneficial nutrients, so some of the effects attributed to dietary fiber may be caused by other factors. Therefore, even after 3 decades of investigation, a reliable estimate of the independent effect of dietary fiber is impossible to make. Nevertheless, the recommendation to eat more fiber-containing foods is prudent, especially because doing so reduces the risk for coronary heart disease and diabetes.

Limit Consumption of Red Meats, Especially Those that are High in Fat and Processed

Evidence for an independent role for diets high in fats and meats—especially red meats (beef, pork, and lamb)—is strongest for colorectal cancers. In several large prospective cohort studies, participants who consumed red meat more frequently had significantly higher risk for colon cancer than those who ate little or no red meat. The effects were not reduced after controlling for intake of energy or fiber or for other known risk factors. Cooking methods that involve intense heat such as charbroiling of meats— especially when they are overcooked— produce or deposit polycyclic aromatic hydrocarbons (from fats) and heterocyclic amines (from proteins) on the meat surfaces. Because many of these compounds are potent carcinogens, cooking methods probably account for some of the association of meats with colorectal cancer. It is prudent not to use these cooking methods with great frequency, and to avoid overcooking.

Epidemiologic studies have long indicated that countries with high per capita fat consumption have higher age-adjusted death rates from cancers of the colon and rectum, prostate, and endometrium than do those with lower fat intakes. Because increased fat consumption tends to be characteristic of more highly developed countries, however, some studies were probably confounded by unmeasured cultural or dietary differences. This may explain why more recent and sophisticated studies failed to confirm an independent association of dietary fat with breast cancer.

Because fats yield 9 kcal per g vs. 4 kcal per g for carbohydrates and proteins, high-fat foods are generally high in energy density, and some associations such as that with breast cancer may be partly or wholly explained by differences in total energy intake. High-fat diets also generally involve consumption of more meats and fewer vegetables, fruits, and grains, and are often associated with higher body weights. These factors probably contribute to the higher cancer risk associated with high-fat diets.

Even though the dietary fat-cancer hypothesis is controversial, the recommendation to reduce fat intake makes a great deal of sense for most Americans. Even if reducing fat to 20% or 30% of energy is not guaranteed to reduce risk for breast cancer, it may do so for colon cancer. Perhaps more importantly, reducing fat intake is often the most efficient way to reduce total energy intake, and if it is accompanied by higher intakes of vegetables, fruits, beans, and grains, it will increase exposure to beneficial nutrients and reduce the risk for overweight or obesity, which is a risk factor for the same cancers that are associated with dietary fat.

Adopt a Physically Active Lifestyle

Evidence is increasing that physical activity is associated with lower risk for cancers of the breast, colon, and prostate gland. It has also been associated with better prognosis in patients who already have breast or prostate cancer. Part of its influence may be through effects on maintenance of a desirable body weight, but it may also act through increasing colonic transit rate, decreasing exposure of the breast to estrogens, improving insulin sensitivity, and decreasing growth factor levels. As discussed in Chapter 1, physical activity has rather global benefits, reducing the risk for diabetes (itself a risk factor for several cancers), hypertension, heart disease, and osteoporosis. Physical activity required to perform daily functions should be distinguished from intentional, scheduled exercise. The former reverses sedentary behaviors and the latter improves body composition and fitness; both confer substantial health benefits. See Chapter 1 for more details.

Maintain a Healthful Weight throughout Life

Balance Caloric Intake with Physical Activity

Obesity was identified at least as early as the 1960s as a risk factor for several cancers. Recent epidemiologic studies have found that obesity increases risk for cancers of the colon and rectum, esophagus, liver, pancreas, kidney, gallbladder, uterus, postmenopausal breast, cervix, ovary, stomach, and prostate gland as well as non-Hodgkin's lymphoma and multiple myeloma. It may be responsible for about 90,000 cancer deaths annually in the United States—as many as 20% of cancer deaths in women or 14% of cancer deaths in men.[2] The mechanisms are thought to involve alterations in hormone metabolism induced by obesity, such as elevated serum insulin, insulin-like growth factor-1, leptin, and androstenedione levels.

As reviewed in more detail in Chapter 17, obese persons are not all at equal risk for the complications of obesity. As with diabetes, hypertension, and heart disease, persons whose excess adiposity is predominantly intra-abdominal are at especially increased risk for endometrial and breast cancer, whereas those with peripheral obesity may not have elevated risk. Although the mechanism for this is not known, it may be caused by differences in hormone metabolism between centrally and peripherally obese persons.

Even when it does not result in obesity, excess energy intake in animals has a profound influence on the appearance of spontaneous or induced cancers. Since the 1930s, studies have demonstrated that allowing rodents to consume food *ad libitum* consistently results in tumor yields at least 25%, and up to 300%, higher than in animals given energy restrictions of only 10% to 25%. The effect of energy restriction is independent of and more potent than that of dietary fat restriction; in fact, in animals mild energy restriction is the most consistent and powerful anticancer "agent" known. Exercising animals to increase energy expenditure or using other methods to alter their body composition also reduces tumor yields, suggesting that absolute energy intake may be less important than the degree to which it matches energy expenditure. It is probable that body composition, energy balance, and the behaviors required to optimize them interact with many of the other nutrients correlated with cancer.

Lose Weight if Currently Overweight or Obese

It has not yet been demonstrated that weight reduction in overweight or obese persons reduces cancer risk. However, energy restriction, physical activity, and weight reduction clearly reverse the hormonal and metabolic alterations that are thought to mediate obesity-related cancer risk. Therefore, in addition to the well-documented beneficial effects on diabetes, hypertension, heart disease, and stroke, overweight or obese persons should be encouraged to adopt behaviors that will enable them to achieve and maintain lower body weights.

If You Drink Alcoholic Beverages, Limit Consumption

Although alcohol is not a carcinogen, it is a promoter of carcinogenesis in several organs. Excess alcohol acts synergistically with cigarette smoking to dramatically increase the risk of oral, pharyngeal, laryngeal, and esophageal cancer. Excessive consumption of alcohol is the major cause of hepatic cirrhosis in the United States, and the incidence of liver cancer is greatly increased in persons with cirrhosis. Risk for colon cancer may be increased as well.

Epidemiologic evidence has also linked even moderate alcohol intake with increased breast cancer incidence in women. In several studies, women who consumed as few as three drinks per week had 50% greater risk of breast cancer than did nondrinkers, especially if they did not have adequate dietary intakes of folic acid. Although this does not indicate that women should abstain from alcohol, especially in light of alcohol's potential cardiovascular benefits, it would be prudent to limit consumption to no more than one drink per day and to consider abstaining if other risk factors for breast cancer, such as a family history of the disease, are present.

Cancer Treatment

It has been observed for centuries that cancer patients frequently suffer from progressive cachexia. With most tumor types, weight loss heralds a poor prognosis, but this is not simply because patients who lose weight have higher tumor burdens; rather, the correlation between total tumor mass and weight loss is poor. The causes of weight loss have been extensively investigated. Elevated resting energy expenditure is a relatively small contributor. Metabolic alterations occur in cancer patients, including activation of cytokines such as tumor necrosis factor and proteolysis-inducing factor, futile metabolic cycles, glucose intolerance, insulin resistance, increased lipolysis, and increased whole-body protein turnover. However, the major cause of weight loss in cancer patients is poor nutrient intake resulting from anorexia, alterations in taste, and other disease- and treatment-related factors. These are summarized in Box 21–2.

The fact that weight loss is associated with poorer survival in cancer patients does not necessarily indicate a cause-effect relationship. If weight loss were the cause, reversing it with sufficient nutrients should improve survival. Although this has been attempted in many randomized trials, the benefits have been minimal and the

---

BOX 21-2   Factors Contributing to Weight Loss
in Cancer Patients

Systemic Disease-Related Effects

Anorexia
Changes in perception of taste and smell
Increased sense of fullness, perhaps resulting from decreased
    digestive secretions, mucosal atrophy, and/or impaired
    gastric emptying
Changes in metabolism, induced by cytokines such as tumor
    necrosis factor and proteolysis-inducing factor

Local Disease-Related Effects

Obstruction of the gastrointestinal tract at any point
Intestinal dysmotility induced by the tumor

Treatment-Related Effects

Surgery affecting the gastrointestinal tract or head and neck
Chemotherapy, causing mucositis, nausea, vomiting, diarrhea
Radiotherapy, causing decreased saliva, taste, and smell;
    occasional radiation enteropathy

Psychological Effects

Depression
Conditioned food aversions related to upcoming therapy

---

risks sometimes substantial, at least when total parenteral nutrition (TPN) is used. Trials that tested TPN as an adjunct to chemotherapy and radiation therapy did not document improvements in survival, tumor response, or tolerance of therapy. Rather, higher sepsis rates were consistently seen in TPN-treated patients as compared with controls, indicating that TPN can produce net harm in these patients, and should not be used routinely.

Enteral feeding trials have produced better results. In some but not all studies enteral feeding—especially with immune-enhancing formulas (see Chapter 23 and Table 13-1)—for 3 to 10 days before or after cancer surgery produced improvements in nutritional status including body weight and quality of life. In some cases (but not uniformly) decreased morbidity (e.g., infections), mortality, and length of postoperative hospital stay were seen. In patients who survived hospitalization, long-term benefits from aggressive nutritional support have not been demonstrated.

In cancer patients who are not undergoing surgical intervention, it is best to take an individualized approach to nutritional support by monitoring nutritional status carefully and intervening aggressively only when clear indications exist. There is no justification for using enteral or parenteral nutrition to prevent weight loss or to treat weight losses of less than 10%. When patients are at risk for losing unacceptable amounts of weight, every effort should be made to use enteral feeding rather than TPN.

Because of general population trends and the cancer risk associated with obesity, increasing numbers of cancer patients are overweight or obese. Although randomized trials have not yet tested the effects of intentional weight reduction in overweight or obese cancer survivors, evidence discussed earlier in this chapter suggests that weight reduction and increased physical activity may benefit overweight or obese patients who have cancers for which obesity is a primary risk factor, particularly postmenopausal breast cancer and prostate cancer.

Although better outcomes from maintaining adequate nutrition during cancer treatment are uncertain, eating and feeling well nourished contribute to an overall sense of well-being. Nutrition, therefore, has an important place in the palliative care of patients with cancer. Paying careful attention to cancer patients' nutritional problems and concerns can help considerably to make them feel stronger and more self-sufficient.

Oral Nutrition

Cancer patients often experience abnormalities in their senses of taste and smell, but because these occur without a predictable pattern, it is best to be aware of individual food preferences and aversions and experiment with various food aromas and seasonings. Cold foods tend to be better tolerated than hot foods, which may increase nausea and vomiting. Acidic foods tend to irritate inflamed mucous membranes. Anorexia and nausea sometimes increase as the day progresses, so breakfast meals may be tolerated best. Small meals with between-meal snacks can augment total food intake. The cancer organization web sites cited at the end of this chapter contain additional useful tips, patient handouts, and recipes to help combat the nutrition-related side effects of cancers and their therapies.

Commercial oral nutritional formulas are very helpful to supplement food intake (see Chapter 13). Some cancer patients are overwhelmed by the sweetness of some oral supplements, and prefer to drink unflavored "tube-only" formulas. To accommodate this, the sweetness of some formulas developed specifically for cancer patients has been muted. Some formulas also contain n-3 fatty acids because of limited evidence that they may help maintain muscle mass and promote weight gain in cancer patients.

Cancer patients and their families are often interested in alternative nutritional therapies for cancer, including megadoses of various vitamins or ingestion of herbs, hormones, antioxidant enzymes, "immune stimulators," exotic juices, "detoxifiers," or special teas. Although well-designed studies to test many alternative therapies have been initiated, none of these approaches has yet been clearly shown to improve any significant outcome variable in cancer patients. However, anorexic cancer patients may become vitamin deficient, so a daily replacement multivitamin is warranted. The possibility of pre-existing deficiencies in patients undergoing medical and surgical therapies should be taken into account as well. Zinc and vitamin C supplementation should be considered in patients with poor wound healing or sepsis.

Enteral Nutrition

When oral intake is inadequate to maintain nutritional status but the intestinal tract is functional, tube feeding should be used as long as it is consistent with the overall treatment plan. Tube feeding can sometimes provide relief for the anorexic patient who is constantly pressured to eat more while experiencing nausea and food aversions. It can be administered at home to reduce the need for hospitalization. Considerations in choosing feeding formulas are the same as in patients without cancer. Unless there is a contraindication, cachectic patients should be given high-protein formulas.

Parenteral Nutrition

Even with the cautions noted above, indications exist for using TPN in cancer patients. Principal among these are intestinal obstruction and major intestinal resection or diversion. Preoperative TPN should be considered for patients who have lost 15% to 20% of body weight, require major surgery, and cannot be fed by any enteral route. The decision to initiate TPN must be consistent with the prognosis and overall treatment objectives. Thus, the ideal candidate is the patient with intestinal obstruction whose prognosis is otherwise reasonably good and for whom additional cancer therapy is planned. However, it is often inappropriate in patients whose malignancies have not responded to therapy and are considered terminal. In these cases maintaining hydration with intravenous fluids usually offers comparable benefits as well as fewer complications and lower costs.

The indications for home parenteral nutrition mirror those for in-hospital use. It can be particularly effective for prolonging the lives of patients with irremediable intestinal obstruction or massive intestinal resection. It can reduce the need for hospitalization during chemotherapy and fistula healing, thus decreasing the total cost of care and improving quality of life. However, as with in-hospital TPN, the appropriateness of its use must be carefully considered in terminal care, in which it may provide no more benefit than maintaining hydration with intravenous fluids would provide.

REFERENCES

1. Jemal A, Murray T, Ward E, et al: Cancer statistics, 2005. CA Cancer J Clin 55:10–30, 2005.
2. Calle EE, Rodriguez C, Walker-Thurmond K, Thun MJ: Overweight, obesity, and mortality from cancer in a prospectively studied cohort of U.S. adults. N Engl J Med 348:1625–1638, 2003.

SUGGESTED READINGS

Brown JK, Byers T, Doyle C, et al: Nutrition and physical activity during and after cancer treatment: An American Cancer Society guide for informed choices. CA Cancer J Clin 53:268–291, 2003.

Byers T, Nestle M, McTiernan A, et al: American Cancer Society guidelines on nutrition and physical activity for cancer prevention (2002). Reducing the risk of cancer with healthy food choices and physical activity. CA Cancer J Clin 52:92–119, 2002.

Eyre H, Kahn R, Robertson RM, et al: Preventing cancer, cardiovascular disease, and diabetes: A common agenda for the American Cancer Society, the American Diabetes Association, and the American Heart Association. CA Cancer J Clin 54:190–207, 2004.

Heber D, Blackburn GL, Go VLW (eds): Nutritional Oncology. New York, Academic Press, 1999.

McCullough ML, Giovannucci EL: Diet and cancer prevention. Oncogene 23:6349–6364, 2004.

World Cancer Research Fund & American Institute for Cancer Research: Food, Nutrition and the Prevention of Cancer: A Global Perspective. Washington, DC, American Institute for Cancer Research, 1997; (new edition due in 2006).

WEB SITES

American Cancer Society, http://www.cancer.org
American Institute for Cancer Research, http://www.aicr.org (specifically focuses on research on diet and cancer prevention)
National Cancer Institute, http://www.cancer.gov

22

Gastrointestinal and Liver Diseases

JAIME ARANDA-MICHEL, MD • ABDULLAH MUBARAK, MD •
REINALDO FIGUEROA, MD

Gastrointestinal Diseases

Because the primary function of the gut is to absorb nutrients (Figs. 22–1 through 22–3 and Table 22–1), it is not surprising that gastrointestinal diseases have an impact on nutrition or that nutritional manipulations are integral to the management of gastrointestinal diseases.

Malabsorption

Many gastrointestinal conditions produce malabsorption, which is a failure of the gastrointestinal tract to absorb ingested nutrients. Malabsorption results from surgical resections and from many types of gastrointestinal disease including pancreatic or biliary insufficiency and primary intestinal conditions such as infiltrative, inflammatory, or neoplastic diseases. It is best to classify malabsorption on the basis of its physiologic effects. Processes that cause malabsorption affect either the intraluminal or the mucosal phase of digestion and absorption.

Intraluminal

The intraluminal phase is the phase in which ingested food is mixed with pancreatic enzymes and bile salts to decrease the sizes of carbohydrates and proteins so they can be absorbed by the mucosa (see Figs. 22–2 and 22–3). Fats are also converted to simpler forms, but bile salts are needed to help them migrate to the

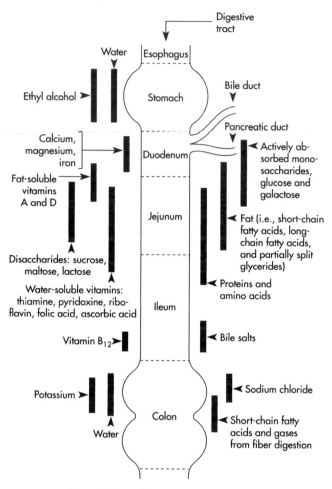

Figure 22–1. SITES OF NUTRIENT ABSORPTION.

intestinal mucosa. This process is disturbed in chronic pancreatitis (in which insufficient pancreatic enzymes are produced) and biliary cirrhosis (in which insufficient amounts of bile salts are excreted). In pancreatic insufficiency, oral replacement of the enzymes can improve digestion, and therefore absorption.

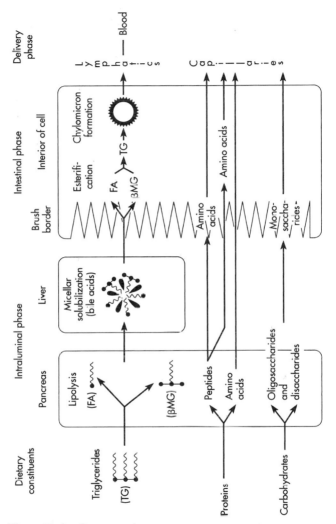

Figure 22–2. DIGESTION AND ABSORPTION OF TRIGLYCERIDES, PROTEINS, AND CARBOHYDRATES. βMC, beta-monoglycerides; FA, fatty acids.

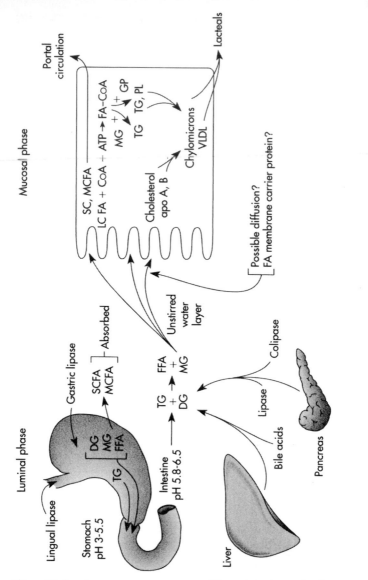

Figure 22–3. FAT DIGESTION AND ABSORPTION. Abbreviated scheme of major steps in fat hydrolysis in the lumen of stomach and intestine and reesterification in the intestinal mucosa. Apo A, apo B, apoproteins A and B; ATP, adenosine triphosphate; CoA, coenzyme A; DG, diglycerides; FFA, free fatty acids; GP, glycerophosphate; LCFA, long-chain fatty acids; MCFA, medium-chain fatty acids; MG, monoglycerides; PL, phospholipids; SCFA, short-chain fatty acids; TG, triglycerides; VLDL, very-low-density lipoproteins.

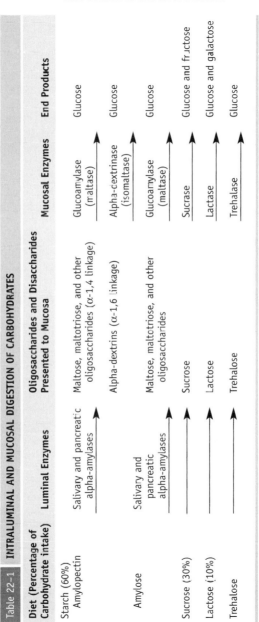

Table 22-1 INTRALUMINAL AND MUCOSAL DIGESTION OF CARBOHYDRATES

Diet (Percentage of Carbohydrate intake)	Luminal Enzymes	Oligosaccharides and Disaccharides Presented to Mucosa	Mucosal Enzymes	End Products
Starch (60%) Amylopectin	Salivary and pancreatic alpha-amylases →	Maltose, maltotriose, and other oligosaccharides (α-1,4 linkage)	Glucoamylase (maltase) →	Glucose
		Alpha-dextrins (α-1,6 linkage)	Alpha-dextrinase (isomaltase) →	Glucose
Amylose	Salivary and pancreatic alpha-amylases →	Maltose, maltotriose, and other oligosaccharides	Glucoamylase (maltase) →	Glucose
Sucrose (30%)	———————	Sucrose	Sucrase →	Glucose and fructose
Lactose (10%)	———————	Lactose	Lactase →	Glucose and galactose
Trehalose	———————	Trehalose	Trehalase →	Glucose

Mucosal

All nutrients must cross the intestinal mucosal surface to enter the circulation, and most do so by specific mechanisms. Anything affecting the length or mass of the intestinal mucosa, such as inflammatory conditions, (e.g., Crohn's disease [regional enteritis]), giardiasis, gluten enteropathy (celiac disease), infiltrative processes, lymphoma, and intestinal resection, will decrease absorption. Problems can also occur when a specific mucosal digestive or transport mechanism is missing or damaged, such as in lactase deficiency. Some types of malabsorption are easily managed when the underlying disease, e.g., giardiasis, gluten enteropathy, and lactase deficiency, is addressed. Others require considerable dietary manipulation, such as those that occur after intestinal resection for intestinal infarction, congenital malformations, inflammatory diseases, cancer, and trauma.

Resection

Gastrointestinal resections can alter the physiology of digestion and absorption in a variety of ways depending on the portion of intestine removed. There may be changes in transit time, reduction in overall surface area, inability to absorb nutrients that require specialized portions of the intestine, and altered bacterial colonization. Resections of the stomach, duodenum, and terminal ileum impair absorption much more than do resections of other parts of the small bowel because of their specific regulatory functions and specialized absorption of nutrients.

Resection of the Stomach

The gastric pylorus normally functions as a gate, retaining the gastric contents until they are isotonic and then releasing them into the duodenum. Most gastric operations alter the pylorus, increasing the rate of gastric emptying. Premature passage of hyperosmolar contents into the upper small intestine can result in rapid shifts of fluid into the small intestine (referred to as dumping syndrome) and maldigestion caused by inadequate mixing with bile and pancreatic secretions.

A total gastrectomy removes the sources of intrinsic factor that are required for ileal absorption of dietary and enterohepatically recirculated vitamin B_{12}, placing the patient at risk for B_{12} deficiency. With decreased gastric acid and pepsin secretion after gastric removal, absorption of heme iron is impaired because its reduction to the ferrous form is hampered. Iron is normally absorbed in the duodenum, but the jejunum can adapt to perform this function if the duodenum is removed.

Resection of the Small Intestine

The signs and symptoms of malabsorption after small intestinal resection depend on the extent and location of the resection and the extent and severity of the underlying disease that led to the resection. Most patients can tolerate resections of less than 50% of the small bowel without any symptoms. When more than 70% of the small bowel has been resected or 100 cm or less of the small bowel remains, most patients have symptoms. Long-term parenteral nutrition is often required when less than 2 feet of jejunum or ileum are intact; when 1 foot or less remains, parenteral nutrition is necessary for survival. For most patients with small bowel resection or disease, steatorrhea (fat loss in the stool) and its consequences are the most significant problems. Although fluids and electrolytes are also absorbed in the jejunum and ileum, and therefore malabsorbed after resection, the colon has a tremendous capacity to absorb what is not absorbed by the small bowel. Table 22–2 lists typical volumes of fluid ingested, secreted, and reabsorbed by specific areas of the gastrointestinal tract. Because the colon is very efficient in reabsorbing fluid, excessive fluid losses or liquid diarrhea are generally not a major problem unless the colon is also damaged or missing.

The most consistent and often the earliest manifestation of steatorrhea is increased stool bulk. Patients may have one to three very large bowel movements a day

Table 22–2	VOLUMES OF FLUID ENTERING AND LEAVING THE INTESTINAL TRACT DAILY	

Ingestion and Secretion		
Fluid	**Volume Entering Lumen (L)**	
Diet	2	
Saliva	1	
Gastric secretion	2	
Bile	1	
Pancreatic secretion	2	
Small intestinal secretion	1	
TOTAL	9	

Reabsorption		
Intestinal Segment	**Volume Reabsorbed (L)**	**Approximate Efficiency of Reabsorption (%)**
Jejunum	4–5 of 9	50
Ileum	3–4 of 4–5	75
Colon	1–2 of 1–2	>90
TOTAL	8–9	

The stool normally contains 100–200 mL of fluid daily. If it contains >300 mL/day, diarrhea is usually present.

rather than small watery stools, and may not complain of diarrhea. Because of their high fatty acid and air contents, the stools may be frothy and float, are often foul smelling, and may be associated with flatulence. Weight loss is a common but inconsistent finding in malabsorption because many patients compensate for poor absorption by increasing their energy intake.

Fat malabsorption can lead to secondary problems. Cramping and paresthesias (numbness and tingling) of the hands and feet are a manifestation of hypocalcemia and/or hypomagnesemia. These conditions develop when unabsorbed free fatty acids form insoluble precipitates (soaps) with calcium and magnesium ions, rendering them unabsorbable. Patients with steatorrhea are at risk for developing calcium oxalate kidney stones, which result from high urinary oxalate excretion (hyperoxaluria).

The latter is caused by enhanced colonic absorption of dietary oxalate resulting from increased free oxalate in the adapted remnant bowel lumen when calcium, which normally binds oxalate and impedes its absorption, is trapped by free fatty acids.

Patients with steatorrhea also malabsorb fat-soluble vitamins A, D, E, and K. Bruising of the skin, especially without trauma, suggests vitamin K deficiency. However, because colonic bacteria produce vitamin K, a deficiency state does not generally develop unless the colonic flora are destroyed by antibiotics. Decreased dark adaptation caused by vitamin A deficiency tends to present initially as reduced visual acuity on entering a dark room such as a theater or when driving at night and looking into the lights of an oncoming car. Bone loss resulting in osteopenia or osteoporosis and increased risk of fractures may result from chronic malabsorption of calcium and vitamin D. Vitamin E deficiency may occur from severe longstanding malabsorption. Dietary carotene is poorly absorbed and serum levels are frequently low, providing a useful diagnostic test to support the impression of fat malabsorption, as long as the patient consumes several servings of carotene per day from yellow and green vegetables and fruits (which many Americans do not).

Digestion and absorption of most nutrients occur primarily in the jejunum; however, the ileum can perform these functions if the jejunum is resected. By contrast, the jejunum cannot replace specific terminal ileal functions such as the active absorption of bile salts and vitamin B_{12}. Diarrhea can develop from the increased amounts of bile salts entering the colon. Both unabsorbed fatty acids and bile acids interfere with colonic sodium and water absorption and may cause fluid secretion and severe diarrhea. This bile acid colitis can usually be managed with bile acid binding resins such as cholestyramine. Bile salt malabsorption also predisposes patients to cholesterol gallstone formation.

Resection or disease of the most distal portion of the ileum prevents the absorption of intrinsic factor-bound vitamin B_{12}. Macrocytic anemia in the setting of malabsorption is strongly suggestive of B_{12} deficiency or folate deficiency. Because physical findings of zinc deficiency may escape notice in patients with malabsorption, blood zinc levels should be monitored and low levels treated because of the potential for altered taste, poor wound healing, and immune compromise.

The presence or absence of the ileocecal valve is a critical determinant of bowel function in individuals with significant intestinal resection or disease. This structure regulates the entrance of small bowel contents into the colon and protects the small intestine from colonization by colonic organisms. If these bacteria enter the small intestine after resection of the ileocecal valve, bacterial overgrowth of the small intestine can occur and produce diarrhea. Regardless of the extent of the small bowel resection, patients with intact ileocecal valves are generally much less symptomatic than are those without them.

Resection of the Colon

The major role of the colon in the digestive process is to absorb electrolytes and water. The electrolyte contents of various body fluids are shown in Table 22–3. Unabsorbed carbohydrates are fermented by colonic bacteria, producing hydrogen, carbon dioxide, and short-chain fatty acids; the colon can absorb these, providing 5.7 kcal/g. However, a large production of short-chain fatty acids decreases the colonic pH to less than 5.5,

Table 22–3	**ELECTROLYTE COMPOSITION OF EXTERNAL LOSSES**		
Fluid	**Na$^+$ (mEq/L)**	**K$^+$ (mEq/L)**	**Cl$^-$ (mEq/L)**
Gastric	20–80	5–20	100–150
Pancreatic	120–140	5–15	90–120
Small intestine	100–140	5–15	90–130
Bile	120–140	5–15	80–120
Ileostomy	45–135	3–15	20–115
Diarrhea	10–90	10–80	10–110
Sweat			
Normal	10–30	3–10	10–35
Cystic fibrosis	50–135	5–25	50–110
Burns	140	5	110

disturbing sodium absorption by the colonic mucosa and tending to cause diarrhea. The presence of these osmotically active fatty acids in the colon also causes diarrhea. Patients who have had extensive resections of both colon and small bowel usually have profuse watery diarrhea. On the other hand, removing the colon protects patients who have had terminal ileum resections against bile acid colitis. Patients with externally draining jejunostomies sometimes have fluid losses large enough to require long-term parenteral nutrition.

Nutritional Management Following Intestinal Resection

Although certain aspects of malabsorption are predictable, no two patients with malabsorption are identical. Survival and rehabilitation after intestinal resection depend on the length, location, and condition of the remaining intestine; the capacity of the intestinal remnant to adapt by increasing its absorptive capacity; and the adequacy of nutritional support. Even after massive intestinal resections, patients with short bowel syndrome often find that they are able to readapt to using oral feeding as their sole nutritional support. However, this result requires judicious use of both parenteral nutrition and a carefully designed oral refeeding regimen to facilitate intestinal adaptation and prevent deficiencies (Fig. 22–4 and Table 22–4).

Nutrition and Bowel Adaptation

Substantial anatomic and physiologic adaptations occur after partial intestinal resection. The remaining bowel dilates, mucosal hyperplasia occurs, crypt length and number increase, and absorption per unit length of bowel increases by as much as several hundred percent. Intestinal motility decreases, maximizing food contact time with the mucosa and enabling better absorption of nutrients. However, this adaptation only takes place when enteral feeding is being used to stimulate the bowel and pancreatic and biliary secretions. Parenteral nutrition without enteral feeding is not sufficient.

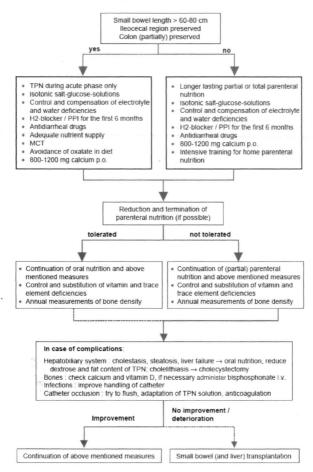

Figure 22–4. ALGORITHM FOR NUTRITIONAL MANAGEMENT AFTER SMALL BOWEL RESECTION. (From Keller J, Panter H, Layer P: Management of the short bowel syndrome after extensive small bowel resection. Best Pract Res Clin Gastroenterol 18:977–992, 2004, with permission.)

After extensive small bowel resections, optimal intestinal function and nutritional status are achieved through a combination of graduated oral feeding and parenteral nutrition. In this way, nutritional needs can be met and weight maintained or gained while the small bowel

Table 22-4	SUPPLEMENTS AND AGENTS FOR PATIENTS WITH MALDIGESTION OR MALABSORPTION	
Agent	**Dosage to Correct Deficiency**	**Maintenance Dose**
Minerals		
Calcium gluconate or Calcium carbonate	IV or po as needed	500 mq po bid to qid
Magnesium gluconate or Magnesium oxide	IV or po as needed	1–4 g po qd to qid
Ferrous sulfate	IV iron dextran or 325 mg qd to tid	325 mg po qd to tid iron dextran 1000 mg IV periodically
Vitamins		
Vitamin A	100,000 U IM	10,000–25,000 U po qd
Vitamin D	10,000–50,000 U po qd	10,000–50,000 U po/day or 50,000 U po 1–3 times weekly
Vitamin E (α-tocopherol)	1000 mg po qd to tid	400–1000 mg po qd
Vitamin K	10 mg IM or IV × 1 to 2	1 mq po qd (rarely required)
Folic acid	1–5 mg qd po or IV	0.4–1 mg po qd
Vitamin B_{12}	1000 µg IM × 1 to 2	100 µg IM or 500 µg nasal gel q month, or 1000 mg po qd
Pancreatic Enzymes		1–3 tabs po with meals, 1 with snacks
Antibiotics		Metronidazole, tetracycline, quinolones
Antidiarrheal Agents		Loperamide 2–4 mg po prn; diphenoxylate + atropine 1–2 tabs qid prn; octreotide
Bile Acid-binding Resin		Cholestyramine 4–8 g po bid to tid

remnant is challenged incrementally with gradual exposure to macronutrients. The intestinal adaptation phase can last 1 to 2 years. To accomplish this goal, the refeeding regimen described in Chapter 12 is recommended for all patients undergoing drastic intestinal resection and for those who have suffered significant weight loss and malnutrition because of malabsorption.

General Nutrition Guidelines

Once the patient has progressed through the refeeding regimen for 1 to 3 weeks, the diet should consist of small frequent meals, avoidance of milk (because of expected lactose intolerance), and restriction of fat (less than 30 g per day). If patients continue to have diarrhea in the early adaptive phase, the causes may include gastric and/or intestinal hypersecretion or bile acid malabsorption, and patients may benefit from treatment with gastric acid inhibitors, cholestyramine, and/or octreotide. Some patients may lose intestinal bicarbonate and develop metabolic acidosis, and thus may need bicarbonate supplementation (e.g., Shohl solution). As intestinal adaptation takes place over 3 to 4 months, intake of fat may be gradually increased to about 40 g per day and then to 50 or 60 g per day. Medium-chain triglyceride (MCT) oil may be supplemented if increased calories are needed. Supplemental enteral formulas can be useful as long as they are lactose-free and low in fat. Although it may be useful to give them a therapeutic trial in difficult cases, special formulas containing pre-hydrolyzed proteins (peptides and/or crystalline amino acids) have no proven advantage in terms of intestinal function or nitrogen balance, and are generally higher in osmolality and cost.

Minerals and Vitamins

When deficiencies of the divalent cations calcium and magnesium exist (as evidenced by hypocalcemia and/or hypomagnesemia), long-term restriction of dietary fat may be helpful. Calcium and vitamin D supplementation are often needed to maintain the serum calcium level but may be inadequate without dietary fat restriction. Hypomagnesemia also dictates a need for fat restriction, because oral magnesium supplements cause diarrhea and are tolerated only in small doses.

Treatment to avoid deficiencies of the fat-soluble vitamins A, D, E, and K should be guided by appropriate blood tests. Large oral doses of vitamins A, D, and E are often needed to sustain normal blood vitamin levels and, in the case of vitamin D, to maintain a normal serum calcium. Vitamin K supplements are not required unless the prothrombin time is prolonged.

Patients with malabsorption usually do not develop deficiencies of most of the water-soluble vitamins since they are efficiently absorbed in even short segments of the small intestine. However, patients with ileal disease or resection usually require periodic injections of vitamin B_{12}. Alternative methods of B_{12} supplementation that are sometimes effective include large oral doses (1000 μg/day) and nasal B_{12} gels. Folate deficiencies sometimes occur in patients with small intestinal disorders and usually respond to supplementation with 1 mg per day. Because maximal iron absorption occurs in the duodenum, iron deficiency is likely only after duodenal bypass such as occurs in bariatric surgery involving gastric bypass with Roux-en-Y. Serum levels of vitamin B_{12}, folate, and iron should be monitored in all patients who have undergone significant gastrointestinal surgeries, and appropriate supplements should be used if they drop to unacceptably low levels.

Patients with hyperoxaluria or a history of oxalate-containing renal stones should be instructed to consume substantial amounts of fluid and oral calcium supplements to increase binding of oxalate in the intestine. Therapeutic multivitamin-multimineral supplements are often helpful in patients with significant malabsorption, especially in those with short bowel syndrome. Examples of these are shown in Appendix C. Individual nutrient supplement recommendations are provided in Table 22-4.

Medications

Several medications commonly used in patients with malabsorption are listed in Table 22-4. Pancreatic enzyme supplements containing high lipase activity may improve fat digestion and steatorrhea in some patients after intestinal resection. Large and frequent doses are usually required, and responses are variable in patients with bowel disease or resections, whereas they are usually effective (and diagnostic) in patients with maldigestion caused by pancreatic insufficiency. In patients who have had the terminal ileum resected, bile acid-induced diarrhea may respond to 8 to 12 g of cholestyramine per day. This binding resin reduces the irritating effects of the bile acids in the colon. In patients with more extensive resections, especially of the colon, cholestyramine is of little help and may aggravate the steatorrhea by further depleting the bile acid pool.

Bacterial colonization of the small bowel can contribute to diarrhea and malabsorption, especially when the ileo-cecal valve is removed. When colonization is suspected, a trial of oral antibiotics such as metronidazole may bring symptomatic improvement.

Gastric acid and fluid hypersecretion commonly occur during the first several weeks after intestinal resection, resulting from gastrin hypersecretion. Proton pump inhibitor drugs are sometimes used in this setting, but hypersecretion is not a constant finding and tends to disappear with time.

Celiac Disease

Celiac disease, also known as celiac sprue and gluten-sensitive enteropathy, is a genetic malabsorptive disorder involving immune-mediated mucosal damage resulting from sensitivity to gluten that occurs naturally in wheat, rye, and barley proteins. It was long felt to be a disease of the young, but with the availability of more sensitive serologic tests, it is being increasingly recognized in older age groups. The clinical manifestations are myriad and include growth failure in children, infertility and miscarriages in women of child-bearing age, fatigue, anemia, weight loss, diarrhea, and overt steatorrhea and malabsorption. Many patients are asymptomatic and undiagnosed for months to years. Some patients exhibit extraintestinal manifestations including diabetes mellitus, dermatitis herpetiformis, asymptomatic elevation of liver enzymes, osteomalacia and osteoporosis, selective IgA deficiency, and even neuropsychiatric illnesses.

Diagnosis is initiated with serologic testing for anti-endomysial and anti-gliadin antibodies, or more recently, the human tissue transglutaminase-based enzyme-linked immunosorbent assay (ELISA). Tissue transglutaminase is the antigen for anti-endomysial antibodies; its high sensitivity (approximately 95%) makes it a cost-effective strategy for identifying both symptomatic and atypical forms of celiac disease. Intestinal biopsy revealing villous atrophy, however, is still required to confirm the diagnosis.

The cornerstone of management is adherence to a gluten-free diet; most compliant patients experience symptomatic relief and histologic improvement. Patients should consult educational web sites (see Web sites at end of this chapter) and a dietitian to learn how to implement the diet. All foods containing wheat, rye, and barley must be eliminated. Soybean or tapioca flours, rice, corn, buckwheat, and potatoes are safe. Prepared foods and condiments should be examined carefully, paying particular attention to additives such as stabilizers or emulsifiers that may contain gluten. Dairy products should be avoided initially because many patients with celiac disease may have secondary lactose intolerance from mucosal atrophy. Consumption of oats is controversial; while pure oats are gluten-free, many commercial oat products are contaminated with gluten from other grains.

All patients with celiac disease should be monitored for micronutrient deficiencies, especially vitamin D deficiency and resulting bone disease. Because patients with celiac disease are at increased risk for small bowel lymphomas, these should be ruled out if abdominal symptoms persist.

Gastrointestinal Problems Without Malabsorption

Many of the common gastrointestinal diseases and conditions do not cause malnutrition, but nutritional management is an important part of their treatment.

Irritable Bowel Syndrome

A very common but poorly understood condition, irritable bowel syndrome can cause abdominal pain, constipation, diarrhea, and abdominal bloating. It is most likely an intestinal motility disorder and it can sometimes be triggered by stress and certain foods. The offending foods, when there are any, vary from patient to patient. Meals that are too large or high in fat may lead to abdominal cramps and diarrhea, as may foods that contain sorbitol or fructose, caffeine, or alcohol. Gas-producing foods (e.g., beans, cabbage, legumes, cauliflower, broccoli, lentils, Brussels sprouts, raisins, onions, and bagels) may produce gas and bloating. Supplementing the diet with up to 30 g per day of fiber benefits many patients.

Constipation

Although constipation can be treated with laxatives and stool softeners, a high-fiber diet can be equally effective, cheaper, and provide added benefits. Whether used for constipation or irritable bowel syndrome, a high-fiber diet must be consistent and accompanied by sufficient fluid intake to be effective. Physical activity may also be helpful.

Gastroesophageal Reflux Disease

Defined as the movement of gastric acid and other gastric contents into the esophagus, gastroesophageal reflux disease can produce pain and "heartburn" and can lead to esophagitis and esophageal strictures. Certain dietary changes can decrease the severity of the reflux. It is important to eliminate caffeine and chocolate from the diet because they relax the lower esophageal sphincter. Even decaffeinated coffee may need to be eliminated because the oils in coffee seem to potentiate reflux.

Liver Diseases

The liver orchestrates a wide variety of major metabolic processes in the body including carbohydrate, fat, and protein metabolism, protein synthesis, and detoxification and excretion of both endogenous and exogenous waste products. The liver has an enormous functional reserve—it can perform satisfactorily when only 20 % of its cells are functioning—and an excellent ability to repair itself after injury. However, severe impairment of any of its functions regardless of the cause can create widespread and diverse metabolic derangements that often affect nutritional status through anorexia, fat malabsorption, depressed protein synthesis, and other mechanisms. Conversely, impairment of nutritional status may further exacerbate abnormal liver function by hampering the liver's ability to regenerate itself. The goal of nutritional therapy in liver disease is to support liver function and optimize the liver's ability to regenerate if the injury is repaired or resolved.

Carbohydrate and Fat Metabolism

The liver plays a central role in blood glucose homeostasis. When exogenous calories fail to meet the body's requirements, the liver initially maintains blood glucose levels by metabolizing glycogen (glycogenolysis). As starvation continues, there is a gradual transition toward synthesis of glucose from amino acids and lipids (gluconeogenesis). In patients with severe hepatic insufficiency, these processes are impaired and hypoglycemia may occur.

The liver also plays an important role in fat metabolism. Fatty acids from both endogenous and exogenous sources are converted to energy via the Krebs cycle. When adapting to starvation, the liver forms ketone bodies, which can be utilized by parts of the body including the brain as an alternative to glucose. By sparing gluconeogenesis and its amino acid substrates, muscle protein is conserved. The liver also synthesizes, packages, and interconverts cholesterol, bile acids, and lipoproteins.

In patients with hepatic injuries, all of these functions may be impaired. Malabsorption of fat and fat-soluble vitamins may occur because of diminished bile salt production and/or excretion by the liver into the bile, where they are needed to facilitate fat absorption.

Protein Metabolism

As with carbohydrate and fat, the liver processes endogenous and exogenous amino acids. Endogenous proteins are continuously hydrolyzed to amino acids and resynthesized into proteins. Through hepatic transamination, amination, and deamination reactions, there is a constant interchange between the amino acids and the energy-producing substrates of carbohydrate and fat metabolism. Ammonia, a byproduct of amino acid catabolism, is converted to urea by the liver for excretion in the urine.

Altered protein metabolism is probably the most significant metabolic disturbance in liver disease (Fig. 22–5). It is characterized by altered plasma amino acid profiles and manifests clinically by muscle wasting and encephalopathy. As hepatic insufficiency develops, the liver provides the body with glucose less efficiently. As a consequence the branched-chain amino acids—leucine, isoleucine, and valine—are utilized locally by several tissues to produce energy, and their blood levels decrease. By contrast, the aromatic amino acids—phenylalanine, tyrosine, and tryptophan—and methionine are not metabolized normally by the liver, and their levels rise, resulting in a low branched-chain amino acid to aromatic amino acid ratio. The ratio of free tryptophan to protein-bound tryptophan in the blood also increases.

Hepatic encephalopathy (a neuropsychiatric disorder manifested by neuromuscular irritability, stupor, and coma) can develop in patients with decompensated liver disease. Usually patients have a precipitating factor such as infection, dehydration, alcohol ingestion, or ingestion of more protein than the liver can handle. The mechanism of hepatic encephalopathy is multifactorial, but it appears to relate at least in part to alterations in amino acid metabolism and the production of false neurotransmitters in the brain. Manipulation of the plasma amino acids to correct this abnormality sometimes improves encephalopathy. Chronic liver disease with superimposed encephalopathy differs metabolically from acute fulminant hepatic failure, in which plasma branched-chain amino acid levels are often normal while those of all other amino acids are increased. This difference may explain the apparent ineffectiveness of manipulation of the plasma amino acids in this condition.

Treatment

Severe hepatic insufficiency places the patient in a difficult nutritional position. Encephalopathy may develop

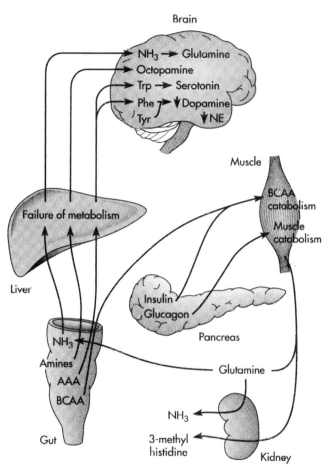

Figure 22–5. PATHOGENESIS OF AMINO ACID IMBALANCES LEADING TO HEPATIC ENCEPHALOPATHY. AAA, aromatic amino acids; BCAA, branched-chain amino acids; NF, norepinephrine; NH_3, ammonia; Phe, phenylalanine; Trp, tryptophan; Tyr, tyramine.

with even normal amounts of protein intake, and inadequate protein synthesis threatens the function of all organ systems as well as immune mechanisms. Therefore, the overall approach in treating liver disease is to meet the estimated energy needs and give enough protein to maintain nitrogen balance without precipitating encephalopathy. Because protein is so important to metabolism and healing, hepatic encephalopathy should be treated appropriately through other means before protein restriction is considered; and if protein restriction is instituted, it should be only temporary. Keeping these principles in mind, the guidelines in Box 22–1 may be used to formulate nutritional support goals.

BOX 22–1   Nutritional Considerations in Liver Disease

Protein energy malnutrition is frequently underdiagnosed in patients with liver disease.

In malnourished patients with any kind of liver disease, look for malabsorption and maldigestion and treat it when present. Also look for causes of hypermetabolism (e.g., infections, ascites, and encephalopathy) and treat them.

Nutritional assessment (see Chapter 10), including energy expenditure and 24-hour urinary urea nitrogen, should be used to estimate energy and protein needs and the level of catabolism (if renal function is stable). Major effort is sometimes required to prevent weight loss.

Sodium restriction (less than 2g/day) is indicated when ascites and/or edema is present.

Fluid restriction is indicated if the serum sodium is below 120 mmol/L.

Standard oral sources of protein and standard enteral and parenteral formulas can usually be used. If there is no history or high likelihood of encephalopathy, a normal protein balance should be maintained. If the patient has a history of protein intolerance or encephalopathy, protein intake can be restricted to about 0.5 to 0.7 g per kg of "dry" body weight per day for only a few days until the encephalopathy is better controlled. It should then be increased judiciously by about 10 to 15 g per day in order to determine protein tolerance.

If encephalopathy develops, and particularly if it does not respond to other therapies, or if mild encephalopathy prevents the intake of adequate protein to maintain nitrogen balance, branched-chain amino acid–enriched formulas can be considered. The formulas designed for enteral use are listed in Table 13-1; preparations for use with parenteral nutrition are also available. Though their usefulness is not universally accepted, adequate doses (1.2 to 1.5 g/kg per day) may result in improvement of encephalopathy.

Dietary fat restriction is unnecessary unless fat malabsorption is symptomatic.

Vitamin and mineral replacement therapy should be initiated and monitored periodically, because deficiencies are common.

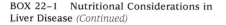

BOX 22-1   Nutritional Considerations in
Liver Disease *(Continued)*

Electrolyte and fluid balance disturbances should be treated as
they are encountered.

In patients with end-stage liver disease, dual-energy x-ray
absorptiometry (DEXA) scans should be performed because
such patients have high incidence of osteopenia and
osteoporosis.

In patients with end-stage liver disease who are awaiting liver
transplantation, aggressive oral supplementation should be
maintained, and nasoenteric feeding tubes should be placed
without delay if oral intake is insufficient.

Periodic nutritional reassessments should be done to evaluate the
effectiveness of the nutritional support regimen.

Acute Pancreatitis

Acute pancreatitis involves inflammation of the pancreas
of varying degrees of severity. Inflammation of the pancreas releases cytokines, produces hypercatabolism, and
leads to various manifestations including systemic
inflammatory response syndrome (SIRS), adult respiratory distress syndrome (ARDS), and rapid depletion of
nutritional stores. Patients have multiple metabolic
derangements including increased resting energy
expenditure, negative nitrogen balance with rapid
turnover of proteins and decreased branched-chain
amino acid to aromatic amino acid ratio, insulin resistance, and glucose intolerance. Hypocalcemia and
micronutrient deficiencies including zinc, thiamin, and
folate are also common, especially in patients with a
history of alcohol abuse.

Apart from general supportive care and management
of dysfunction in organs other than the pancreas, the
traditional standard of care for patients with pancreatitis
has been gut rest with intravenous fluids or parenteral
nutrition. However, there is now clinical evidence that
early initiation of enteral nutrition is beneficial in patients
with moderate to severe pancreatitis. Total parenteral

nutrition increases the vigor of the inflammatory response and impairs cell-mediated and humoral immunity. Bowel rest can lead to hypoplasia of the intestinal mucosa and to bacterial translocation, and increases the incidence of bacterial infections in critically ill patients, including those with acute pancreatitis.

By contrast, jejunal feeding that bypasses pancreatic stimulation from food in the duodenum is preferable in patients with acute pancreatitis. Meta-analyses comparing enteral and parenteral nutrition in patients with acute pancreatitis have concluded that jejunal feeding, and perhaps even nasogastric feeding, initiated within 48 hours of admission to the hospital results in better outcomes. Patients fed enterally had fewer infections and surgical interventions, shorter lengths of hospital stay, and overall decreased costs of medical care.[2]

REFERENCES

1. Keller J, Panter H, Layer P: Management of the short bowel syndrome after extensive small bowel resection. Best Pract Res Clin Gastroenterol 18:977–992, 2004.
2. Marik PE, Zaloga GP: Meta-analysis of parenteral nutrition versus enteral nutrition in patients with acute pancreatitis. BMJ 328: 1407–1412, 2004.

SUGGESTED READINGS

Florez DA, Aranda-Michel J: Nutritional management of acute and chronic liver disease. Semin Gastrointest Dis 13:169–178, 2002.
Schiff L, Schiff E (eds): Diseases of the Liver, 9th ed. Philadelphia, Lippincott, 2003.
Sleisenger M, Fordtran J (eds): Gastrointestinal Disease, 7th ed. Philadelphia, WB Saunders, 2002.

WEB SITES

American Association for the Study of Liver Diseases, http://www.aasld.org/
American Gastroenterological Association, http://www.gastro.org/
Celiac.com, http://www.celiac.com/
Gluten Intolerance Group, http://www.gluten.net

23

Critical Illness

LAURA E. NEWTON, MA, RD • DOUGLAS C. HEIMBURGER, MD

Various critical illnesses, especially those resulting from trauma or severe sepsis, share many metabolic and nutritional features. Regardless of whether they are septic, many critically ill patients exhibit a constellation of systemic inflammatory responses that impair immune function and tissue healing and can lead to lung, kidney, and liver dysfunction (multiple organ failure syndrome), prolonged hospitalization, and high mortality.

Metabolic Response to Injury and Infection

Since the 1930s, scientists and clinicians have been aware of the marked catabolic response involving breakdown of body tissues that occurs in injured patients even when they are receiving what appears to be adequate nutritional support. In fact, injury and infection induce the most accelerated breakdown of body tissues observed in the practice of medicine, with burns and head injuries representing the most severe forms of catabolism. Fortunately, there is documentation that the rapid mobilization of the body's fuel and tissue reserves can be offset (though not diminished or halted) by aggressive and appropriate nutritional intervention.

The three major components of the metabolic response to injury and infection are hypermetabolism, proteolysis with nitrogen loss, and accelerated gluconeogenesis and glucose utilization (Box 23–1). The most evident metabolic change is a shift from storage to utilization of protein, fat, and glycogen reserves. The degree of substrate mobilization is closely related to the extent and

---

BOX 23-1   Metabolic Features of Injury and Infection

Hypermetabolism
↑ Metabolic rate
↑ Oxygen consumption

Proteolysis and Nitrogen Loss
↑ Proteolysis and use of amino acids for energy production
↑ Ureagenesis and urinary nitrogen excretion
↑ Hepatic synthesis of acute phase proteins
↓ Hepatic production of albumin and prealbumin (transthyretin)

Gluconeogenesis and Glucose Utilization
↑ Glycogenolysis
↑ Gluconeogenesis
↑ Blood glucose levels

---

severity of the insult and is mediated largely through the release of cytokines and counterregulatory hormones—tumor necrosis factor, interleukins 1 and 6, catecholamines (epinephrine and norepinephrine), glucagon, and cortisol. These hormones are counterregulatory to the effect of insulin, the primary hormone of anabolism. Although circulating levels of insulin tend to be high in patients in a stressed state, tissue responsiveness is severely blunted (especially in skeletal muscle) as a result of insulin resistance caused by the other hormones. Regardless of the nutritional support, only when the critical illness has subsided do the hormone levels return to normal.

Hypermetabolism

Hypermetabolism (increased energy expenditure) occurs in proportion to the severity and duration of a critical illness (see Fig. 9–2). Because it is a systemic response, even when an injury is localized to one area of the body, increased oxygen consumption occurs throughout the body, including the skeletal muscle, splanchnic bed, and kidneys. The increase in metabolic rate is partly a result of the inefficiency with which glucose is utilized in the area of injury or infection. Glucose becomes the sole source of energy and is converted to lactate via anaerobic glycolysis under hypoxic conditions in the unstructured "front-line" of repair where blood perfusion is limited. Lactate is then returned to the liver where it is converted back to glucose and returned to the injured area (Cori cycle). In effect, the localized area of injury or infection represents an energy drain on the rest of the body, and hence contributes to the hypermetabolic state.

Proteolysis and Nitrogen Loss

Hypercatabolism (accelerated proteolysis) is common in critically ill patients. It derives largely from muscle and can be measured as increased urea nitrogen excretion in the urine. It reflects a systemic stress response and not simply protein release from injured tissues. Like energy expenditure (see Fig. 9–2), nitrogen excretion is proportional to the severity of the insult. The glucocorticoids are a major mediator of protein catabolism, accelerating the movement of amino acids from skeletal muscle to the liver where they serve as sources of glucose and acute-phase proteins for host defense. Alanine is the major precursor of glucose for the production of ATP in the hypermetabolic response. Glutamine also plays a role in the glucogenic process by contributing nitrogen to the kidneys for the synthesis of ammonia, which neutralizes the acid load produced by rapid protein degradation. Production of visceral proteins synthesized by the liver, such as albumin and prealbumin, is decreased in critical illness.

Gluconeogenesis and Glucose Utilization

Glucose is considered the fuel of reparation because it is the major fuel used by injured tissues and by the cells involved in repair and immune processes. For example, polymorphonuclear leukocytes receive their energy from glycolysis, particularly during phagocytosis; fibroblasts, which in their immature stage are active in the healing process, are also pure glycolyzers; and all cells functioning under anaerobic conditions such as poorly perfused wound sites are dependent on glucose as their sole source of fuel. Fat cannot be metabolized in the absence of oxygen, and fatty acids cannot be converted to glucose.

Glycogen stores are generally depleted in 12 to 24 hours. As this occurs, the body catabolizes protein to provide amino acids for gluconeogenesis. Exogenous glucose administered to a critically ill patient produces little, if any, reduction in the rate of protein breakdown, suggesting that it is a basic survival response that serves the organism at a time when food intake is not possible. By contrast, even small amounts of exogenous glucose markedly reduce protein catabolism in nonstressed, fasting individuals.

For example, under the influence of the counterregulatory hormones, hepatic glucose production increases from normal rates of about 200 g per day to approximately 400 g per day in patients with bacteremia. Hyperglycemia often results, and the high circulating concentrations of glucose can be preferentially provided to the reparative tissues. Because of insulin resistance, little glucose is utilized by resting skeletal muscle. Instead, fatty acids become the main fuel used by skeletal muscle and the liver and are therefore a major energy source, justifying their use in nutritional support of critically ill patients.

Nutritional Consequences of Injury and Infection

Circulating Proteins

Physiologic stress results in both catabolism and decreased synthesis of proteins. Thus, reduced circulating levels of proteins such as albumin and transferrin (or total iron binding capacity) are expected consequences of critical illness. Hypoproteinemia may complicate an illness and its treatment and has been associated with reduced wound healing, wound dehiscence, formation of pressure sores, reduced immune responsiveness, delayed gastric emptying, and reduced small intestinal motility and absorption. Hypoproteinemia is not necessarily an indication of malnutrition but a reflection of the severity of metabolic stress. As the stress subsides, it is only with adequate nutritional support that protein synthesis can return circulating levels to normal.

Body Composition

Without adequate nutritional support, profound weight loss and erosion of essential body compartments accompany critical illness. Loss of more than 10% to 20% of body weight that occurs rapidly in the setting of acute illness can seriously compromise physical performance, impair respiratory, cardiac, and immune functions, and increase operative morbidity and mortality.

Weight loss in patients with physiologic stress cannot be justified by the assumption that it primarily reflects loss of body fat reserves. In fact, in the presence of stress, lean body mass is likely to be the largest component wasted. For example, without nutritional support a septic individual with a resting energy expenditure (REE) of 1.4 times normal and with total nitrogen losses of 16 g per day is catabolizing about 0.4 kg of muscle protein vs. only 0.3 kg of adipose tissue per day (see Chapter 9). Accompanying the loss of muscle are proportional losses of potassium, phosphorus, magnesium, and zinc.

Nutritional Support of the Critically Ill Patient

The goals of nutritional support in the critically ill patient are to minimize weight loss, attain nitrogen equilibrium or, ideally, positive nitrogen balance to aid healing, and to provide nutrients to support the immune system. The traditional belief that injury is accompanied by about 6 weeks of catabolism, only after which nutritional repletion may take place, is no longer valid. With improved understanding and modern techniques of nutritional support, it is now possible to achieve energy and nitrogen balance in many patients throughout critical illness, and by doing so improve survival and reduce the length and cost of hospital stay.

Enteral vs. Parenteral Nutrition

The advantages of enteral over parenteral nutrition discussed in Chapter 11 are particularly relevant to the critically ill patient. Enteral feeding may maintain a healthier intestinal mucosa and thus prevent the translocation of intestinal bacteria and toxins and reduce the risk of multiple organ failure syndrome. Parenteral nutrition frequently contributes to hyperglycemia in already insulin-resistant patients, and through this and perhaps other mechanisms, may be immunosuppressive. Enteral feeding is the method of choice in critically ill patients.

Energy and Protein Requirements

Determining energy needs in the critically ill patient is challenging, but it is important to do so because of the deleterious effects of overfeeding or underfeeding (see Chapter 11). Overfeeding calories can result in respiratory impairment, hyperglycemia, and hepatic steatosis. Fat accumulation also increases the production of tumor necrosis factor (TNF) and other pro-inflammatory cytokines. Underfeeding may contribute to impaired immune function and poor wound healing.

The most accurate method to determine calorie requirement is to measure energy expenditure with indirect calorimetry. Various equations may also be used to predict energy expenditure (see Chapter 11). The energy requirements of most injured or septic patients are in the range of 1.1 to 1.4 times their calculated basal energy expenditure (BEE). Only in cases of extensive injury such as burns covering more than 40% of total body surface area (TBSA) do energy requirements generally exceed this range. Equations used to estimate energy needs may overestimate the needs of patients who are heavily sedated, paralyzed, or mechanically ventilated. Pharmacologic paralysis, frequently used in mechanically ventilated patients, can decrease energy expenditure by up to 30%. Propofol, a sedative commonly given to mechanically ventilated patients, is suspended in a 10% lipid vehicle. Treatment with propofol, therefore, simultaneously provides calories and reduces energy expenditure. Fat calories delivered with propofol, the rate of which often varies from day to day, must be included in assessing overall caloric intake.

Protein requirements are best calculated using the 24-hour urinary urea nitrogen (UUN) excretion (see Chapter 10). Although carbohydrate calories do not suppress nitrogen mobilization in the stress state, sufficient energy intake is necessary for ingested protein to be used to replace nitrogen losses and promote protein synthesis rather than to meet energy needs. To ensure positive protein balance, the goal for protein intake should be about 10 g per day higher than protein loss.

Micronutrient Requirements

Early in the course of stressful illnesses, serum levels of many micronutrients decrease significantly because they are either consumed, excreted, or sequestered in the liver and reticuloendothelial system.[1] Zinc is sequestered in the liver, zinc and vitamin A are excreted in the urine, and vitamin C is consumed at an accelerated rate. Because zinc and vitamins C and A figure importantly in immune competence and the healing of wounds, it is prudent to supplement them.

In general, avoid iron supplementation in acutely ill patients. Their serum iron levels are often low because the body sequesters iron in the reticuloendothelial system in response to stress (not because it is lost from the body). Therefore, the serum iron level is an unreliable indicator of iron status in this setting (see Chapter 26). Since the iron binding capacity is frequently low in the stress state as well, treatment with iron can result in the circulation of unbound iron, making it more available for bacterial uptake and thus infection. Patients with anemia should be treated with transfusions during acute illness, and investigation of iron deficiency should be postponed until after the stress resolves.

Nutritional Support in Specific Critical Illnesses

Burns

Burn injuries result in many hormonal, immunologic, metabolic, and nutritional alterations. Burn size and depth are the primary determinants of prognosis and the degree of hypermetabolism and hypercatabolism. Aggressive nutritional support is necessary to aid wound healing and improve immunocompetence. Post-burn energy expenditure exceeds that of any other form of traumatic injury or disease. Energy demands usually peak about 5 to 12 days after injury, but a hypermetabolic state remains until wound coverage is achieved. Multiple equations exist for estimation of energy needs in burn patients. Two of the most common are shown in Box 23–2. These formulas often incorporate data such as weight and body surface area burned. Many things affect energy expenditure, and the data used in equations may change. Also, advances in medical and surgical care after the formulas were developed, such as early excision of burns and wound closure, have reduced the severity and duration of hypermetabolism. Thus, older formulas may overestimate energy needs, making serial indirect calorimetry important in burned patients.

Extensive nitrogen losses, proportional to burn size, occur in patients with burns, so protein repletion is

---

BOX 23–2   Estimating 24-Hour Energy Expenditure in Burn Patients (kcal/day)

Harris-Benedict equation – BEE (see Chapter 11 for equations)
  = BEE × 1.1 − 1.4 (for ≤40% TBSA)
  = BEE × 2 (for >40% TBSA)
Modified Curreri formula (for ≤40% TBSA)
  = (25 × Wt) + (40 × % TBSA)
where:
Wt = Body weight in kilograms
TBSA = Percent total body surface area burned (*whole number*, not decimal)

BEE, basal energy expenditure.

critical for recovery from burn injury. Protein intake should be monitored and adjusted according to nitrogen balance studies, using UUN equations modified as shown in Box 23-3 to account for protein lost directly through the burned skin. It is generally necessary to provide 20% to 25% calories as protein to patients with greater than 25% TBSA burns.

Supplemental nutritional support is often necessary for burns exceeding 20% to 25% TBSA. Enteral feeding should be initiated as soon as practicable. Gastric ileus sometimes prevents gastric feeding, therefore transpyloric placement of a feeding tube is often indicated. Clinical studies have shown that supplemental glutamine results in a decreased incidence of bacteremia, improvement in wound healing, and reduction in length of stay.[2-4]

Trauma

After traumatic injury, a cascade of metabolic and systemic events occurs, including increased oxygen consumption, hypermetabolism, and hypercatabolism. Hyperglycemia often results from insulin resistance and increased glucagon/insulin ratio. Under normal circumstances, oxygen delivery to the viscera exceeds oxygen consumption, but after trauma, splanchnic blood flow

---

BOX 23-3   Estimating Protein Catabolic Rate in Burn Patients

$= (UUN + 4 + [0.2 \text{ g} \times \%3°] + [0.1 \text{ g} \times \%2°]) \times 6.25$
where:
UUN = Measured urinary urea nitrogen in grams
%3° = Percent body surface area with 3 (full thickness) burns (*whole number*, not decimal)
%2° = Percent body surface area with 2 (partial thickness) burns (*whole number*, not decimal)
Example: for a patient with 35% 3° burns, 15% 2° burns, and 24 hr UUN of 13 g,
$= (13 + 4 + [0.2 \times 35] + [0.1 \times 15]) \times 6.25$
$= 159$ g protein catabolized

is decreased, making the viscera vulnerable to ischemic injury. This makes it possible that enteral feeding could exacerbate the potential for ischemia, but it could also protect the mucosa in this low-flow state. Numerous studies in trauma patients have demonstrated reductions in the incidence of infections, intra-abdominal abscesses, and septic morbidity in patients fed enterally compared to through parenteral nutrition. Although gastrointestinal ileus, gut wall edema, and abdominal distention are common after traumatic injury, feeding in the small bowel is generally well tolerated within 12 to 24 hours after injury. Therefore, enteral nutrition is preferred over parenteral, but it should be started only after appropriate resuscitation and consideration of the feeding location and rate if the patient is hemodynamically unstable.

Several studies have shown decreased infection rates, decreased abdominal abscess formation, and shortened length of stay in patients who were fed immune-enhancing formulas (see section "Specialized Nutritional Support" later in the chapter and Table 13–1). Further study is needed to define more clearly the optimal indications, contraindications, and durations of use of these formulas.

Neurologic Injury

Injury to the central nervous system, whether from head injury or spinal cord injury, can have a significant impact on a patient's nutritional status. Closed head injury often triggers a cascade of systemic and local metabolic responses that result in a hypermetabolic and especially hypercatabolic state comparable to that following burns. Nitrogen excretion can be extremely high. Energy expenditure is dependent on infections, body temperature, alterations in intracranial pressure (ICP), medications, motor activity, and other injuries sustained. Neuromuscular blockade, which is often used when the ICP is high, can decrease energy expenditure by 20% to 50%.

Head-injured patients are at particularly high risk for aspiration pneumonia because of gastroparesis (impaired gastric motility) and suppressed gag and cough reflexes. Gastroparesis, most common when the injury is severe and ICP is increased, results in poor tolerance of gastric enteral feeding. Postpyloric placement of feeding tubes is recommended.

Spinal cord injuries (SCIs) produce many nutritional concerns, both in the acute and chronic phase of injury (Box 23–4). The metabolic rate of SCI patients is dependent on the severity, location, and time phase of the injury. In the acute phase, energy expenditure is increased from the stress of the injury. Chronically, metabolic rate reduces below the BEE; over the long term, this increases risk for obesity. Due to paralysis, risk is high for developing pressure sores. Hypercalciuria and hypercalcemia are common because of immobilization and bone resorption. Restricting dietary calcium does not reduce urinary calcium excretion or serum calcium, and it could accelerate bone loss. Intravenous (IV) fluids, diuretics, oral phosphates, and calcitonin are some methods used to treat hypercalciuria and hypercalcemia.

Pancreatitis

Mild acute pancreatitis typically results in an uneventful recovery with a few days of bowel rest and IV fluids. In its severest form, pancreatitis may lead to SIRS, which can result in organ failure and death. Severe pancreatitis causes marked hypermetabolism and hypercatabolism. The goals of nutrition support are to meet the increased metabolic needs as well as limit stimulation of pancreatic secretions. Historically, parenteral nutrition and bowel rest have been used to treat severe acute pancreatitis

---

BOX 23–4 Nutritional Consequences of Spinal Cord Injury
Decreased energy expenditure Negative nitrogen balance Decreased muscle mass Hypercalciuria, hypercalcemia, and osteoporosis Pressure sores and poor wound healing Neurogenic bladder and bowel resulting in constipation

because of concern that enteral feeding may stimulate pancreatic secretions. However, as with other critically ill states, these patients are at increased risk for hyperglycemia and catheter-related sepsis associated with parenteral nutrition. Several studies have shown that jejunal enteral feeding was well tolerated and resulted in fewer septic events and overall complications as compared to parenteral nutrition.[5] The cephalic and gastric phases of exocrine pancreatic stimulation are avoided by feeding into the jejunum. There is no general consensus on the type of enteral formula to use in patients with acute pancreatitis. Early studies found that pancreatic secretions were reduced using low-fat, hydrolyzed protein formulas as compared to polymeric formulas that were higher in fat. Later studies demonstrated that polymeric formulas could be safely given when fed jejunally.

If parenteral nutrition is necessary, lipid emulsions (along with dextrose and amino acids) are usually well tolerated. Serum triglyceride levels should be measured at baseline and after lipid emulsion starts to assure adequate lipid clearance. IV lipid should be withheld in patients with a triglyceride level exceeding 400 mg/dL.

Specialized Nutritional Support

Much research has gone into developing nutritional formulas specially designed for critically ill patients. A number of intriguing findings from basic and clinical research have been explored to determine whether alterations in the intake of specific nutrients will provide benefits beyond those of basic macronutrient and micronutrient support. However, before specialized formulas are put into practice, clinical trials must demonstrate superior outcomes that justify their inevitably higher costs.

Glutamine is a conditionally essential amino acid that is mobilized in large quantities from skeletal muscle and lung in patients with critical illnesses. It is used directly as an energy source by enterocytes; contributes to ammoniagenesis (counteracting acidosis); and supports lymphocyte and macrophage proliferation, hepatic gluconeogenesis and ureagenesis, and fibroblast function in healing wounds. A trial of glutamine-enriched parenteral nutrition showed improved nitrogen balance, a lower incidence of clinical infection, and a shortened hospital stay in bone marrow transplant patients.[6] Another study in severely burned patients found that glutamine supplementation significantly reduced the incidence of gram-negative bacteremia.[2] A study of trauma patients found that enteral glutamine supplementation significantly decreased the incidence of sepsis, pneumonia, and bacteremia.[7]

Glutamine is absent from standard parenteral solutions and is typically present only in small quantities in standard enteral feedings. It is relatively unstable in solution unless it is bound to protein, but it is stable and available in powdered form or in small-peptide enteral formulas. The addition of 20 to 40 g per day of glutamine has been found to be safe and well tolerated by adults. Glutamine use may be contraindicated in patients with hyperammonemia or hepatic or liver failure, as supplementation in these patients may contribute to excess ammonia production.

Because small peptides are more rapidly absorbed by the gastrointestinal tract than whole proteins, and critically ill patients often have intestinal dysfunction including mucosal atrophy, a number of enteral formulas containing small peptides from hydrolyzed proteins have been promoted. Although efficient absorption has been well documented, clinical trials have not demonstrated improved outcomes such as faster nutritional recovery, shorter intensive care unit or hospital stays, or lower mortality rates.

Fish oils contain high levels of omega-3 fatty acids from which eicosapentaenoic acid (EPA) and docahexaenoic acid (DHA) are derived. EPA and DHA enhance lymphocyte function. Supplemental omega-3 fatty acids have a positive effect on the immune system by reducing the inflammatory response and enhancing neutrophil function. Studies have shown improved length of stay and infection rate following burn injury in patients supplemented with omega-3 fatty acids.

Arginine is a conditionally essential amino acid with immune-enhancing properties. Arginine is a precursor in the nitric oxide pathway. Nitric oxide is important for immune function and regulation of blood pressure and organ blood flow. Other effects of arginine include the promotion of normal T lymphocyte growth and response to antigen. Supplementation improves nitrogen balance in critically ill patients and has been found to improve wound healing in healthy elderly subjects.

Several other nutrients and dietary substances have been reported to improve immune function and reduce infection rates in injured animals, by stimulating lymphocyte proliferation, enhancing macrophage and

---

BOX 23–5   Recommendations of the U.S. Summit on Immune-Enhancing Enteral Therapy

Patients Who Should Receive Immune-Enhancing Enteral Therapy
Moderately malnourished patients (albumin <3.5 mg/dL) undergoing major elective gastrointestinal surgery
Severely malnourished patients (albumin <2.8 mg/dL) undergoing lower gastrointestinal surgery
Trauma patients with Injury Severity Score of 18 or higher
Patients with Abdominal Trauma Index of 20 or greater

Patients Who Could Potentially Benefit from Immune-Enhancing Enteral Therapy, but Where Additional Research is Needed
Patients with chronic obstructive pulmonary disease and prolonged need for mechanical ventilation
Ventilator-dependent, non-septic medical and surgical patients at risk of infectious morbidity
Malnourished patients who are undergoing major head and neck surgery
Patients with a Glasgow Coma Scale <8 and abnormal head computed tomography
Patients with third-degree burns covering 30% or more of total body surface area

From Kudsk KA, et al: Consensus recommendations from the U.S. Summit on Immune-Enhancing Enteral Therapy. J Parenter Enteral Nutr 25:S61–S62, 2001.

killer-cell function. So-called immune-enhancing enteral formulas containing these nutrients are available. Several meta-analyses have concluded that their use ("immunonutrition") may reduce infectious complications but was not associated with an overall improvement in mortality. Some studies found that patients with sepsis at initiation of formula use may actually have increased mortality with immune-enhancing formulas. A summit on immune-enhancing enteral therapy made specific recommendations for the use of immune-enhancing formulas (Box 23–5). Further study is needed before recommending widespread use of these formulas in the critically ill patient population.

Monitoring the Patient

As with other patients, the main parameters to be tracked during nutritional support of patients with critical illness are glucose control, body weight, nutrient delivery, nitrogen balance, and serum proteins. Tight glucose control is critical in this patient population, as it reduces the incidence of sepsis, morbidity, and mortality. Common sense dictates the frequency of measurement and interpretation of changes in body weight, but it is helpful to measure it 2 to 3 times weekly. If available, indirect calorimetry should be used to measure energy expenditure periodically. Dietary records of energy and protein intake should be reviewed daily. The 24-hour UUN should be measured 1 to 2 times weekly to monitor nitrogen balance. Serum albumin, prealbumin, or other circulating proteins should be monitored weekly. Although in stressed patients the albumin level falls acutely, roughly in proportion to the severity of the injury, its nadir generally occurs within 7 to 10 days of the initial insult. A gradual upward trend thereafter usually reflects adequate nutritional support. Failure to rise and/or periodic declines in the albumin level suggest persistent or intercurrent stress or inadequate nutritional support. Additional information is obtained from serial measurements of electrolytes, BUN, creatinine, phosphorus, magnesium, and anthropometrics.

REFERENCES

1. Louw JA, Werbeck A, Louw MEJ, et al: Blood vitamin concentrations during the acute-phase response. Crit Care Med 20:934–941,1992.
2. Wischmeyer PE, Lynch J, Liedel J, et al: Glutamine administration reduces gram-negative bacteremia in severely burned patients: A prospective, randomized, double-blind trial versus isonitrogenous control. Crit Care Med 11:2075–2080, 2001.
3. Garrel D, Patenaude J, Nedelec B, et al: Decreased mortality and infectious morbidity in adult burn patients given enteral glutamine supplements. A prospective, controlled, randomized clinical trial. Crit Care Med 10:2444–2449, 2003.
4. Peng X, Yan H, You Z, et al: Effects of enteral supplementation with glutamine granules on intestinal mucosal barrier function in severely burned patients. Burns 30:135–139, 2004.
5. Marik PE, Zaloga GP: Meta-analysis of parenteral nutrition versus enteral nutrition in patients with acute pancreatitis. Brit Med J 328(7453):1407, 2004.
6. Ziegler TR, Young LS, Benfell K, et al: Clinical and metabolic efficacy of glutamine-supplemented parenteral nutrition after bone-marrow transplantation: A randomized, double-blind, controlled study. Ann Intern Med 116:821–828, 1992.
7. Houdijk APJ, Rijnsburger ER, Jan Sen J, et al: Randomized trial of glutamine-enriched nutrition on infectious morbidity in patients with multiple trauma. Lancet 352:772–776, 1998.

SUGGESTED READINGS

American Society for Parenteral and Enteral Nutrition, Shikora SA, Martindale RG, Schwaitzberg SB (eds): Nutritional Considerations in the Intensive Care Unit: Science, Rationale, and Practice. Dubuque, Iowa, Kendall/Hunt, 2002.
Gottschlich MM (ed): Nutrition support of specific states. In The Science and Practice of Nutrition Support. Dubuque, Iowa, Kendall/Hunt, 2001.

WEB SITES

American Society for Parenteral and Enteral Nutrition (ASPEN), http://www.clinnutr.org/
Society of Critical Care Medicine, http://www.sccm.org/

24

Pulmonary Disease

LAURA E. NEWTON, MA, RD • SARAH L. MORGAN, MD

Patients with acute and chronic respiratory failure are at high risk for developing malnutrition. Malnutrition is common among patients with chronic obstructive pulmonary disease (COPD), especially those with emphysema, who frequently have reduced weight-for-height and triceps skinfold measurements, midarm muscle circumferences, and creatinine/height indexes. Factors contributing to malnutrition in COPD patients include high resting energy expenditure (REE) due to increased work of breathing, reduced dietary intake, and effects of medications such as corticosteroids and $\beta 2$-agonists. The degree of weight loss generally correlates with reduced air flow as measured by spirometry. Thus, COPD can create a cycle in which respiratory dysfunction promotes weight loss, and weight loss further hinders respiratory function.

When patients with COPD are hospitalized for ventilatory failure, clinical outcomes are affected by nutritional support. The most significant effect of nutritional support documented by research is that patients who receive adequate nutritional support are more readily weaned from mechanical ventilators than those whose diets are deficient in protein and energy.

Nutritional Effects on the Respiratory System

Nutrition impacts patients with pulmonary disease at several levels. Nutritional status affects all components of the respiratory system, including central hypoxic and hypercapnic drives, respiratory muscles, and lung tissues (parenchyma). The amount and composition of energy intake affect the metabolic rate, O_2 consumption, and CO_2 production. Hypophosphatemia can have a profound effect on ventilation. Nutritional status is also important to the integrity of the immune system.

Ventilatory Drive

Ventilatory drive (the body's increase in minute ventilation in response to hypoxia or hypercapnia) is closely associated with metabolic rate. When the metabolic rate increases, as it does during exercise, tissue oxygen levels drop (hypoxia), producing a compensatory increase in ventilation. However, in patients who are underfed (e.g., receiving only 5% dextrose infusions), the ventilatory response to hypoxia is depressed, impairing the ability to maintain adequate ventilation. Fortunately, these changes tend to normalize with refeeding and are prevented if semistarvation is initially avoided. Therefore, underfeeding a patient with pulmonary disease is detrimental to the respiratory drive.

Respiratory Function

As body weight decreases, there is a proportional reduction in the weight and strength of the diaphragm and the function of respiratory muscles. In emphysema, the hyperinflated lungs alter the fiber length of the respiratory muscles and impair their efficiency. With malnutrition, the diaphragm, intercostal, and accessory muscles are catabolized for energy, resulting in a decrease in inspiratory capacity. Infection, inflammation, and decreased protein intake lead to a drop in serum albumin, which lowers the oncotic pressure and results in pulmonary edema. Undernutrition also affects the pulmonary parenchyma by diminishing collagen synthesis and increasing proteolysis. This may manifest as decreased surfactant production and alveolar collapse.

Metabolism, O_2 Consumption, and CO_2 Production

One of the hallmarks of respiratory insufficiency is abnormal gas exchange, with resultant hypoxemia and/or hypercapnia. Patients with pulmonary failure often have limited capacities to expire CO_2, so it is retained. Because total energy intake and the macronutrient composition of the diet affect the body's CO_2 production and O_2 consumption, nutrient intake can be altered to influence metabolism and gas exchange favorably.

Energy Intake

Giving excess energy to acutely ill patients with respiratory insufficiency can increase the metabolic rate, and thus O_2 consumption and CO_2 production. The synthesis of fat from excessive carbohydrate calories is also associated with production of a large amount of CO_2. In patients with limited pulmonary reserves, this may precipitate respiratory failure from CO_2 retention. Remember that hypermetabolic, stressed patients respond differently to excessive calories than semi-starved patients or normal persons (see Chapter 11).

Carbohydrate/Fat Mix

The oxidation of carbohydrate, fat, and protein to yield energy requires O_2 and produces CO_2 and H_2O, in proportions unique to each substrate. The ratio of moles of CO_2 produced to moles of O_2 consumed—the respiratory quotient (RQ)—is 1.0 for carbohydrates, 0.7 for fat, and approximately 0.8 for protein. The synthesis of fat from carbohydrate, which can occur during overfeeding, yields an RQ of greater than 1.0. Thus, the oxidation of carbohydrate generates more CO_2 per unit of energy produced than does fat or protein, and overfeeding can dramatically increase CO_2 production by increasing both metabolic rate and the conversion of carbohydrate to fat. Respiratory quotients dictate that if the predominant nonprotein energy source in the diet is carbohydrate, the amount of CO_2 that must be expired is greater than if the predominant source is fat. Reducing CO_2 production by substituting fat for carbohydrate may prevent the need for mechanical ventilation and facilitate weaning from the ventilator. Conversely, relying on carbohydrate can worsen respiratory failure or make ventilator weaning more difficult. Of the two effects, overfeeding has a greater impact on CO_2 production than does the carbohydrate/fat mix, so it is very important not to exceed a patient's estimated energy requirements during the weaning process.

Hypophosphatemia

Hypophosphatemia has a particularly deleterious effect on respiratory muscle function, by impairing diaphragmatic contractility. Hypophosphatemia with decreased 2,3-diphosphoglycerate in red blood cells and diminished levels of adenosine triphosphate (ATP) may complicate acute respiratory failure by impairing tissue oxygen delivery and respiratory muscle function, respectively. Therefore, hypophosphatemia should be prevented and, when present, treated vigorously (see Chapter 11).

Immune Function

Because chronic lung disease is often complicated by pneumonia and sepsis, impairment of the immune system from malnutrition adversely affects recovery. Epidemiologic studies have found a strong link between malnutrition and pneumonia. Malnutrition depresses clearance of bacteria from the lungs and predisposes to pulmonary infection. It is also associated with decreased cell-mediated immunity, altered immunoglobulin production, and impaired resistance of the tracheobronchial mucosa to bacterial infections (see Chapter 29).

Nutritional Support in Pulmonary Disease

Guidelines for nutritional support in patients with pulmonary disease are summarized in Box 24–1. Nutritional evaluation is important in order to detect malnutrition and make appropriate plans for feeding.

Optimization of total energy intake is the cardinal principle in therapy; both overfeeding and underfeeding should be avoided. Generally, giving 1.1 to 1.4 times estimated REE is adequate; cachectic patients with pulmonary disease should be refed with particular care

---

BOX 24-1   Nutritional Support of Patients with
Pulmonary Disease

Perform a complete nutritional assessment.
Evaluate energy needs and provide an appropriate amount;
   do not overfeed or underfeed.
Ensure protein balance.
Monitor fluids and electrolytes, especially phosphorus.
Evaluate vitamin and mineral status as indicated.
Consider high-fat, low-carbohydrate feedings in patients with
   persistent hypercapnia.

(see Chapter 11). When there is a question about energy requirements or the effects of nutritional support on gas exchange, indirect calorimetry should be performed. The data generated from indirect calorimetry indicate the REE as well as the RQ, and can be used to tailor nutritional support. Reduction of energy intake to a level equal to or below the REE may facilitate weaning, but should be avoided in highly catabolic patients and never prolonged. If weight gain is desired and the patient is stable and ambulatory, intake may be increased to 2 times the REE, as long as it does not impair respiratory function.

In patients who are not hypercapnic, calories may be distributed conventionally, with 50% to 60% as carbohydrate, 20% to 30% as fat, and 15% to 20% as protein. For patients with hypercapnia, whether ambulatory or ventilator-dependent, giving 25% to 30% of calories as carbohydrate and 50% to 55% of calories as fat may be beneficial. Intake should be individualized to determine the lowest percentage of fat that maintains an acceptable pCO_2 level. Remember that providing an appropriate amount of energy is more important than fine-tuning the balance of fat and carbohydrate.

Acute Respiratory Distress Syndrome

Acute respiratory distress syndrome (ARDS) is a form of acute lung injury characterized by bilateral infiltrates and progressive hypoxemia. These abnormalities are associated with an increase in inflammatory mediators such as the arachidonic acid metabolites (prostanoids and leukotrienes). Numerous studies have examined the effects of altering fatty acid intake on the inflammatory response. Two studies of ventilated patients fed a formula with borage and fish oil, gamma-linolenic acid (GLA), eicosapentenoic acid (EPA), and antioxidants found that patients fed the specialized formula had significant improvements in oxygenation, fewer days on mechanical ventilation, and decreased ICU length of stay as compared with the control patients.[1]

Cystic Fibrosis

Cystic fibrosis (CF) is a genetic disorder characterized by multisystem organ involvement including the pancreas, lungs, and gastrointestinal tract. Pancreatic enzyme replacement is necessary to promote adequate digestion of nutrients. Nutritional status has a strong impact on the survival of patients with CF; deterioration of pulmonary function correlates with the severity of malnutrition. Contributing to malnutrition in this patient population are high energy demands from increased work of breathing, increased nutrient losses from maldigestion, and decreased intake. Energy requirements are 120% to 150% of the recommended daily allowance (RDA), or up to 200% of the RDA in patients unable to maintain their weight. A high-fat diet (30% to 40% of energy) is encouraged for CF patients due to fat's high energy density and the low RQ associated with its oxidation. Fat-soluble vitamins should be supplemented because of their impaired digestion and absorption.

Additional complications of CF that are influenced by nutrition include osteoporosis and cystic fibrosis–related diabetes (CFRD). Bone density is typically decreased in CF patients due to their small body size, maldigestion of nutrients including calcium and vitamins D and K, use of corticosteroids, and limited physical activity. Weight-bearing activity should be encouraged along with calcium and vitamin D supplements. CFRD occurs in about 5%

to 6% of CF patients in North America and Europe.[2] Treatment of CFRD includes insulin therapy along with appropriate meal timing and carbohydrate counting. Because of the importance of adequate nutrition for growth in children and weight maintenance in adults, nutritional recommendations for CF take precedence over typical diabetic dietary recommendations in this patient population.

REFERENCES

1. Gadek JE, De Michele SJ, Karlstad MD, et al: Effect of enteral feeding with eicosapentenoic acid, γ-linolenic acid, and antioxidants in patients with acute respiratory distress syndrome. Crit Care Med 27:1409–1420, 1999.
2. Moran A, Hardin D, Rodman D, et al: Diagnosis, screening and management of cystic fibrosis related diabetes mellitus: A consensus conference report. Diabetes Res Clin Pract 45:61–73, 1999.

SUGGESTED READINGS

Mallampalli A: Nutritional management of the patient with chronic obstructive pulmonary disease. Nutr Clin Pract 19:550–556, 2004.
Olson DL, Schwenk WF: Nutrition for patients with cystic fibrosis. Nutr Clin Pract 19:575–580, 2004.
Talpers SS, Romberger DJ, Bunce SB, Pingleton SK: Nutritionally associated increased carbon dioxide production. Excess total calories vs high proportion of carbohydrate calories. Chest 102:551–555, 1992.

WEB SITES

American Lung Association, http://www.lungusa.org/
American Society for Parenteral and Enteral Nutrition (ASPEN), http://www.clinnutr.org/
American Thoracic Society, http://www.thoracic.org/
Society of Critical Care Medicine, http://www.sccm.org/

25

Kidney Disease

LAURA E. NEWTON, MA, RD

The kidneys play a crucial role in maintaining the body's physiologic milieu by excreting, secreting, synthesizing, regulating, and degrading metabolic substances and participating in erythropoiesis (formation of blood) and the metabolism of hormones. When these functions deteriorate as a result of kidney disease, various metabolic abnormalities occur that impinge on nutritional status, including the following:

- Impaired clearance of urea and other nitrogenous products of protein metabolism
- Impaired regulation of sodium, potassium, phosphorus, calcium, magnesium, water, and hydrogen ions
- Impaired vitamin D metabolism
- Anorexia and loss of body mass

The severity of these changes reflects the type and duration of kidney disease (acute or chronic) and the degree of catabolic stress the patient experiences. The role of nutritional support in kidney disease is to prevent or reverse associated malnourished states, minimize the adverse effects of substances that are inadequately excreted, and favorably affect the progression and outcome of kidney disease.

Chronic Kidney Disease

Chronic kidney disease is caused by a variety of prolonged renal insults such as diabetes mellitus, hypertension, and primary renal diseases such as glomerulonephritis. Diabetes is the most prevalent cause of kidney failure in the United States and accounts for half of all new cases of irreversible kidney failure each year. The stages of

Table 25-1	STAGES OF CHRONIC KIDNEY DISEASE	
Stage	Description	Glomerular Filtration Rate (GFR) (mL/min/1.73 m²)
1	Kidney damage with normal or increased GFR	≥90
2	Kidney damage with mildly decreased GFR	60–89
3	Moderately decreased GFR	30 59
4	Severely decreased GFR	15–29
5	Kidney failure	<15 (or dialysis)

From National Kidney Foundation Kidney Disease Outcomes Quality Initiative: Clinical practice guidelines for nutrition in chronic renal failure. Am J Kidney Dis 35:S1–S140, 2000; available at http://www.kidney.org/professionals/kdoqi/guidelines_updates/doqi_nut.html.

chronic kidney disease, developed by the National Kidney Foundation Kidney Disease Outcomes Quality Initiative (NKF-K/DOQI) are illustrated in Table 25-1.[1] With the Medicare End-Stage Renal Disease (ESRD) Program paying about $14 billion annually to support and treat ESRD patients, end-stage renal disease is a major consumer of U.S. health care dollars.

The broad spectrum of abnormalities in chronic kidney disease correlates with the number of functioning nephrons. More than 50% of normal renal function must be lost before the serum creatinine level begins to rise and nutritional interventions are needed. Patients with 20% to 50% of normal renal function (stage 3 or 4 kidney disease) usually have serum creatinine levels between 2 and 5 mg/dL, mild anemia, and mild retention of sodium, potassium, magnesium, phosphorus, and water. For these patients, nutritional regulation is paramount. Progressive chronic renal failure produces anorexia and increased protein catabolism, resulting in wasting of lean body mass, reduced growth rates in children, and diminished synthesis of proteins including albumin. Careful dietary management may make it possible to stabilize the progression of chronic kidney disease and avoid or postpone dialysis. Nutrient recommendations for chronic kidney disease are summarized in Table 25-2.

Table 25-2	NUTRITIONAL RECOMMENDATIONS FOR PATIENTS WITH CHRONIC KIDNEY DISEASE				
Nutrient	Predialysis	Hemodialysis	Peritoneal Dialysis	Continuous Renal Replacement Therapy	Post-transplant
Calories	30–35 kcal/kg IBW	30–35 kcal/kg IBW	20–35 kcal/kg IBW, subtract kcal absorbed from dialysate	30–35 kcal/kg IBW	30–35 kcal/kg IBW
Protein	0.6–1.0 g/kg IBW	1.1–1.4 g/kg IBW	1.2–1.5 g/kg IBW	1.5–2.0 g/kg IBW	1.3–2.0 g/kg IBW
Sodium	1–3 g/day	2–3 g/day	2–4 g/day	Individualized based on fluid balance.	2–4 g/day
Potassium	Individualize according to lab values.	40–70 mEq/kg IBW, adjust to serum levels.	Typically unrestricted, adjust to serum levels.	Adjust to serum levels.	Unrestricted
Phosphorus	8–12 mg/kg IBW; individualize	≤17 mg/kg IBW	≤17 mg/kg IBW	≤17 mg/kg IBW; individualize	Unrestricted
Fluid	Individualize	500–750 mL + urine output; if anuric, 1,000 mL/day	Generally unrestricted	Individualize	Unrestricted

IBW, ideal body weight.
From Wiggins K: Guidelines for Nutrition Care of Renal Patients, 3rd ed. Chicago, American Dietetic Association, 2001.

These should be individualized for each patient, because over-restriction of nutrients can result in inadequate energy intake and protein-energy malnutrition.

In patients with ESRD who have less than 10% of normal renal function (serum creatinine greater than about 7 mg/dL), nutritional regulation is not usually sufficient to control uremic symptoms, and dialysis is often required. Nutritional management is still important after dialysis has begun, but the restrictions are less rigorous.

Acute Renal Failure

Patients with acute renal failure have an abrupt and marked decrease in renal glomerular filtration rate caused by a variety of insults to the kidney such as infection, trauma, dehydration, shock, and exposure to exogenous nephrotoxins such as drugs. Acute renal failure occurs in approximately 5% of hospitalized patients and is associated with a high mortality rate. Urine output may be normal (nonoliguric), reduced (oliguric), or absent (anuric). Fluid and electrolyte balances become rapidly deranged through defective renal regulation. A patient with acute renal failure is often highly catabolic because of the underlying disease process.

Using dialysis, the fluid and electrolyte abnormalities of acute renal failure can be regulated and uremic symptoms reduced. However, the ravages of catabolism including poor wound healing, infections, and increased mortality cannot be prevented by dialysis alone. Nutritional support must be used to maintain nutritional status until the acute renal failure improves. In a sense, dialysis relieves renal excretory insufficiency so that nutritional support can be administered. Dialysis options include hemodialysis, peritoneal dialysis, and continuous renal replacement therapy (CRRT), including continuous venovenous hemodiafiltration (CVVHD). CRRT is administered 24 hours per day in patients unable hemodynamically to tolerate hemodialysis. It is typically reserved for the critical care setting.

Nutritional Assessment in Kidney Disease

In chronic kidney disease it is particularly important to monitor nutritional status. In early disease, simple assessments such as weight, triceps skinfold, and calculation of BMI on a regular basis are sufficient to detect significant changes in body composition. Assessment of nutritional status in patients with oliguria is rendered difficult by variability in hydration status and demands special caution in interpreting anthropometric and biochemical parameters. The characteristics of patients at high risk for malnutrition listed in Chapter 10 apply to patients with kidney disease. Additionally, the K/DOQI Clinical Practice Guidelines for Nutrition in Chronic Renal Failure[1] recommend that for individuals with a glomerular filtration rate (GFR) less than 20 mL/min, protein-energy nutrition status should be evaluated by serial measurements of a panel of markers including at least one value from each of the following:

- Serum albumin
- Edema-free actual body weight, percent of standard body weight or subjective global assessment
- Normalized protein nitrogen appearance (nPNA) performed by urea kinetic modeling in hemodialysis patients or dietary interviews and diaries to assess overall intake.

In ESRD, serum albumin levels below 3.5 g/dL are associated with increased mortality.[2] Therefore, it is reasonable to give greater weight to albumin when using the previously mentioned criteria. A desirable goal level for albumin is greater than 4.0 g/dL. Dietary records or recall are the only practical techniques for estimating energy intake in outpatients. However, it should be noted that these methods may underestimate or overestimate intake by considerable amounts.

Nutritional Support in Kidney Disease

The general principles of nutritional support discussed in Chapter 11 apply to patients with kidney disease.

Tables 25-2 and 12-1 summarize specific dietary recommendations for this population.

Energy

Although most patients with renal insufficiency require about 25 to 40 kcal/kg of their ideal body weight or 1.1 to 1.4 times the calculated basal energy expenditure, these guidelines must be applied with caution because physical activity varies substantially among individuals. For many kidney disease patients, maintaining sufficient energy intake to avoid weight loss may be difficult when other nutrients are restricted. By contrast, peritoneal dialysis provides a significant amount of glucose, and thus calories, to the patient via the dialysate. Depending on the amount of dialysate infused, the dwell time, and the concentration of dextrose, as many as 500 to 1000 calories may be absorbed each day. For these reasons and because vigilance is required to sustain good dietary habits, the help of a dietitian is invaluable in the management of these patients. Because environmental factors such as poverty and disability commonly interfere with food availability, an interdisciplinary approach is highly recommended.

Protein

Under normal conditions the renal glomeruli filter amino acids and up to 30 g of intact protein each day, virtually all of which is reabsorbed in the proximal tubules. Renal disease often increases the glomerular permeability to proteins and/or decreases tubular reabsorption, resulting in proteinuria. Urea is also filtered and only about half is reabsorbed; the excretion of the remaining urea is one of the most important functions of the kidneys. As the glomerular filtration rate (GFR) decreases, urea is not adequately filtered and the blood urea nitrogen (BUN) level rises. The term *uremia* refers to the constellation of signs and symptoms associated with chronic kidney disease, regardless of cause or of BUN level.

The once common practice of restricting protein intake in patients with chronic kidney disease to about

0.6 g/kg per day to control uremic symptoms or delay the onset of ESRD was shown in a multicenter trial to provide only small benefit,[3] so slightly more generous guidelines can be recommended (see Table 25–2). However, because Americans' average protein intake is around 100 g per day or 1.5 g/kg per day, much more than is required, some dietary adjustments are almost always needed. Changes in diet are also required for treating the most common underlying causes of chronic kidney disease, diabetes, and hypertension (see Chapters 18 and 19). Protein losses are higher in patients receiving peritoneal dialysis or continuous renal replacement therapies, dictating higher dietary protein requirements.

In stage 4 chronic kidney disease patients (GFR <25 mL/min) who are not on dialysis, very low-protein diets (0.28 g/kg per day) in combination with essential amino acid or ketoacid supplementation have been shown to reduce uremic symptoms and stabilize BUN levels while maintaining nitrogen balance.[3] The limited protein intake may enhance nitrogen recycling from ammonia by urea-splitting bacteria in the gut. However, no delay in the development of ESRD or death has been demonstrated with this approach.[3] Compliance with this diet is also difficult to achieve. In patients with acute renal failure, limitation of nonessential amino acids is not beneficial because they are required for the synthesis of acute-phase proteins and the repair of the kidneys themselves. Randomized trials using essential amino acid formulas have shown that they do not improve the resolution of acute renal failure or survival rates in patients with acute renal failure.

Therefore, a balanced mixture of essential and nonessential amino acids is recommended for treatment of both chronic kidney disease and acute renal failure. When enteral or parenteral feeding is used, a formula that meets the patient's energy and protein needs should be chosen. The objective is for the patient to take only as much protein as necessary to meet protein require-ments. Because patients with larger-than-average body mass, those under physiologic stress, or those receiving steroid treatment (e.g., after renal transplantation) may require more protein than other patients, each patient's needs should be documented and tracked using measurements of 24-hour urine urea nitrogen (UUN) to determine the actual protein requirement (see Chapter 10). In patients whose urine output is minimal or absent and/or whose BUN levels are changing, the 24-hour UUN is unreliable. Calculation of urea nitrogen appearance (UNA), including measurement of UUN in any urine produced, provides a suitable estimate of individual protein needs (see Chapter 10). UNA is best calculated using the changes in BUN and body water during one- to three-day periods between dialyses.

It is often assumed that in stressed patients with renal disease, dietary protein intake should not be increased to meet protein requirements calculated by UUN or UNA; there is a fear that doing so will increase ureagenesis, tax the kidneys further by increasing the renal urea load, and raise the BUN level. However, if protein intake only matches and does not exceed protein requirements, it does not increase ureagenesis. On the contrary, negative nitrogen balance is as deleterious to patients with renal impairment as it is to others and should be avoided.

Replacement of protein lost in the urine of a patient with the nephrotic syndrome does not correct disordered plasma or tissue protein pools; protein supplementation increases glomerular permeability, exacerbating urinary albumin losses. Therefore, protein requirements in these patients should be estimated as they are in other patients with renal disease, without adjusting for the proteinuria.

Lipids

Hypertriglyceridemia is quite common in patients with chronic kidney disease primarily because of defective catabolism of lipoproteins. In the nephrotic syndrome, other factors contribute to increased triglyceride-rich very-low-density lipoprotein (VLDL) levels. Aggressively lowering triglycerides has not been shown to reduce morbidity or mortality, but a lipid-lowering diet (see Table 12–1 and Chapter 20) is recommended for use with non-uremic patients to prevent coronary artery disease, the leading cause of death in patients with ESRD.

Because hypertriglyceridemia may impair a patient's tolerance of intravenous lipid emulsions, triglyceride levels should be monitored in kidney disease patients treated with parenteral nutrition. Fat emulsions do not need to be restricted unless serum triglyceride levels consistently exceed 350 mg/dL.

Fluids and Electrolytes

Sodium and Water

Normally, sodium and water are filtered by the renal glomeruli and reabsorbed by the tubules and/or collecting ducts (sodium actively and water passively). When the GFR is reduced in patients with either chronic or acute renal failure, filtration is impaired and reabsorption is fixed and therefore unable to adapt to changes in sodium intake. The resulting retention of sodium and water may produce edema, hypertension, and congestive heart failure. In this instance, restriction of sodium and water intake is appropriate depending on the level of renal impairment and urine volume. A suitable starting point is sodium intake of 1 to 3 g per day and a fluid intake 500 mL greater than the urine output, to account for insensible water losses. Adjustments can be made according to body weight and serum sodium levels to eliminate edema and normalize blood pressure and serum sodium levels. In patients with nephrotic syndrome, sodium restriction is always indicated.

In contrast, when the primary defect is in the renal tubule, ineffective reabsorption of sodium and water sometimes results in dehydration, hypotension, and further reduction in the GFR. Restriction of sodium and water is inappropriate in this circumstance, and their judicious addition may be required.

Potassium

Like sodium, potassium is filtered by the renal glomeruli and reabsorbed mainly in the proximal tubules. It is then actively secreted into the late distal tubules and collecting ducts for excretion. Renal tubular damage from acute renal failure or chronic kidney disease often impairs potassium filtration. This can lead to hyperkalemia, which can result in fatal arrhythmias. Potassium should be restricted to about 60 mEq per day when this occurs. Hyperkalemia is especially likely if acidosis, oliguria, or catabolism is present.

Phosphorus and Calcium

When renal glomerular filtration of phosphorus is hampered in chronic kidney disease, the serum level rises, leading to depression of serum calcium. This stimulates parathyroid hormone, which restores homeostasis by obtaining more calcium from bone, intestines, and kidneys and increasing renal phosphorus clearance. This can lead eventually to hyperparathyroidism and progressive loss of bone (renal osteodystrophy). Hyperphosphatemia and hyperparathyroidism may not only cause morbidity, they may themselves inflict further renal damage.

Therefore, patients should be instructed as soon as possible about dietary phosphate restriction (see Table 25–2) and use of phosphate-binding antacids to keep the serum phosphorus level as low as possible, even prior to its first elevation. Calcium carbonate is the preferred antacid because although aluminum hydroxide antacids bind phosphorus more strongly, aluminum accumulation in the brain and bone can lead to dementia and osteomalacia. In addition, calcium carbonate (which is best given between meals) provides needed supplemental calcium and corrects mild acidosis. Sevelamer, a non-absorbed phosphate-binding polymer that does not contain calcium or aluminum, may also be prescribed.

Magnesium

Magnesium is also normally excreted by the kidney, but it is often retained in patients with both acute and chronic kidney disease. Dietary restriction of the other nutrients discussed usually reduces magnesium intake sufficiently.

Magnesium-containing antacids, enemas, or laxatives should be avoided because they can result in dangerously high magnesium levels.

pH

Metabolic acidosis is often present in patients with acute and chronic kidney disease who are not on dialysis because of retention of metabolic acids and/or renal loss of bicarbonate. It can produce profound malaise, promote muscle proteolysis, and increase bone dissolution, and should therefore be vigorously treated. Calcium carbonate is useful for treating mild acidosis, but sodium bicarbonate is necessary when acidosis is severe. Dialysis is indicated if these measures are ineffective in controlling acidosis. When patients require total parenteral nutrition (TPN), using acetate as the anion to accompany sodium and/or potassium helps to ameliorate acidosis.

Vitamins

Water-soluble vitamin deficiencies are common in patients with chronic kidney disease because of poor oral intake, decreased renal reabsorption (e.g., of vitamin B_6), and losses from dialysis. Patients with chronic kidney disease on or off dialysis should receive supplements that provide at least the Recommended Daily Allowances (RDAs) of all water-soluble vitamins and additional amounts of folic acid (0.8 to 1 mg) and vitamin B_6 (5 mg off dialysis and 10 mg on dialysis).

Because a diseased kidney may not adequately remove retinol binding protein from circulation, hypervitaminosis A may occur in patients with chronic kidney disease; therefore, vitamin A supplements should be avoided. Functional vitamin D deficiency can occur in chronic kidney disease patients because the renal hydroxylation of 25-hydroxycholecalciferol (calcifediol) to the metabolically active 1,25-dihydroxycholecalciferol (calcitriol) is impaired. This results in reduced intestinal calcium absorption and exacerbates the derangement in bone metabolism and the hypocalcemia caused by phosphorus retention. Vitamin D deficiency can be prevented by supplementing the patient with calcitriol, starting with a dose of 0.25 to 0.50 μg/day. Calcitriol can cause hypercalcemia and hyperphosphatemia, so serum calcium and phosphorus levels must be closely monitored.

Trace Elements

Iron deficiency is common in chronic kidney disease patients because of poor oral intake and intestinal absorption of iron, occult gastrointestinal bleeding, phlebotomy for laboratory tests, and hemodialysis. Oral or intravenous iron supplementation is often used in conjunction with the human recombinant form of erythropoietin (epoetin alpha) to treat anemia. Although some studies indicate that the use of zinc sulfate in doses of about 220 mg daily may improve taste acuity, appetite, and sexual dysfunction, it has not been firmly established that patients with kidney disease should be routinely supplemented with zinc.

Intradialytic Parenteral Nutrition

Intradialytic parenteral nutrition (IDPN) involves infusion of dextrose, amino acids, and/or lipids during hemodialysis sessions through the venous dialysis drip chamber. It is sometimes used in malnourished maintenance hemodialysis patients when intensive counseling, oral supplementation, and tube feeding have failed to improve nutritional status. The use of IDPN is controversial because well-designed, large-scale prospective studies have not been done to confirm whether it positively affects outcome. Medicare coverage of outpatient IDPN is very tightly controlled and multiple criteria must be met for approval.[4]

REFERENCES

1 National Kidney Foundation Kidney Disease Outcomes Quality Initiative: Clinical practice guidelines for nutrition in chronic renal failure. Am J Kidney Dis 35:S1–S140, 2000; available at http://www.kidney.org/professionals/kdoqi/guidelines_updates/doqi_nut.html.

2. Owen WF, Jr., Lew NL, Liu Y, et al: The urea reduction ratio and serum albumin concentration as predictors of mortality in patients undergoing hemodialysis. N Engl J Med 329:1001–1006, 1993.
3. Klahr S, Levey AS, Beck GJ, et al: The effects of dietary protein restriction and blood-pressure control on the progression of chronic renal disease. N Engl J Med 330:877–884, 1994.
4. Moore E, Celano J: Challenges of providing nutrition support in the outpatient dialysis setting. Nutr Clin Pract 20:202–212, 2005.

SUGGESTED READINGS

Kopple JD: Nutrition, diet, and the kidney. In Shils ME, Shike M, Ross AC, (eds): Modern Nutrition in Health and Disease, 10th ed. Baltimore, Lippincott Williams & Wilkins, 2005.
McCann L: Pocket Guide to Nutrition Assessment of the Patient with Chronic Kidney Disease, 3rd ed. New York, Council on Renal Nutrition, National Kidney Foundation, 2002.

WEB SITES

National Kidney Foundation, http://www.kidney.org
National Kidney Foundation's Clinical Practice Guidelines for Nutrition in Chronic Renal Failure, http://www.kidney.org/professionals/kdoqi/guidelines_updates/doqi_nut.html

26

Anemias

SARAH L. MORGAN, MD • JOSEPH E. BAGGOTT, PhD

Anemia is a deficit of circulating red blood cells (RBCs) associated with diminished oxygen-carrying capacity of the blood. Anemia is diagnosed when the hemoglobin concentration is less than 12 g/dL in adult females or less than 13.0 or 13.5 g/dL in adult males, or when the hematocrit is less than 36% in females or less than 41% in males. Hemoglobin levels do not change significantly in healthy older adults between the ages of 60 and 98 years.

Signs and Symptoms

Anemia is a multisystem disorder whose symptoms often depend less on its severity than on the pace of its development. Thus, symptoms are more likely to occur from acute gastrointestinal bleeding than from long-term occult blood loss from, for example, aspirin use. If the anemia onset is gradual, a person may not be symptomatic until the hemoglobin level is less than 8 g/dL. Symptoms of severe anemia include easy fatigability and poor exercise tolerance. In iron deficiency, exercise tolerance is further impaired by lack of iron for myoglobin synthesis and for the function of energy-releasing heme-containing proteins in mitochondria. Resting tachycardia with a pulse rate greater than 100 beats per minute reflects the body's attempt to compensate for diminished oxygen-carrying capacity in the blood. Other symptoms may include palpitations, dizziness, syncope (loss of consciousness), or amenorrhea (absence of menstrual periods). Pallor of the mucous membranes (conjunctivae, buccal mucosa, and tongue) and skin may provide a clue to the presence of anemia, but pallor does not correlate closely with the hematocrit. Other signs of anemia can include a wide pulse pressure, systolic ejection murmurs, a cardiac venous hum, and a slick tongue.

Nutritional anemias are often accompanied by deficiencies of other vitamins and minerals. Because vitamin C and folic acid coexist in many foods, patients with folate-deficiency anemia may also have signs of scurvy. Additionally, anemia is not usually an isolated finding. A nutritional deficiency that limits RBC production usually affects other cells with high turnover rates such as leukocytes, platelets, and enterocytes. Therefore, reddening and soreness of the tongue, loss of lingual papillae, and megaloblastic changes in the intestinal tract accompany most cases of megaloblastic anemia.

Etiologies

The major hematopoietic nutrients are iron, vitamin B_{12}, and folic acid. Because of the particular steps in hematopoiesis where these nutrients function, the causes of nutritional anemias are suggested by the morphologic appearance of cells in peripheral blood or bone marrow smears. The mean corpuscular volume (MCV) provides the first clue to the etiology of anemias (Table 26–1). Anemias are classified as microcytic (small-cell) when the MCV is less than 80 fl. The major nutritional cause of microcytic anemias is iron deficiency, and minor ones are pyridoxine and copper deficiencies. Normocytic anemias (MCV 80 to 96 fl) are common in patients with protein-energy malnutrition (PEM) and various chronic diseases, and macrocytic anemias (MCV greater than 96 fl) can be caused by vitamin B_{12} or folic acid deficiencies. Microcytic and macrocytic cells can coexist; for example, a patient can have both iron and folate deficiencies. In these cases, the MCV may be deceptively normal and suggest a normocytic anemia, but the blood smear shows a dimorphic population of RBCs. The diagnosis of a nutritional anemia is confirmed by measuring the blood level of the suspected nutrient and sometimes by examination of the bone marrow.

Table 26-1	DIFFERENT DIAGNOSIS OF NUTRITIONAL ANEMIAS BY RED BLOOD CELL MEAN CORPUSCULAR VOLUME	
Mean Corpuscular Volume Category	**Nutritional Causes**	**Other Causes**
Microcytic (<80 fl)	Iron deficiency (common)	Chronic diseases, thalassemias
	Copper deficiency (uncommon)	Hemoglobin E disorders
	Pyridoxine deficiency (uncommon)	Sideroblastic anemia (lead toxicity)
Normocytic (80–96 fl)	Protein-energy malnutrition	Chronic diseases
Macrocytic (>96 fl)	Folic acid deficiency (common)	Alcoholism, liver disease
	Vitamin B_{12} deficiency (common)	Hemolysis

Final proof of the diagnosis is provided by a therapeutic response to replacement of the deficient nutrient. Table 26-1 also lists non-nutritional conditions that can cause anemias of each morphologic type.

Anemias have many etiologies, so underlying causes must be investigated. Three basic mechanisms are involved: (1) diminished erythropoiesis (RBC production), usually caused by nutritional deficiencies or bone marrow failure; (2) blood loss; and (3) increased hemolysis (RBC destruction), either hereditary or acquired. Thus, anemia is a manifestation of not only nutritional deficiencies, but many different conditions. An anemia is considered nutritional in origin when one or more nutrients essential to RBC formation is deficient. Such deficiencies may occur with normal dietary intake if increased requirements (e.g., pregnancy, hemolysis, or alcohol abuse) or external losses (e.g., chronic gastrointestinal blood loss) exist. The major mechanisms by which an individual becomes nutrient deficient include inadequate ingestion, malabsorption, impaired utilization, elevated requirements, increased excretion, or increased destruction.

Diagnostic Steps

The investigation of anemia requires a thorough history and physical examination. It is important to elicit whether the patient has a history of drug exposure, because many medications interfere with nutrient metabolism and erythropoiesis (see Chapter 15). During physical examination, look for signs of gastrointestinal or genitourinary blood loss, ecchymoses, petechiae, or purpura. Laboratory data including complete and differential blood cell counts and examination of the blood smear are mandatory. A count of reticulocytes (immature cells recently released from the bone marrow) is also helpful. A high reticulocyte count (>1.5%) suggests the presence of hemolysis or hemorrhage. The red blood cell distribution width (RDW) quantifies variability in the size of red blood cells. In deficiencies of iron, vitamin B_{12}, and folic acid, the RDW is elevated, indicating a wide range in the size of rRBCs. In contrast, thalassemia and anemia of chronic disease tend to have normal RDWs. A variety of other tests such as vitamin and mineral levels can provide important evidence about etiology. A bone marrow aspirate and/or biopsy is often necessary to make a definitive diagnosis.

Microcytic Anemias

Microcytic anemias are characterized by small cells and MCVs less than 80 fl caused by retarded maturation of the cytoplasm. Although the major nutritional cause is iron deficiency, other conditions including copper and pyridoxine deficiencies can cause microcytic anemia (see Table 26–1).

Iron Deficiency

Iron deficiency anemia can result from inadequate intake, inadequate absorption, or excessive losses (bleeding); the latter is most often the cause in the United States. Iron deficiency anemia is the most common nutritional anemia and perhaps the most common nutritional deficiency in the world.

Pathophysiology

Iron is present in the body in functional and storage forms. In its functional form, Iron is incorporated into heme and myoglobin and is part of many enzymes. A small amount is found in plasma, bound to transferrin and other iron-binding proteins. Its storage form is ferritin and hemosiderin.

Dietary iron is composed of heme iron, which is mainly from meat, and nonheme iron, which is principally from vegetables and cooking vessels. Both forms are largely absorbed in the upper small intestine, especially the duodenum. Heme iron is about 20% bioavailable, whereas nonheme iron is only 3% bioavailable. Between the two forms, net absorption is about 10%. The absorption of nonheme iron can be enhanced up to threefold by the simultaneous ingestion of high-quality protein and 25 to 75 mg of vitamin C. Vitamin C aids in the conversion of ferric (Fe^{+3}) iron to the more readily absorbed ferrous (Fe^{+2}) form. Absorption of heme iron is unchanged by these factors. When necessary, (e.g., in pregnancy, after blood loss, or in anemic states), mucosal cells of the upper small intestine can respond to the body's need for more iron by increasing its absorption. However, it is not always possible to meet these requirements through diet alone. Therefore, daily supplementation of iron during pregnancy is recommended (see Chapter 4).

Each day in normal adults, about 1% of the red blood cell mass is destroyed, releasing about 30 mg of iron into the reticuloendothelial system and then into circulation for transport to the bone marrow. Of the 30 mg released, about 29 mg is salvaged and utilized for the synthesis of new hemoglobin and only 1 mg must be replaced. In adult males, nutritional equilibrium is maintained by the absorption of about 1 mg per day from a diet containing the Recommended Dietary Allowance (RDA) of 8 mg iron. Menstruating women need an additional 0.5 mg per day to compensate for menstrual losses, or approximately a total of 1.5 mg per day to maintain equilibrium. Therefore, the RDA for women aged 14 to 50 years is 18 mg per day; it increases to 27 mg per day during pregnancy and drops to 9 to 10 mg per day during lactation.

The greatest risk for iron deficiency occurs during the following four stages of the life cycle: (1) between 6 months and 4 years of age, (2) in early adolescence, (3) during the menstruating years, and (4) during pregnancy. When iron deficiency occurs during growth and development, it usually results from inadequate iron intake rather than increased losses. In adults who are not pregnant, blood loss is most often the cause of iron deficiency, so it is crucial to find and correct the source of blood loss as well as to replace the iron deficit. Large doses of aspirin or other nonsteroidal anti-inflammatory drugs frequently cause gastrointestinal blood loss, as does alcohol abuse. Blood loss in premenopausal women is usually from menstruation, so if the patient's history and physical examination provide no other clues, it is justifiable to recommend a 30-day therapeutic trial of oral iron supplementation without searching for additional sources of blood loss. However, this method of treatment is almost never justified in males, in whom iron deficiency is most often caused by chronic, occult blood loss from the gastrointestinal tract. Multiple stool specimens should be tested for occult blood, and complete examination of the gastrointestinal tract with x-rays and/or endoscopy is often indicated. In hospitalized patients, repeated blood sampling for laboratory tests may lead to iron deficiency anemia. One unit of donated blood (450 mL) contains about 225 mg of iron, which may require 2 to 4 months to replace. Because nonheme iron requires an acid pH for optimal absorption, the use of histamine-2 receptor blocker and proton pump inhibitor drugs, *Helicobacter pylori* infection, and gastric achlorhydria are frequently associated with iron deficiency. Subtotal gastrectomy and gastric bypass surgery for obesity also frequently cause iron deficiency.

Diagnosis

In addition to physical findings generally associated with anemia, patients with iron deficiency sometimes exhibit glossitis and (infrequently) koilonychia (spooning of the nails). Pica, especially a craving to chew ice, very commonly follows iron deficiency.

Table 26-2 presents characteristic laboratory findings in patients with nutritional anemias. Iron deficiencies occur in stages: first, the bone marrow iron is depleted; next, the serum iron level drops and the total iron-binding capacity (TIBC) increases; finally, the MCV and hemoglobin levels drop. The diagnosis of iron deficiency should be considered when the RBCs are small (microcytic) and pale (hypochromic). Low MCV and mean corpuscular hemoglobin concentration (MCHC) usually indicate iron deficiency, but they can also be caused by thalassemias, which are particularly common among persons of African, Asian, and Mediterranean descent. The diagnosis of iron deficiency is supported by low serum iron and high TIBC levels. The serum iron level is normally 15% that of the TIBC; lower values indicate that the available binding sites on transferrin are not saturated and suggest the patient may have iron deficiency. A high TIBC is important for distinguishing iron deficiency from other causes of low serum iron such as PEM, injury, infection, or chronic inflammatory disease (Table 26-3), which can lower both iron and TIBC levels and produce a variable effect on percent saturation of TIBC. Severe physiologic stress such as from burns and sepsis can result in serum iron levels as low as zero, even when iron stores are normal. This occurs because the body sequesters iron in ferritin, especially in the reticuloendothelial system, with the benefit of reducing the risk of infections by inhibiting infectious organisms from using free iron for growth.

Another laboratory finding that suggests the diagnosis of iron deficiency is a serum ferritin level less than 40 ng/mL; a level less than 12 ng/mL is virtually diagnostic. With ferritin levels between 12 and 100 ng/mL, patients may have iron deficiency, anemia of chronic disease, or both types of anemia. Caution must be used in interpreting ferritin levels when the patient also has liver disease or acute stress, because they can raise the

Table 26-2	MORPHOLOGIC FINDINGS AND LABORATORY VALUES IN NUTRITIONAL ANEMIAS			
			Deficiency	
	Normal	Iron	Folic Acid	Vitamin B$_{12}$
RBC morphology	Normocytic	Microcytic, hypochromic	Macrocytic	Macrocytic
MCV (fl)	80–96	<80	>96	>96
MCHC (g/dL)	32–36	<32	>32	>32
Hypersegmented neutrophils	Absent	Absent	Present	Present
Bone marrow morphology	Normal	Normoblastic	Megaloblastic	Megaloblastic
Bone marrow iron	Normal	Absent	Normal/High	Normal/High
Serum iron (µg/dL)	30–170	<30	Normal/High	Normal/High
Serum TIBC (µg/dL)	240–450	>450	Normal/High	Normal/High
Serum ferritin (ng/mL)	12–500	<12	Normal/High	Normal/High
Plasma folate (ng/mL)	5–40 (3–5 is marginal)	5–40	<3	Normal/High
RBC folate (ng/mL)	280–900	280–900	<280	280–900
Plasma vitamin B$_{12}$ (pg/mL)	200–900 (200–299 is marginal)	200–900	Normal/High	<200
Serum homocysteine (µmol/L)	4–12	4–12	>12	>12
Serum methylmalonic acid (µmol/L)	0–0.4	0–0.4	0–0.4	>0.4

MCHC, mean corpuscular hemoglobin concentration; MCV, mean corpuscular volume; RBC, red blood count; TIBC, total iron-binding capacity.

Table 26-3	CONDITIONS AFFECTING IRON PARAMETERS		
Laboratory Findings	Injury, Infection, Chronic Inflammation	Iron Deficiency	Protein-energy Malnutrition
Serum iron	Low	Low	Generally low
Serum TIBC	Normal or low	High	Low
Serum ferritin	Normal or slightly high	Low	Generally low
Marrow and liver iron stores	Present	Absent	Low to absent

TIBC, total iron-binding capacity.

ferritin level as an acute phase reactant even when iron deficiency is present. A ferritin level up to 70 ng/mL in the presence of these conditions does not rule out iron deficiency. The gold standard for diagnosing iron deficiency is a bone marrow with greatly diminished or absent iron stores. When both iron and TIBC levels are low and the ferritin level is equivocal, examination of the bone marrow is the only way to establish the diagnosis. Bone marrow examination also helps identify rare cases of iron-loading (e.g., sideroblastic) anemia and thalassemia, in which patients have hypochromic and/or microcytic anemia but adequate or excessive stores of iron.

Dietary Sources

About 10% to 15% of the iron in the American diet comes from heme sources such as meats and seafood, and 85% to 90% comes from nonheme sources including dried beans and peas, leafy green vegetables, enriched breads and cereals, dried fruits, and egg yolks. Non-food sources include cooking vessels, water pipes, iron tablets, and multiple vitamins. Phytates, polyphenols, calcium, oxalates, and tannins decrease nonheme iron absorption, while ascorbic acid, amino acids, and animal proteins increase it.

Treatment

Iron deficiencies can usually be treated effectively with iron preparations such as ferrous sulfate given orally in doses of 325 mg (60 mg elemental iron) 1 to 3 times daily with meals. Therapy should be continued for 4 to 6 months to restore normal hemoglobin levels and iron stores. Depending on the cause of deficiency, long-term low-dose therapy may be required. Modification of the diet to include meats, vitamin C, iron-fortified foods such as enriched grains and cereals, and foods cooked in cast-iron cookware and avoidance of iron binders such as phytates can also improve iron status. However, these modifications produce smaller effects than are achieved with iron supplements.

When oral supplementation is ineffective in correcting iron deficiency, such as in patients with malabsorption, iron can be given intravenously. It is available as iron dextran, sodium ferric gluconate complex, or iron sucrose. A small test dose should be given initially to detect hypersensitivity. Total iron replacement can be effected with a single, slow intravenous infusion of iron dextran using the following calculation: total dose (mL) = 0.0442 × (desired hemoglobin − observed hemoglobin) × weight (kg) + (0.26 × weight [kg]).

Macrocytic Anemias

Macrocytic (large-cell) anemias are characterized by MCV greater than 96 fl. When caused by a deficiency of folic acid or vitamin B_{12}, they are also called megaloblastic anemias because large, immature red cell precursors (megaloblasts) accumulate in the bone marrow. Not all macrocytic anemias are megaloblastic; in those associated with alcoholism, liver disease, and hemolysis, the red cells are large for other reasons, and megaloblasts are not present in the bone marrow. In addition, artifactual macrocytosis without anemia can be caused by cold agglutinins, hyperglycemia, and marked leukocytosis.

Vitamin B_{12} Deficiency

Vitamin B_{12} deficiency anemia is most often caused by impaired absorption rather than inadequate intakes.

It is common in geriatric populations, where prevalences have been estimated between 3% and 40%.

Pathophysiology

Most vitamin B_{12} originates from bacterial synthesis, which occurs particularly in the rumen of ruminant animals; therefore, meat and animal proteins are good sources. Upon entry into the stomach, vitamin B_{12} is bound to proteins called R-binders secreted by the salivary glands and stomach. After passing into the small intestine, pancreatic enzymes remove vitamin B_{12} from the R-binders, and it is then bound to intrinsic factor (IF), a glycoprotein secreted by the acid-producing parietal cells of the stomach. Vitamin B_{12} must be bound to IF to be absorbed at specific receptor sites in the distal ileum. Vitamin B_{12} is transported in plasma and intracellularly bound to transcobalamin. Because it is excreted in the bile but is very efficiently reabsorbed in the distal ileum (enterohepatic recirculation), it takes many years for an individual to deplete vitamin B_{12} stores on a vitamin B_{12}-free (i.e., vegan) diet, as long as the intestinal and hepatobiliary systems are intact. The total body pool of vitamin B_{12} in normal adults is about 2500 μg; the largest storage site is the liver.

Because of the small amounts required and the efficiency with which the body manages its vitamin B_{12} stores, anemia resulting from inadequate vitamin B_{12} intake is uncommon. Strict vegetarians who consume no dairy products, eggs, or meat are at increased risk for deficiency, but even bacterial and insect contamination of food provides some protection against B_{12} deficiency. Vegetables and drinking water contaminated by feces of ruminant animals may actually serve as a source of dietary vitamin B_{12} for vegetarians living in poor areas of the world.

Malabsorption of food-bound vitamin B_{12} is felt to be the most common cause of B_{12} deficiency in older adults. Risk for this is increased by the presence of atrophic gastritis, *H. pylori* infection, and treatment with histamine-2 receptor blocker and proton pump inhibitor drugs, which are common in the elderly. It is recommended that individuals older than 50 obtain adequate B_{12} by eating foods fortified with it or by taking a vitamin B_{12}-containing supplement.

Another cause of vitamin B_{12} deficiency is pernicious anemia (PA), a condition affecting primarily elderly white persons of Northern European ancestry in which gastric secretion of IF becomes markedly reduced, leading to vitamin B_{12} malabsorption. Intestinal disorders can also cause vitamin B_{12} deficiency even when dietary intake is adequate. Absorption is disrupted by gastrectomy or gastric bypass surgery because the site of IF secretion is eliminated. Regional enteritis (Crohn's disease), bacterial overgrowth of the small bowel (which occurs in a variety of intestinal disorders), and ileal resection interfere with vitamin B_{12} by impairing or eliminating the site of absorption. Severe pancreatic disease and total pancreatectomy hinder vitamin B_{12} absorption by decreasing the transfer of cobalamins from R-binders to IF. Use of metformin, colchicine, cholestyramine, histamine-2 receptor proton pump inhibitors, and anti-convulsants can cause malabsorption of vitamin B_{12}. Additional medications that can impair vitamin B_{12} absorption are listed in Chapter 15.

Diagnosis

In addition to the general physical findings associated with anemia, prolonged vitamin B_{12} deficiencies affect the central and peripheral nervous systems, causing loss of vibratory and position sense, numbness and tingling in the hands and feet, unsteadiness, and even delusions and psychosis.

In vitamin B_{12} and folic acid deficiencies, the morphologic appearance of cells in peripheral blood and bone marrow are indistinguishable. Macrocytes and hyper-segmentation of neutrophils are found on the peripheral smear; there is hypersegmentation if 5% of the neu-trophils have more than 5 lobes, or if the average number of lobes per cell exceeds 3.5. Hypersegmentation may also be congenital or caused by chronic renal failure or pyruvate kinase deficiency. Macrocytes are also present in hypothyroidism, reticulocytosis, and liver failure.

Vitamin B_{12} deficiency should be considered when the plasma vitamin B_{12} concentration is less than about 200 pg/mL. However, not all patients with low cobalamin levels are vitamin B_{12} deficient, and conversely, serum cobalamin levels are normal in a significant minority of patients with vitamin B_{12} deficiency. Some individuals who are not deficient may have low plasma vitamin B_{12} levels because of low vitamin B_{12} transport proteins (transcobalamins) or the presence of plasma inhibitors of intrinsic factor that interfere with the vitamin B_{12} assay, giving falsely low results. Additional causes of falsely low vitamin B_{12} levels are folate deficiency, use of oral contraceptive pills, and excessive vitamin C intake. Causes of falsely normal plasma vitamin B_{12} levels in spite of deficiency include liver disease, alcoholism, lymphoma, and myeloproliferative disorders.

Serum homocysteine and methylmalonic acid levels, which are elevated in the presence of vitamin B_{12} deficiency, are useful in distinguishing true deficiencies. Methylmalonic acid levels are particularly useful in older individuals who present with neuropsychiatric abnormalities of vitamin B_{12} deficiency without hematologic findings.

In evaluating macrocytic anemias, it is important to check both vitamin B_{12} and folate status and to confirm the diagnosis of PA. If vitamin B_{12} deficiency is mistakenly treated with folic acid, the anemia can improve, but degeneration of the posterolateral columns of the spinal cord will progress. Because of this risk of masking PA with large doses of folate, the folic acid content of over-the-counter vitamin supplements is limited to 400 μg per pill. Concerns were expressed that fortification of foods with folate, which was required by the U.S. Food and Drug Administration in 1998, would produce similar masking of vitamin B_{12} deficiency. However, at the present time there is no evidence that folate food fortification has had such an effect.

The presence of IF antibodies in the serum of a patient with a low serum vitamin B_{12} level is diagnostic of PA, and makes further investigation unnecessary. However, the classic and sometimes still used method of diagnosing of PA was the Schilling test, which compares the intestinal absorption of vitamin B_{12} bound to IF with that of unbound vitamin B_{12} after a vitamin B_{12} injection of 1000 µg is given to saturate plasma-binding sites. PA patients absorb the IF-bound vitamin B_{12} normally, as demonstrated by urinary excretion of more than 10% of the isotope in 24 hours, but do not absorb the unbound vitamin B_{12} normally. If neither isotope is absorbed well, intestinal dysfunction (not PA) is the likely cause; it is important to perform both stages of the test in order to make this distinction. Not all patients with PA have abnormal Schilling tests, because some patients can absorb the crystalline vitamin B_{12} (cyanocobalamin) used in the test, but not vitamin B_{12} associated with food proteins. This has led to the use of a "food" Schilling test in some patients.

The development of vitamin B_{12} deficiency occurs in stages. The first stage is characterized by a negative vitamin B_{12} balance, during which the plasma vitamin B_{12} level is marginal, and only vitamin B_{12} carriers in the plasma (transcobalamins) may be abnormally low. Subsequently, the plasma vitamin B_{12} level falls. When the level reaches 100 to 150 pg/mL, neutrophils begin to appear hypersegmented. Finally, macroovalocytes appear, the MCV is elevated, and the hemoglobin level drops. Anemia develops in the later stages of vitamin B_{12} deficiency as it does with iron deficiency.

Dietary Sources

Vitamin B_{12} is found only in foods of animal origin. Most meats and dairy products contain some vitamin B_{12}; beef liver is an especially rich source.

Treatment

Remission of the signs and symptoms of vitamin B_{12} deficiency begins with a single intramuscular injection of 100 to 1000 µg of cyanocobalamin or hydroxycobalamin. Daily administration of 100 µg for several days is advisable. Reticulocytosis, indicating hematologic response, begins after 5 to 7 days. For PA patients and others who need continued parenteral therapy, injections of 100 µg every month are generally adequate. Large oral doses of 500 to 2000 µg daily or nasal gel doses of 500 µg monthly may suffice for maintenance of normal levels after they are attained with injections. Therapy should be individualized according to the patient's hematologic response and plasma B_{12} levels.

Folic Acid Deficiency

In contrast to vitamin B_{12}, where inadequate intake is rarely a cause of deficiency, folic acid deficiency from insufficient intake is common when folate-rich foods are not consumed regularly or when pregnancy increases requirements. In addition to anemia, suboptimal folate intake during pregnancy even without frank deficiency is a major risk factor for congenital neural tube birth defects. To prevent this, mandatory folic acid fortification of grain and cereal products began in the United States in 1998. Fortification has produced higher blood folate levels and lower serum homocysteine levels in the U.S. population.

Pathophysiology

Folate is the generic term for folic acid coenzymes in the body. They consist of a pteridine ring, a para-aminobenzoic acid moiety, and a polyglutamate side chain. Folate acts as a coenzyme in numerous one-carbon transfer reactions, including the methylation of homocysteine to form methionine; serine, glycine, and histidine metabolism; the synthesis of purines; and the formation of deoxythymidylate from deoxyuridylate.

Folic acid is present in foods in the form of polyglutamates with numerous glutamate side chains linked in a gamma carboxy amide linkage. Absorption occurs in the upper small intestine after the polyglutamate side chains are hydrolyzed by conjugase to form the monoglutamate. Folate stores in the liver are estimated to be 5 to 10 mg. Dietary folate equivalents (DFE) take into account differences in the bioavailability of synthetic folic acid and food folates. One DFE equals 1 µg of food folate, 0.5 µg of folic acid taken on an empty stomach, or 0.6 µg of folic acid taken with a meal.

Persons who rarely consume green leafy vegetables or other sources of folate can exhibit low plasma folate levels in a few weeks and signs of deficiency after several months. Folate malabsorption is associated with a variety of intestinal disorders such as Crohn's disease, celiac disease, and tropical sprue. Alcoholics are also commonly deficient. The average plasma folate levels of cigarette smokers are lower than those of nonsmokers, partly from poor diets but probably also from smoke-induced destruction of folate.

Folate-deficiency anemia can also result from inter-actions with drugs, including alcohol (see Chapter 15). Abnormal utilization of folate has been observed with certain anticonvulsants (phenytoin, phenobarbital), diuretics (triamterene), antibiotics (trimethoprim, sulfasalazine), and antimalarials (pyrimethamine) as well as methotrexate, a folate antimetabolite widely used in the treatment of autoimmune diseases and cancer.

Diagnosis

The hematologic characteristics of folate-deficient anemia in both the peripheral blood and bone marrow are indistinguishable from those of vitamin B_{12}-deficient anemia. Folic acid deficiency is indicated by a plasma folate level less than 3 ng/mL. However, because plasma folate levels fluctuate with recent dietary intake, the RBC folate level is a more reliable indicator of tissue stores; levels less than 140 ng/mL indicate deficiency. The serum homocysteine level is also elevated in patients with folic acid deficiency, indicating an inability to remethylate homocysteine to form methionine.

Like iron and vitamin B_{12} deficiencies, folate deficiency develops in stages. The first stage is charac-terized by negative folate balance, manifest by a low serum folate level. Next, the RBC folate level decreases and neutrophils appear hypersegmented.

Finally, macroovalocytes appear, the MCV is elevated, and the hemoglobin level drops.

Dietary Sources

Folic acid is widely distributed in yeast, liver and other organ meats, legumes, leafy vegetables, fresh fruits, and fortified grains and cereal products (flour, corn meal, grits, breads, rice, and pasta). Orange juice is the highest contributor of food folic acid to the American diet. Between 50% and 90% of the folate in foods can be destroyed by prolonged cooking and processing.

Treatment

Folic acid deficiency is readily corrected in most patients with a 1 mg daily oral supplement. Folic acid supplements are also frequently used in patients taking antifolates such as methotrexate, to reduce their toxicity. In patients with malabsorption, initial treatment with parenteral folate is advised, but thereafter maintenance with oral therapy usually suffices. Plasma and RBC levels should be used to guide therapy. As noted earlier, folic acid supplements given to vitamin B_{12}-deficient patients can ameliorate the hematologic signs of vitamin B_{12} deficiency while the neurological signs progress.

Other Nutritional Anemias

Although less common, anemia can be caused by deficits of other trace elements and vitamins, some of which are involved in the normal metabolism and utilization of iron, folate, and vitamin B_{12}. For example, copper is essential for normal iron metabolism and the production of hemoglobin; copper deficiency leads to hypochromic anemia and low serum iron levels. Vitamin A deficiency may also produce anemia and low serum iron levels. Riboflavin deficiency has been reported to cause reversible aplasia of RBC precursors in the bone marrow. An atypical sideroblastic anemia responsive to vitamin B_6 (pyridoxine) has also been described.

SUGGESTED READINGS

Clarke R, Refsum H, Birks J, et al: Screening for vitamin B_{12} and folate deficiency in older persons. Am J Clin Nutr 77:1241–1247, 2003.

Dharmarajan TS, Adiga GU, Norkus EP: Vitamin B_{12} deficiency: Recognizing subtle symptoms in older adults. Geriatrics 58:30–34, 37–38, 2003.

Stanger O: Physiology of folic acid in health and disease. Current Drug Metabolism 3:211–223, 2002.

Yates JM, Logan ECM, Steward RM: Iron deficiency anaemia in general practice: Clinical outcomes over three years and factors influencing diagnostic investigations. Postgrad Med J 80:405–410, 2004.

27

Eating Disorders

BONNIE A. SPEAR, PhD

Eating disorders are considered psychiatric conditions, but they are remarkable for their nutritional and medical complications, which can sometimes be life-threatening. As a general rule, they are characterized by abnormal eating patterns and cognitive distortions related to food and body weight, which adversely affect nutritional status and lead to medical complications and impaired health status and function. About 85% of eating disorders begin during adolescence.

Diagnostic criteria for anorexia nervosa (AN), bulimia nervosa (BN), and eating disorders not otherwise specified (EDNOS) based on psychological, behavioral, and physiologic characteristics are defined in the *Diagnostic and Statistical Manual of Mental Disorders* (DSM-IV) (Box 27-1).

Features and Interventions in Eating Disorders

The Treatment Team

Because of the complex biopsychosocial nature of eating disorders, an interdisciplinary team consisting of professionals from medical, nursing, nutritional, and mental health disciplines with expertise in treating eating disorders provides the optimal assessment and management of these conditions. Team members can work in different facilities in the community, but the key is that they must communicate about plans and goals for the patient.

Anorexia Nervosa

AN occurs in approximately 1% to 2% of young adult women, with 85% of patients having onset during

541

BOX 27–1 Diagnostic Criteria for Eating Disorders

Anorexia Nervosa (Diagnostic Code 307.10)

A. Refusal to maintain body weight at or above a minimally normal weight for age and height, e.g., weight loss leading to maintenance of body weight less than 85% of that expected; or failure to make expected weight gain during period of growth, leading to body weight less than 85% of that expected.

B. Intense fear of gaining weight or becoming fat, even though underweight.

C. Disturbance in the way in which one's body weight, size, or shape is experienced, undue influence of body weight or shape on self-evaluation, or denial of the seriousness of the current low body weight.

D. Amenorrhea in postmenarcheal females, i.e., the absence of at least three consecutive menstrual cycles. (Women are also considered to have amenorrhea if their periods occur only following hormone, e.g., estrogen, administration.)

Specific Type

Restricting type: During the current episode of anorexia nervosa, the person has not regularly engaged in binge eating or purging behavior (i.e., self-induced vomiting or the misuse of laxatives, diuretics, or enemas).

Binge-eating/Purging type: During the current episode of anorexia nervosa, the person has regularly engaged in binge eating or purging behavior (i.e., self-induced vomiting or the misuse of laxatives, diuretics, or enemas).

Bulimia Nervosa (Diagnostic Code 307.51)

A. Recurrent episodes of binge eating. An episode of binge eating is characterized by both of the following:

  1. Eating, in a discrete period of time (e.g., within any 2-hour period), an amount of food that is definitely larger than most people would eat in a similar period of time under similar circumstances.

  2. A sense of lack of control over eating during the episode (e.g., a feeling that one cannot stop eating or control what or how much one is eating).

B. Recurrent inappropriate compensatory behavior in order to prevent weight gain, such as self-induced vomiting; misuse of laxatives, diuretics, enemas, or other medications; fasting or excessive exercise.

C. Both the binge eating and inappropriate compensatory behaviors occur, on average, at least twice a week for 3 months.

BOX 27–1   Diagnostic Criteria for Eating
Disorders *(Continued)*

Bulimia Nervosa (Diagnostic Code 307.51) *(Continued)*

D. Self-evaluation is unduly influenced by body shape and weight.
E. The disturbance does not occur exclusively during episodes
of anorexia nervosa.

Specific Type
Purging type: During the current episode of bulimia nervosa,
the person has regularly engaged in self-induced vomiting
or the misuse of laxatives, diuretics, or enemas.
Nonpurging type: During the current episode of bulimia nervosa, the person has used other inappropriate compensatory behaviors, such as fasting or excessive exercise, but
has not regularly engaged in self-induced vomiting or the
misuse of laxative, diuretics, or enemas.

Eating Disorders Not Otherwise Specified (EDNOS) (Diagnostic Code 307.5)

The Eating Disorders Not Otherwise Specified category is for
disorders of eating that do not meet the criteria for any
specific eating disorders. Examples include:
1. Females who meet the criteria for anorexia nervosa but
have regular menses.
2. Individuals who meet the criteria for anorexia nervosa
including significant weight loss, but the current weight
is in the normal range.
3. Individuals who meet the criteria for bulimia nervosa
except that the binge eating and inappropriate compensatory behaviors occur less than twice a week or for a
duration of less than 3 months.
4. The regular use of inappropriate compensatory behaviors by an individual of normal body weight after eating
small amounts of food (e.g., self-induced vomiting after
the consumption of two cookies).
5. Repeatedly chewing and spitting out but not swallowing
large amounts of food.
6. Binge eating disorder: Recurrent episodes of binge eating
in the absence of the regular use of inappropriate compensatory behaviors characteristic of bulimia nervosa.

Binge Eating Disorder (Research Criteria of EDNOS)

A. Recurrent episodes of binge eating. An episode of binge
eating is characterized by both of the following:
1. Eating, in a discrete period of time (e.g., within any
2-hour period), an amount of food that is definitely

Box continued on following page

> **BOX 27–1   Diagnostic Criteria for Eating Disorders** *(Continued)*
>
> **Binge Eating Disorder (Research Criteria of EDNOS)** *(Continued)*
>
>   larger than most people would eat in a similar period of time under similar circumstances.
>
>   2. A sense of lack of control over eating during the episode (e.g., a feeling that one cannot stop eating or control what or how much one is eating).
>
> B. The binge eating episodes are associated with three or more of following:
>   1. Eating much more rapidly than normal.
>   2. Eating until feeling uncomfortably full.
>   3. Eating large amounts of food when not feeling physically hungry.
>   4. Eating alone because of embarrassment over how much one is eating.
>   5. Feeling disgusted with oneself, depressed, or very guilty after overeating.
>
> C. Marked distress regarding binge eating is present.
> D. The binge eating occurs, on average, at least 2 days a week for 6 months.
> E. The binge eating is not associated with the regular use of inappropriate compensatory behaviors (e.g., purging, fasting, excessive exercise) and does not occur exclusively during the course of anorexia nervosa or bulimia nervosa.
>
> ---
>
> *From American Psychiatric Association: Diagnostic and Statistical Manual of Mental Disorders, 4th ed, text revised. Washington, DC, American Psychiatric Association, 2000 (10).

the adolescence. In the pathogenesis of AN, dieting or other purposeful changes in food choices contribute enormously to the course of the disease because the physiologic and psychological consequences of starvation perpetuate the disease and impede progress toward recovery. Higher prevalence rates among specific groups, such as athletes and patients with diabetes mellitus, support the concept that increased risk occurs with conditions in which dietary restraint or control of body weight is considered important. However, only a small proportion of individuals who diet or restrict intake develop an eating disorder.

Physical Features

Essential to the diagnosis of AN is that patients weigh less than 85% of that expected. There are several ways to determine the 85th percentile. For adults older than 20 years of age, a body mass index (BMI) of 17.5 or less could make AN an appropriate diagnosis. For children and young adults up to the age of 20, the percent of average weight-for-height can be calculated by using Centers for Disease Control and Prevention growth charts or body mass index charts. Because children are still growing, the BMI increases with age in children and therefore BMI percentiles must be used, not the absolute BMI. Individuals with BMIs below the 10th percentile are considered underweight and BMIs below the 5th percentile indicate risk for AN. In all cases, the patient's body build, weight history, and stage of development (in adolescents) should be considered.

Physical characteristics include lanugo hair on face and trunk, brittle listless hair, cyanosis of hands and feet, and dry skin. Cardiovascular changes include bradycardia (less than 60 beats/min), hypotension (systolic blood pressure below 90 mmHg), and orthostatic hypotension. Many patients as well as some health providers attribute the low heart rate and low blood pressure to their physical fitness and exercise regimen. However, AN patients with bradycardia and hypotension exhibit altered cardiovascular responses to exercise. A reduced heart mass has also been associated with the reduced blood pressure and pulse rate. Cardiovascular complications have led to mortality in AN patients.

AN can also significantly affect the gastrointestinal tract and brain mass. Self-induced starvation can lead to delayed gastric emptying, decreased gut motility, and severe constipation. There is also evidence of structural brain abnormalities (tissue loss) with prolonged starvation, which appears early in the disease process and may be of substantial magnitude. While some reversal of brain changes occurs with weight recovery, it is uncertain whether complete reversal is possible. To minimize the potential long-term physical complications of AN, early recognition and aggressive treatment is essential.

Amenorrhea, a primary characteristic of AN, is associated with a combination of hypothalamic dysfunction, weight loss, decreased body fat, stress, and excessive exercise. The amenorrhea appears to be caused by an alteration in the regulation of gonadotropin-releasing hormone. In AN, gonadotropins revert to prepubertal levels and patterns of secretion.

Osteopenia and osteoporosis, like brain changes, are serious and possibly irreversible medical complications of AN. It may be serious enough to result in vertebral compression and stress fractures. Results indicate that some recovery of bone may be possible with weight restoration, but compromised bone density has been evident 11 years after weight recovery for individuals who had onset during the adolescent period. Unlike other conditions in which low estrogen levels are associated with bone loss (e.g., postmenopausal), providing exogenous estrogen has not been shown to preserve or restore bone mass in patients with AN. Adequate calcium intake may help to lessen bone loss, but calcium supplementation alone (1500 mg/d) or in combination with estrogen has not been observed to promote increased bone density. Only weight restoration has been shown to do so.

In patients with AN, laboratory values usually remain in normal ranges until the condition is far advanced; however, true laboratory values may be masked by chronic dehydration. Some of the earliest abnormalities include bone marrow hypoplasia with varying degrees of leukopenia and thrombocytopenia. Despite consuming low-fat and low-cholesterol diets, patients with AN often have elevated cholesterol and abnormal lipid profiles. Reasons for this include mild hepatic dysfunction, decreased bile acid secretion, and abnormal eating patterns. Additionally, serum glucose tends to be low due to a deficit of precursors for gluconeogenesis and glucose production. Patients with AN may have recurrent episodes of hypoglycemia.

Despite dietary inadequacies, vitamin and mineral deficiencies are rarely seen in AN. This has been attributed to a decreased metabolic need for micronutrients in a catabolic state. Additionally, many patients take vitamin and mineral supplements. Despite low iron intakes, iron deficiency anemia is rare, perhaps because of decreased needs due to amenorrhea, absence of anabolism, and hemoconcentration from altered hydration. Prolonged malnutrition leads to low levels of zinc, vitamin B_{12}, and folate. Low nutrient levels should be treated appropriately with food and supplements as needed.

Medical and Nutritional Management of Anorexia Nervosa

Outpatient therapy. In AN the goals of outpatient treatment are to focus on nutritional rehabilitation, weight restoration, cessation of weight reduction behaviors, improvement in eating behaviors, and improvement in psychological and emotional state. Weight restoration alone does not indicate recovery, and forcing weight gain without psychological support and counseling is contraindicated. Typically, the patient is terrified of weight gain and may be struggling with hunger and urges to binge, but the foods he/she allows himself/herself are too limited to enable sufficient energy intake. Individualized guidance and a meal plan that provides a framework for meals and snacks and food choices (but not a rigid diet) is helpful for most patients. The team should work together to determine the individual caloric needs and, with input from the patient, develop a nutrition plan that allows the patient to meet them. In the early treatment of AN, this may be done by incrementally increasing the caloric prescription to reach the desired energy intake. Nutrition counseling should be targeted at helping the patient understand nutritional needs, make wise food choices by increasing variety in the diet, and practice appropriate food behaviors. One effective counseling technique is cognitive behavioral therapy, which involves challenging erroneous beliefs and thought patterns with more accurate perceptions and interpretations regarding dieting, nutrition, and the relationships between starvation and physical symptoms.

Physical activity recommendations should be based on medical status, psychological status, and nutritional intake. Physical activity may need to be limited or initially eliminated with the compulsive exerciser with AN so that weight restoration can be achieved. Counseling should deliver the message that exercise is an activity undertaken for enjoyment and fitness rather than a way to expend energy and promote weight loss. Supervised low-weight strength training is less likely to impede weight gain than are other forms of activity, and it may be psychologically helpful for patients.

During early refeeding, the patient should be monitored closely for signs of refeeding syndrome. Refeeding syndrome (see Chapter 11) is characterized by sudden and sometimes severe hypophosphatemia, glucose intolerance, hypokalemia, hypomagnesemia, gastrointestinal dysfunction, and cardiac arrhythmias. Water retention during refeeding should be anticipated and discussed with the patient. Guidance with food choices to promote normal bowel function should be provided as well. A weight gain goal of 1 to 2 pounds per week for outpatients and 2 to 3 pounds per week for inpatients is recommended.

Inpatient therapy. Although many patients respond to outpatient therapy, some do not. Underweight is only one index of malnutrition, and body weight should not be used as the only criterion for hospital admission. Most patients with AN are knowledgeable enough to falsify weights through such strategies as excessive intake of water or other fluids, potentially leading to acute hyponatremia or dangerous degrees of unrecognized weight loss. All criteria for inpatient admission (Box 27–2) should be considered together.

The goals of inpatient therapy are the same as for outpatient management, but the intensity increases. If the patient is hospitalized for medical instability, medical and nutritional stabilization, frequently on a medical unit, is the initial goal of treatment. This is often necessary before psychological therapy can be optimally effective.

BOX 27-2   Severe Malnutrition*

Dehydration
Electrolyte disturbances
Physiologic instability
    Severe bradycardia (<45/min)
    Hypotension
    Hypothermia (<36° C)
    Orthostatic pulse and blood pressure changes
Cardiac dysrhythmia (including prolonged QT)
Acute medical complication (e.g., syncope, seizures,
    cardiac failure, pancreatitis, etc.)
Arrested growth and development
Failure of outpatient treatment
Acute food refusal
Uncontrollable bingeing and purging
Acute psychiatric emergencies (e.g., suicidal ideation,
    acute psychoses)
Comorbid diagnosis that interferes with the treatment of the
    eating disorder (e.g., severe depression, obsessive compulsive
    disorder, severe family dysfunction)

---

*Weight <75% expected weight/height.

The nutrition plan should help the patient as quickly as possible to consume a diet that is adequate in energy intake and nutritionally well balanced. As with outpatient therapy, medical nutrition therapy should focus on helping the patient to understand nutritional needs and begin to make wise food choices by increasing variety in diet and by practicing appropriate food behaviors. In very rare instances, enteral or parenteral feeding is necessary. However, risks associated with aggressive nutrition support in these patients are substantial, including hypophosphatemia, edema, cardiac failure, seizures, aspiration of enteral formula, and death (see Chapter 11). Reliance on foods rather than on enteral or parenteral nutrition as the primary method of weight restoration contributes significantly to successful long-term recovery. The overall goal is to help the patient normalize eating patterns and learn that behavior must involve planning and practicing with real food.

Bulimia Nervosa

BN occurs in approximately 2% to 5% of the population, and covers a wide diversity of socioeconomic status. Most patients with BN are of normal weight or moderately overweight, and are therefore usually undetectable by appearance alone. The age of onset is most often between mid-adolescence and the late 20s. Individuals at risk for BN are often prone to depression that may be exacerbated by a chaotic or conflicting family as well as the stress of social expectations. This group tends to have higher body weights.

The diagnostic criteria for this disorder focus on the binge/purge behavior; however, many persons with BN restrict their dietary intake. The dietary restriction can be the physiologic or psychological trigger to subsequent binge eating. Also, the trauma of "breaking the rules" by eating something other than or more than what was intended may lead to self-destructive binge/purge eating behavior. Any sensation of stomach fullness may trigger purging. Common purging methods consist of self-induced vomiting (with or without the use of syrup of ipecac), laxative use, diuretic use, and excessive exercise.

Physical Features

Muscle weakness, fatigue, cardiac arrhythmias, dehydration, and electrolyte imbalances can be caused by purging, especially by self-induced vomiting and laxative abuse. Hypokalemia and hypochloremic alkalosis are common. Additionally, esophagitis and less commonly esophageal or gastric rupture can occur. Some patients may have calluses on one or both hands around the knuckles, from contact with the teeth during self-induced vomiting. Dental erosion from self-induced vomiting can be quite serious. Although laxatives are used with the intent to purge calories, they are quite ineffective at doing so. Chronic ipecac use can cause skeletal myopathy, electrocardiographic changes and cardiomyopathy with consequent congestive heart failure, arrhythmia, and sudden death.

Medical and Nutritional Management of Bulimia Nervosa

As with AN, interdisciplinary team management is essential. Most patients with BN are treated as outpatients. Indications for inpatient hospitalization include severe disabling symptoms that are unresponsive to outpatient treatment or additional medical problems such as uncontrolled vomiting, severe laxative abuse withdrawal, metabolic abnormalities or vital sign changes, or suicidal ideations.

The main goal of nutrition therapy is to help the patient develop normal eating habits. Any weight loss that is achieved should result from prudent eating patterns and the elimination of bingeing. Helping patients combat food myths often requires specialized nutrition knowledge. Bulimic patients with normal or excess body weight often present with a history of attempts to control weight through severe caloric restriction. Foods become categorized as "good" or "bad" or "safe" or "forbidden." Food intake patterns are usually quite rigid, and the patient often believes that this seemingly controlled intake is healthy and is the only way to lose or maintain weight. These unrealistic dietary restrictions need to be met with clear guidelines that promote satiety, thereby reducing the risk of bingeing. Meal planning consists of three meals a day with one to three snacks per day prescribed in a structured fashion to help break the chaotic eating pattern that continues the cycle of bingeing and purging. Caloric intake should initially be based on weight maintenance to help prevent hunger, because hunger substantially increases the susceptibility to bingeing. One of the principal challenges in normalizing eating patterns is to expand the diet to include the patient's self-imposed "forbidden" or "feared" foods. Cognitive behavioral therapy provides a framework for exposing patients to these foods, moving from the least feared to the most feared in a safe, structured, supportive environment. This step is critical in breaking the all-or-none behavior that goes along with the deprive-binge cycle.

Fluid retention commonly follows the cessation of purging. The patient must be taught that continual purging or other methods of dehydration such as restricting sodium or using diuretics or laxatives may prolong the fluid retention. If the patient is laxative dependent, a protocol for laxative withdrawal should be implemented to prevent bowel obstruction. The patient should be instructed on a high-fiber diet with adequate fluids while laxatives are gradually withdrawn.

Eating Disorders Not Otherwise Specified

EDNOS accounts for about 50% of eating disorders. Although patients with EDNOS do not meet the diagnostic criteria for either AN or BN, if the disordered behaviors continue, they may progress to frank BN or AN. The nature and intensity of the medical and nutritional problems and the most effective treatment modality depend on the severity of impairment and the symptoms. For example, some patients may have met all criteria for AN with the exception of missing three consecutive menstrual periods, or they may be of normal weight and purge without bingeing. Although patients may not present with medical complications, they often present with medical concerns.

EDNOS also includes binge eating disorder (BED), which entails bingeing behavior without the compensatory purging seen in BN. Although many patients with obesity exhibit hyperphagia, frank BED is estimated to affect only 1% to 2% of the population. Binge episodes must occur at least twice a week and have occurred for at least 6 months. Most patients diagnosed with BED are overweight and suffer the same medical problems faced by the nonbingeing obese population such as diabetes, high blood pressure, high blood cholesterol levels, gallbladder disease, heart disease, and certain types of cancer. The patient with binge eating disorder often presents with weight management concerns rather than eating disorder concerns. Although researchers are still trying to find the treatment that is most helpful in controlling BED, many treatment recommendations utilize the cognitive behavioral therapy model shown effective for BN.

The Adolescent Patient

Eating disorders rank as the third most common chronic illness in adolescent females, with an incidence of up to 5%. The prevalence has increased dramatically over the past 3 decades. Large numbers of adolescents who have eating disorders do not meet the strict DSM-IV criteria for either AN or BN but can be classified as EDNOS. In one study, more than half of the adolescents evaluated for eating disorders had subclinical disease but suffered a similar degree of psychological distress as those who met strict diagnostic criteria. Diagnostic criteria for eating disorders, such as those in DSM-IV, may not be entirely applicable to adolescents. The wide variability in the rate, timing, and magnitude of both height and weight gain during normal puberty and the absence of menstrual periods in early puberty along with the unpredictability of menses soon after menarche limit the application of diagnostic criteria to adolescents.

Because of the potentially irreversible effects of eating disorders on physical and emotional growth and development in adolescents, intervention in adolescents should occur earlier (before all diagnostic criteria are met) and with greater intensity than may be appropriate in adults. Medical complications in adolescents that are potentially irreversible include growth retardation if the disorder occurs before closure of the epiphyses, pubertal delay or arrest, and impaired acquisition of peak bone mass during the second decade of life, increasing the risk of osteoporosis in adulthood.

SUGGESTED READINGS

Committee on Adolescence, American Academy of Pediatrics: Identifying and treating eating disorders. Policy statement. Pediatrics 111:204–210, 2003.

Rome ES, Ammerman S: Medical complications of eating disorders: An update. J Adolesc Health 33:418–426, 2003.

WEB SITES

National Eating Disorders Association, http://www.edap.org

National Association of Anorexia Nervosa and Associated Disorders, http://www.anad.org

28

Metabolic Bone Disease

SARAH L. MORGAN, MD • BETH KITCHIN, MS, RD

Osteoporosis

Definition and Classification

Osteoporosis is a skeletal disorder characterized by compromised bone strength predisposing a person to an increased risk of fracture.[1] Bone strength primarily reflects the integration of bone density and bone quality. When measured by dual energy x-ray absorptiometry (DEXA), bone mineral densities 2.5 or more standard deviations below that of a "young normal" standard indicate osteoporosis. Bone densities between 1.0 and 2.5 standard deviations below this standard are termed *osteopenia*. Osteoporosis is a silent disease with no outward symptoms with fractures occur. It is the most common cause of fractures in the United States, resulting in an estimated 1.5 million fractures a year.[2] The aging of the population is expected to result in an increased incidence of osteoporosis, with an estimated 1 in 2 Americans having or at risk of developing the disease by the year 2020. Caring for osteoporotic fractures is expensive; the estimated annual direct cost is $12 billion to $18 billion and is likely to increase over time.[2]

Osteoporosis can be classified as primary (no clear cause) or secondary (related to a specific cause, such as hypogonadism, hyperparathyroidism, vitamin D deficiency, or corticosteroid use), and has both high- and low-turnover forms, reflecting the activity of osteoblasts and osteoclasts. Typical fracture sites include the hip, vertebrae, humerus, forearm, tibia, and pelvis.

Pathophysiology

Osteoporosis is the end result of defects in the bone remodeling cycle. Bone remodeling is a dynamic process during which older bone is resorbed by osteoclasts, osteoblasts are recruited, and osteoid bone matrix is deposited and ultimately calcified. When bone resorption outpaces formation, bone mineral density declines. Osteoporosis involves either a high or low bone turnover state. In high-turnover disease, there is accelerated bone resorption. In low-turnover disease resorption exceeds formation, without a net increase in bone turnover. Both bone quality and bone strength are important factors for fracture risk. At present they are not directly measured, but they are positively correlated with bone density, which is measured with DEXA.

Risk Factors for Low Bone Mass and Fracture

A number of factors related to lifestyle, genetics, hormones, and medical conditions and therapies affect the risk for osteoporotic fractures (Table 28–1).

Age

Bone mass increases until about age 30, with the majority being achieved during late adolescence and young adulthood. After a period of stabilization, age-related bone loss begins in both females and males. Bone loss is associated with aging, partly due to a decline in intestinal calcium absorption. However, osteoporosis is not a certain consequence of aging.

Gender

Females are more affected than males because bone loss accelerates when estrogen levels decline at menopause. Postmenopausal women may experience bone loss at a rate of 3% to 5% each year during the 5 years after the onset of menopause.

Table 28–1	**RISK FACTORS FOR OSTEOPOROTIC FRACTURES**

Nutrition and Lifestyle
Low lifetime dietary calcium and/or vitamin D intake
Excessive caffeine, alcohol, or salt intake
Lack of weight-bearing exercise
Smoking

Genetics
Female gender
Lactose intolerance
Small, lean body habitus
Family history of osteoporosis
White or Asian ethnicity

Hormones and Life Cycles
Advanced age
Early menopause (surgical or natural)
Postmenopausal estrogen deficiency
Prolonged amenorrhea
Late menarche
Hypogonadism (low testosterone levels in males)

Medical Comorbidities
Gastric or intestinal resection, malabsorption, long-term parenteral
    nutrition
Eating disorders
Renal failure, dialysis
Cardiopulmonary or renal transplantation
Cushing's syndrome
Diabetes mellitus
Prolactinoma
Hyperparathyroidism
Hyperthyroidism
Rheumatoid arthritis
Frailty
Personal history of insufficiency fracture
Impaired eyesight
Very low bone mineral density

Medications
Corticosteroids, cyclosporine A
Anticonvulsants
Excessive thyroid replacement therapy
Gonadotropin-releasing hormone agonists
Heparin
Methotrexate

Peak Bone Mass

Peak bone mass, which occurs in the third decade of life, is one of the most important modifiers of risk for osteoporosis. If greater absolute bone mass is attained, bone reserve is greater, and more can be lost during the aging process or as a result of other factors before symptoms of osteoporosis (i.e., fractures) occur. Therefore, a person with low peak bone mass at age 30 is at greater risk for osteoporotic fractures.

Heredity

The quantity and quality of bone mass attained by maturity are associated with numerous inherited factors. Reduced bone mass is associated with being female, white or Asian, lean, or having long-term lactose intolerance or a family history of osteoporosis. Conversely, being male, black, or obese is correlated with higher bone mass.

Nutrition

Bone mass is related to calcium intake throughout life, but especially during the first 30 years, when peak bone mass is developing. Recommended calcium intakes are outlined according to age and gender in the Dietary Reference Intakes (see Table 3–2). Unfortunately, calcium intake in many age groups of both males and females in the United States is substantially below these levels; among adult females it averages approximately 700 mg per day.

Excessive protein intake (as might occur with high-protein fad diets) stimulates calcium excretion in the urine and places a burden on calcium balance. However, studies have shown that calcium supplementation resulted in the greatest bone density in subjects with the highest protein intake. Because the elderly, who are most at risk for osteoporosis, often have low protein intakes, reducing dietary protein is not advisable as a general guideline.

Excessive sodium intake, which is common among Americans, can lead to negative calcium balance by increasing urinary calcium excretion. Data also suggest that *excessive* caffeine intake can have an adverse effect on calcium balance.

Recent studies have suggested that excessive vitamin A intake (as little as twice the RDA) can increase fracture risk. This increased risk has not been found with beta-carotene, a precursor of vitamin A, which is widely available in fruits and vegetables. Patients should be advised to avoid daily vitamin A supplementation that exceeds the RDA.

Vitamin K plays important roles in bone metabolism and in the biochemistry of the bone matrix. Preliminary data suggest that poor vitamin K status may increase fracture risk. However, further study is required before vitamin K supplementation can be recommended.

Other Lifestyle Habits

Excessive alcohol intake and tobacco have adverse effects on bone mass, as does a sedentary lifestyle. Exercise throughout life, especially weight-bearing exercise, helps to maintain the health of the skeleton. However, exercising so heavily that amenorrhea results is detrimental to skeletal health. For persons who already have osteoporosis, avoiding falls has a significant influence on fracture risk.

Hormonal Factors

Normal sex hormone status is one of the most important factors in maintaining bone mineral density. Hypogonadism in males can cause osteoporosis. The decline in estrogen at menopause greatly accelerates the rate of bone loss in the early postmenopausal period. Estrogen loss at younger ages due to early menopause, anorexia nervosa, or excessive physical exercise can contribute to bone loss in younger women.

Medical Conditions and Medications

Many medical and/or surgical conditions and drug therapies have adverse effects on bone mineral density and can increase fracture risk (see Table 28–1). These include resection or restriction of the stomach (including bariatric surgery), malabsorption, renal failure, hyperparathyroidism, hyperthyroidism, long-term use of corticosteroids or anticonvulsants, and excessive thyroid hormone replacement.

Diagnosis

The diagnosis of osteoporosis is made by combining historical data, clinical examinations, laboratory tests, plain radiographs, and specialized radiographic procedures.

History and Physical Examination

When completing a patient's history, information should be obtained about genetic and lifestyle risk factors, medical conditions, and medications that can affect bone mineral density. Height should be measured with a stadiometer, placed in the patient's record, and compared to the patient's height at age 18 or the height on the driver's license. Because clinical manifestations of osteoporosis can be silent, posture, skeletal deformities, and gait are important factors to note. Characteristic changes in posture result from vertebral fractures, including loss of height, a humped back (the dowager's hump), loss of waistline contour, and a protuberant abdomen. Vertebral fractures may be painful just after they occur, but subsequent pain is generally from paraspinous muscle tenderness.

Laboratory Tests

In patients with normal renal and liver function, serum 25-hydroxyvitamin D is the preferred measure of vitamin D status. However, serum 25-hydroxyvitamin D ranges reported as normal by many clinical laboratories may be too wide to detect vitamin D deficiency sensitively. Recent research shows that secondary hyperparathyroidism may occur with vitamin D levels in these lower "normal" ranges. Therefore, it is prudent to keep 25-hydroxyvitamin D levels above 32 to 35 ng/mL (80 nmol/L).

Laboratory tests are indicated to rule out secondary causes of osteoporosis such as thyrotoxicosis, metastatic bone cancer, and hyperparathyroidism, as well as to quantify the rate of bone turnover. A reasonable battery of laboratory tests includes a complete blood count with differential count, erythrocyte sedimentation rate, chemistry panel, and serum and urine protein electrophoresis if malignancy is suspected. Free thyroxine and thyroid-stimulating hormone levels can rule out thyrotoxicosis or excessive thyroid replacement. Luteinizing hormone, follicle-stimulating hormone, estradiol, and testosterone levels can help detect hypogonadism. Parathyroid hormone levels are measured to diagnose hyperparathyroidism. A variety of specialized markers for bone formation is available. Serum osteocalcin and bone specific alkaline phosphatase serve as markers of bone formation. Pyridinoline, deoxypyridinoline, and the N-telopeptide of type I collagen (NTX) can serve as markers of bone resorption. Measurement of 24-hour urinary calcium and creatinine excretion helps detect impaired calcium absorption and hypercalciuria.

Radiographic Procedures

Plain radiographs are useful in evaluating underlying disorders such as rheumatoid arthritis, the morphology of bones, and the presence of fractures. Because standard radiographs can only detect losses of bone density greater than 30%, they are relatively insensitive indicators of bone mass. A lateral radiograph of the spine is useful to check for vertebral compression fractures.

Bone density is measured by a variety of methods, such as single-energy x-ray absorptiometry (SEXA), DEXA, quantitative computed tomography (QCT), and radiographic absorptiometry (RA). DEXA is currently the most common method. It generates a T-score that relates the bone density to that of a "young normal," and a Z-score that compares it to that of an "age-matched" control. Current approved indications for DEXA include low-impact fractures, parathyroid disease, chronic corti-costeroid therapy, incidental osteopenia noted on plain films, hypogonadism, and to assess the effect of a U.S. Food and Drug Administration approved therapy.

Bone Histomorphometry and Biopsy

Bone biopsy is another useful test for establishing the diagnosis of metabolic bone disease in challenging cases. If the patient takes tetracyclines before the biopsy, the rate of bone formation can be assessed.

Treatment Guidelines

In addition to addressing all modifiable risk factors, treatment of established osteoporosis includes prevention of falls and often includes drug therapy.

Lifestyle

Smoking, excessive alcohol intake, and inactivity should be addressed. Weight-bearing exercise and modified weight training are especially useful in increasing and/or maintaining bone mass. Premenopausal women who have amenorrhea should be evaluated and treated appropriately. Women with eating disorders should be referred to an eating disorders specialist.

Diet

A rational approach to achieving adequate calcium intake is to maximize dietary sources and, if necessary, take supplements. Because bone health is influenced by other nutrients as well as calcium, a good diet is the cornerstone of both prevention and therapy. Dairy products, canned salmon with bones, collard and turnip greens, broccoli, and cooked dried beans (e.g., kidney, lima, and navy) all contribute calcium to the diet. While spinach is a source of calcium, high levels of oxalic acid prevent much of the calcium's absorption. If dairy products are used, low-fat ones are preferred to minimize the intake of saturated fat and cholesterol. Lactose-reduced (e.g., cultured or lactase-treated) products can be used by individuals who have lactose intolerance. Calcium-fortified products such as calcium-fortified orange juice and cereals can also add calcium to the diet.

Nutritional Supplements

The amounts of calcium contained in commonly used supplements are listed in Table 28–2. The most commonly used one, calcium carbonate, is available in numerous commercial preparations that contain a variety of doses. Preparations that contain bone meal or dolomite can be contaminated with heavy metals and should not be used. To optimize absorption, it is recommended that no more than 500 to 600 mg of elemental calcium be consumed at one time. Because calcium carbonate requires hydrochloric acid for absorption, these supplements should be consumed with food. Calcium citrate supplements do not require hydrochloric acid for absorption, so they can be taken with or without food. Because of this, it may be prudent to advise patients who take histamine-2 receptor blocker or proton pump inhibitor drugs to use calcium citrate supplements.

Adequate vitamin D status is essential for calcium absorption. *The Dietary Reference Intakes* for vitamin D are based on Adequate Intake because data are not conclusive enough to set RDAs. Recent research suggests that intake levels of 800 to 1000 IU (20 to 25 µg) may

Table 28–2	ELEMENTAL CALCIUM CONTENT OF COMMONLY PRESCRIBED SUPPLEMENTS	
Preparation	**Percent Elemental Calcium**	**Amount (mg) Providing 500 mg Elemental Calcium**
Calcium carbonate (various)	40	1250
Calcium phosphate tribasic (Posture)	39	1280
Calcium acetate (Phos-Ex, PhosLo)	25	2000
Calcium citrate (Citracal)	21	2380
Calcium lactate (various)	13	3850
Calcium gluconate (various)	9	5550
Calcium glubionate (Neo-Calglucon)	6.5	7700

be necessary to maintain adequate levels in patients with osteoporosis. Patients can easily achieve this level of intake through a combination of a daily multivitamin (most contain 400 IU), vitamin D–containing calcium supplements, and vitamin D–fortified milk and juices. Unfortified foods are insufficient for achieving these levels of intake.

Drug Therapy

Several drug therapies are now available for treating established osteoporosis. Many of them reduce the rate of bone resorption. Calcitonin can be injected subcutaneously or inhaled nasally. Because of its analgesic effect, calcitonin is especially useful in treating recent compression fractures. Another class of drugs, bisphosphonates, becomes integrated into the hydroxyapatite crystal and downregulates osteoclast activity. Thiazide diuretics can be prescribed to treat hypercalciuria. Many promising new medications are being investigated, including anabolic agents such as injectable parathyroid hormone.

Osteomalacia

Definition

Osteomalacia and rickets are disorders of mineralization of bone osteoid. Rickets occurs in growing bones and involves the epiphyses as well as trabecular and cortical bone. Osteomalacia occurs after growth has ceased.

Pathophysiology

The major causes of rickets and osteomalacia are deficiencies of vitamin D, calcium, and phosphorus. Recent research suggests that vitamin D deficiency is more prevalent in the United States than previously thought. It occurs when (1) there is insufficient sun exposure to produce calciferol in the skin, (2) dietary vitamin D intake is inadequate, or (3) patients are provided total parenteral nutrition (TPN) that is not supplemented with vitamin D.

Vitamin D deficiency causes inadequate calcium and phosphorus absorption from the intestine, which causes secondary hypocalcemia. Hypocalcemia increases the secretion of parathyroid hormone, which in turn increases bone resorption by osteoclasts to normalize serum calcium and phosphorus concentrations. Increased parathyroid hormone levels also increase renal calcium reabsorption and phosphorus excretion.

Diagnosis

When obtaining the patient's history, focus on the intake of vitamin D, the amount of sun exposure, phosphorus and calcium in the diet, and circumstances in which these nutrients could become deficient. Clinical findings commonly seen in patients with rickets include muscle weakness, bowing deformities of the long bones, and prominence of the costochondral junction (rachitic rosary). Patients may also have kyphosis, lordosis, pelvic deformities, and a waddling gait. The most common complaint in patients with osteomalacia is diffuse bony pain.

Biochemical findings in osteomalacia tend to be highly variable. Serum calcium and phosphorus levels may be normal or low. Alkaline phosphatase levels are frequently elevated. A low serum 25-hydroxyvitamin D level is diagnostic of vitamin D deficiency. As noted previously for patients with osteoporosis, it is recommended that 32 to 35 ng/mL (80 nmol/L) be considered the lower limit of normal serum 25-hydroxyvitamin vitamin D.

Radiographs show thinning of the cortex and disappearance of cartilaginous calcification. Stress fractures perpendicular to the bone shaft may be seen. DEXA shows diminished bone mass.

Treatment

Treatment is aimed at correction of the underlying cause. Calcium, phosphorus, and vitamin D should be supplemented as needed. Useful vitamin D preparations include ergocalciferol (vitamin D_2), cholecalciferol (vitamin D_3), and calcitriol (1,25-dihydroxycholecalciferol). Doses of vitamin D must be tailored to the cause of the deficiency. For example, a patient with renal disease who cannot hydroxylate 25-hydroxyvitamin D requires therapy with the 1,25-dihydroxy form (see Chapter 25). Patients with malabsorption require a higher dose of vitamin D than those with intact gastrointestinal tracts. A commonly used treatment regimen for uncomplicated vitamin D deficiency is ergocalciferol (50,000 IU) once a week for 2 to 3 months. Vitamin D, calcium, and phosphorus levels must be monitored to ensure they are in the normal range.

REFERENCES

1. NIH Consensus Development Program, Statement 111: Osteoporosis Prevention, Diagnosis, and Therapy. NIH Consensus Statement Online March 27–29, 2000; 17:1–36; available at http://consensus.nih.gov/cons/111/111_statement.htm.
2. U.S. DHHS: Bone Health and Osteoporosis: A Report of the Surgeon General, 2004; available at http://www.surgeongeneral.gov/library/bonehealth/.

SUGGESTED READINGS

American Society for Bone and Mineral Research: Primer on the Metabolic Bone Diseases and Disorders of Mineral Metabolism, 5th ed. New York, Raven Press, 2003.
Holick MF, Dawson-Hughes B (eds): Nutrition and Bone Health. Totowa, NJ, Humana Press, 2004.
Saag K, Morgan S, Cao X: Osteopenic bone diseases. In Koopman WJ (ed): Arthritis and Allied Conditions, 15th ed. Baltimore, Lippincott Williams & Wilkins, 2004, pp 2473–2541.

WEB SITES

UAB Osteoporosis Prevention and Treatment Clinic Tone Your Bones site, http://www.ToneYourBones.com
National Osteoporosis Foundation, http://www.nof.org/

29

Human Immunodeficiency Virus Infection

DONALD P. KOTLER, MD • GABRIEL IONESCU, MD

Nutritional alterations are common in individuals with human immunodeficiency virus (HIV) and have adverse effects on morbidity and mortality. In the absence of highly active antiretroviral therapy (HAART), protein energy malnutrition is the main outcome, and is related to a combination of comorbid conditions, HIV infection, and the complications of immune deficiency. Severe malnutrition is typically limited to patients with acquired immunodeficiency syndrome (AIDS), which represents the final stage of a prolonged illness. Both micronutrient and macronutrient deficits have been demonstrated. In contrast, successfully treated patients are more likely to demonstrate nutritional and metabolic alterations similar to those in patients with metabolic syndrome, a condition termed HIV-associated lipodystrophy. Nutritional management in the former circumstance involves prevention of macronutrient and micronutrient deficiencies as well as reversing the adverse nutritional effects of disease complications. With lipodystrophy, the goals are similar to those of preventive cardiology. Both topics have generated clinical and research interest, and the published results suggest that proper nutritional management has beneficial effects in HIV-infected patients.

Effects of Protein Energy Malnutrition on Immune Function

Severe protein-energy malnutrition (PEM) is frequently associated with immune deficiency, both humoral and cell-mediated, which reverses after effective nutritional repletion. Impaired cutaneous responses to antigens that evoke delayed-hypersensitivity responses (anergy) are frequently seen. In addition, absolute numbers of circulating lymphocytes expressing the CD4 molecule, as well as the ratio of CD4 to CD8 cells, are depressed in malnourished subjects, as are the number of antibody-producing cells and the amounts of secreted, though not circulating, immunoglobulins. Children with kwashiorkor and marasmus in developing countries may suffer the same types of infections as those that plague patients with AIDS in the United States. The similar effects of PEM and AIDS on immunity suggest that the development of wasting in patients with AIDS could exacerbate the already diminished T cell–mediated immune response.

Nutritional Issues in HIV Patients

Micronutrient Deficiencies

During HIV infection, nutrient requirements are increased to sustain immune cell turnover. It has been hypothesized that vitamin and micronutrient deficits impair cell function and energy balance, contributing to poor immune status in HIV-infected subjects.

In particular, deficiencies of vitamin A, zinc, and iron adversely affect immune function through different mechanisms, and their correction can restore immune function, though they do not compensate for T lymphocyte depletion, such as occurs in HIV infection. Iron is a key component of cytochromes that mediate cellular energy metabolism, as well as of important enzymes, potentially influencing immune cell turnover. Zinc is important in the activity of many enzymes, DNA-binding proteins, and the thymic hormone, thymulin, and its deficiency impairs lymphocyte function. The active metabolite of vitamin A, retinoic acid, affects the production of immunologically significant cytokines such as gamma-interferon and interleukin-4, and influences the ability of cells to respond to these cytokines. There are reports of low serum vitamin A in up to 11 % of HIV-infected homosexual men, and in up to 60 % of pregnant women in developing countries. Vitamin A deficiency specifically impairs the ability of CD4 cells to respond to antigenic stimulation, particularly to bacterial antigens. In addition, low levels of 1,25-dihydroxyvitamin D and vitamin E have been reported in various HIV-infected populations. Deficiencies in B-vitamins can also compromise immune function by virtue of their roles as cofactors in many enzymes, including those involved in nucleic acid synthesis. Vitamin B_{12} deficiency was very prevalent in the pre-HAART era and was related to absent intrinsic factor secretion and to abnormal ileal B_{12} absorption. Serum levels of other water-soluble vitamins also have been reported to be low, despite apparent normal intake, whereas fat-soluble vitamin deficiencies occur in subjects with diarrhea and malabsorption.

An effective response to HIV and other pathogens is dependent on intact energy-generating mechanisms and on adequate protection from ongoing oxidative stress. Depletion of antioxidant nutrients (e.g., vitamins E and C, and selenium) and of various regulatory molecules, such as reduced glutathione and nitric oxide, impairs immune responsiveness and allows greater oxidative damage to immune and other cell types. Selenium deficiency has been associated epidemiologically with increased mortality risk, while autopsy studies have shown low myocardial concentrations of selenium in HIV-infected subjects. Low levels of reduced glutathione in CD4 lymphocytes were documented in HIV-infected subjects with CD4 counts below 200, compared to HIV-infected subjects with CD4 counts above 200 and HIV-uninfected controls, reflecting increased antioxidant requirements. In a randomized trial of supplementation with the pro-drug N-acetyl cysteine, normal levels of reduced glutathione were restored.[1] In addition, it was noted that survival rates were higher in HIV-infected subjects with higher baseline levels of reduced glutathione in CD4 lymphocytes. These results indicate a possible influence of oxidative stress on the progression of HIV infection.

Macronutrient Deficiencies

Few nutritional studies have been reported in asymptomatic patients at an early stage of disease, but mild weight loss may be noted. More evidence of metabolic and nutritional alterations has been gathered in the intermediate and late stages of HIV disease, particularly during and after opportunistic infections. Early studies documented disproportionate depletion of body cell mass in AIDS patients with clinical complications. Body cell mass depletion was associated with variable amounts of fat depletion, and with expansion of the extracellular space. Patients with malabsorptive illnesses demonstrated depletion of total body water. Weight loss and body cell mass depletion in HIV infection are associated with shortened survival and diminished quality of life.

Biochemical Indicators of Nutritional Status

Biochemical measures have received little study in HIV wasting. An acute phase response to infection during early and intermediate stage HIV infection may be inferred from reports of elevations in some indices, such as copper, and decreases in others, such as zinc. Subnormal serum Vitamin A, albumin, and prealbumin concentrations have been reported repeatedly. However, in the absence of opportunistic infections, body weight and albumin levels are generally normal. An acute phase response may be observed in AIDS patients with opportunistic infections or tumors, as would be expected in HIV-negative patients.

Energy Expenditure and Nutrient Intake

In early stages of HIV infection, body weight, including fat-free mass, is maintained. However, there is increased fat oxidation and a mild increase in resting energy expenditure (REE), compared to healthy controls. In the absence of clinically evident infection, increased interleukin-6, as part of the acute phase response, and a predominance of sympathetic tone have been hypothesized as causes of elevated REE. In the intermediate stage, active HIV replication and the resultant acute phase response are associated with decreased protein synthesis, mild-to-moderate depletion of body cell mass, and mild elevations in resting energy expenditure, without a compensatory increase in caloric intake. However, wasting is uncommon until serious disease complications develop.

Pathogenesis of Protein-Energy Malnutrition

Nutritional deficiencies may be severe and progressive in the late stage of HIV infection (AIDS) and are multifactorial in etiology, evolving from alterations in food intake, nutrient absorption, or intermediary metabolism, or combinations of these.

Decreased Nutrient Intake

Food intake remains relatively normal throughout most of the course of HIV infection. However, in symptomatic late stages, appetite and food intake may be suppressed by the cytokine response to opportunistic infections or in response to intestinal dysfunction. Decreased food intake is the strongest predictor of short-term weight loss in AIDS patients with opportunistic infections. Oropharyngeal or esophageal pathology, medications, and psychosocial and economic factors may act alone or in combination to reduce food intake.

Malabsorption

Patients with malabsorptive disorders were most prevalent in the pre-HAART era. Chronic malabsorption was limited to patients with severe immune depletion and opportunistic infections, and ranged from occult to clinically severe. The hallmark pathologic change is jejunal villous atrophy and crypt hyperplasia, which has been correlated in some studies with malabsorption parameters. In one study, the degree of D-glucose absorption was correlated with serum albumin, body mass index (BMI), and CD4 counts, and was at its lowest in pathogen-positive diarrhea.[2] In the pre-HAART era, water-borne infections such as cryptosporidiosis, microsporidiosis, and isosporiasis were among the most common intestinal organisms found in malnourished AIDS patients with diarrhea, and caused small intestinal injury with primary damage to the villous epithelial cell. Mycobacterium avium-intracellulare complex organisms promote malabsorption by an alternative mechanism: Infected macrophages infiltrate lamina propria, submucosa and intestinal lymphatics leading to an exudative enteropathy characterized by marked fat malabsorption. Enteroadherent bacteria have been associated with diarrhea and ileal dysfunction, but in 15% to 25% of evaluations for malabsorption, no pathogenic organisms are found. It has been suggested that some of the small intestinal alterations may be mediated by infected CD4 lymphocytes, the so-called *HIV enteropathy*. Inflammatory conditions such as cytomegalovirus colitis may lead to chronic diarrhea with weight loss, but they do not cause malabsorption.

Nutrient Losses and Increased Requirements

Nutrient losses and electrolyte and acid-base disturbances are common when HIV nephropathy is present, but this is limited to a small proportion of HIV-infected individuals. Proteinuria is common in these patients, leading to excess losses of albumin and retinol-binding protein. Requirements for energy and some micronutrients, such as vitamins B and C, increase during HIV infection as evidenced by low serum nutrient levels, increased energy expenditure, and oxidative stress. However, there is no evidence that ingestion of megadoses of vitamins is beneficial.

HIV Lipodystrophy

HIV lipodystrophy emerged when HAART was introduced in 1996. It is characterized by body composition changes including loss of subcutaneous fat and accumulation of fat in the intra-abdominal (visceral) and retroperitoneal compartments. In addition, metabolic abnormalities similar to those found in metabolic syndrome, such as dyslipidemia and insulin resistance, are encountered. It is not clear how the various components of the syndrome are linked, and some studies have suggested that the sizes of the subcutaneous and visceral compartments are independent of one another. In contrast, body cell mass and muscle mass are normal or slightly increased.

Epidemiologic studies have found multiple associations with the various components of lipodystrophy, related to the host, the infection, and the treatment. The strongest associations are between the development of lipoatrophy and the use of certain nucleoside reverse transcriptase inhibitors. However, the levels of greatest immune depletion and repletion have also shown independent effects, implying some relationship to immune activity.

Hyperinsulinemia with peripheral and hepatic insulin resistance has been observed and is partially due to a direct effect of certain protease inhibitors on glucose metabolism. However, insulin resistance also occurs in patients who are not treated with these drugs. The results of *in vitro* and *in vivo* studies have suggested that proinflammatory cytokines such as interleukin-6 and tumor necrosis factor-alpha may play pivotal roles in altered glucose and lipid metabolism as well as in lipolysis and peripheral fat loss.

Preventing Malnutrition in HIV Patients

Preventing and Treating Opportunistic Infections

Because opportunistic infections are a common cause of significant weight loss, effective care of the underlying HIV infection and prevention of opportunistic infections is the best way to prevent weight loss. Similarly, the key to minimizing or reversing weight loss related to opportunistic infections is to treat the infections effectively. The development of effective drug regimens to prevent and treat infections has been singularly important in prolonging the lives of AIDS patients. A contributing factor to enhanced survival is also maintenance of lean body mass. As discussed in Chapters 9, 11, and 23, nutritional interventions can reduce the loss of lean body mass during metabolic stress, but no intervention can prevent it altogether.

Nutrition Education and Intervention

Nutrition assessment, education, and appropriate nutrition interventions should be integrated upon diagnosis into the preventive health care planning and medical treatment of patients with HIV infection (see Chapter 10). The evaluation should include assessment of weight and of lean body mass, if possible, as a benchmark against which to monitor subsequent changes in body weight and composition. Active interventions should be implemented through periodic nutrition education and counseling that addresses healthful eating principles and how to achieve them, risks from foodborne pathogens, alternative feeding methods (e.g., making foods more palatable or nutrient-dense, and using oral nutritional supplements), and guidelines for evaluating the nutritional value of foods. Counseling should also address unfounded food fads and nutritional "therapies" that are often attractive to patients with HIV infection.

Nutritional Support

Vigorous nutritional support strategies including enteral and parenteral feeding sometimes become necessary when frank AIDS develops, but they are not necessary in the stable patient. The rationale for providing nutritional support to HIV-infected patients is that malnutrition produces adverse effects in this disease and that improvements in nutritional status benefit the patient clinically. While improved nutritional status reverses the immune dysfunction associated with PEM, there is no evidence that this occurs in HIV-infected individuals. The specific indications for nutritional support in HIV-infected patients include progressive wasting producing objective evidence of morbidity with little likelihood of self-correction, in patients with the potential for prolonged, comfortable life. The most straightforward approach involves treating the underlying disease complication responsible for malnutrition, an approach that was shown to be successful in treating both the underlying HIV infection and opportunistic infections. An important clinical corollary is that nutritional supplementation may be futile in the presence of untreated serious disease complications.

There are two broad approaches to nutritional therapy. The first is intended to promote nutritional repletion chiefly by providing a balanced diet, whereas the second employs supraphysiologic or pharmacologic doses of specific macronutrients or micronutrients in an attempt to affect the underlying disease process. In the former case, nutritional therapies may be food-based or provided as formulas, orally or non-volitionally by enteral or parenteral routes. Food-based strategies of nutritional support are intended to provide 25 to 35 kcal/kg/day body weight through a diet composed of the individual's own food preferences, provided that intake is not hindered by active disease complications. In the latter case, because studies of micronutrient supplementation have been fragmentary and inconclusive, supplements should be used in physiologic doses to correct deficiencies rather than in supraphysiologic or megadoses.

Oral Supplements

Several types of supplements have been studied in HIV infection. An elemental diet containing medium-chain triglycerides (MCT) and hydrolyzed whey protein produced improvements in fat and nitrogen balance, accompanied by weight maintenance and decreased diarrhea.[3] The use of high-protein/high-calorie supplements in AIDS patients is associated with weight gain, provided there are no active opportunistic infections. The use of these supplements is usually associated with a convergent change in body cell mass, leading to the conclusion that weight maintenance in subjects with intact gastrointestinal tract and free of opportunistic infections is related to general caloric intake.

Because of its putative anti-cytokine effects, special consideration has been given to supplementation with omega-3 fatty acids. Their inclusion in enteral formulas that also contain peptides, MCT, beta carotene, vitamins and minerals, and soluble fiber may decrease hospitalization rates in HIV-positive patients, without affecting weight or immune function.

Micronutrient deficiency has been directly linked with mortality in HIV disease. As with macronutrient deficiencies, the association is statistical and it is unclear whether micronutrient deficiencies are a direct cause of poor outcomes or only a correlate. This is especially true of zinc and selenium, as serum concentrations may fall as a result of the acute phase response, implying extravascular sequestration rather than deficiency. However, the results of several studies suggest a causal link. Neuropsychological abnormalities associated with low serum vitamin B_{12} concentrations improved after specific supplementation.[4] High doses of vitamin A were shown to stabilize CD4 cells in an inner-city intravenous drug use population.[5] In African cohorts, multivitamin or B-vitamin supplementation reduced the risk of progression to AIDS and death, while improving immunologic parameters.[6,7]

Oxidative stress, induced by the production of reactive oxygen species, contributes to HIV replication through NF-kB activation. *In vitro* addition of antioxidant vitamins to experimental systems blocks this activation and inhibits HIV replication. Supplementation with vitamins C and E produced a significant decrease in oxidative stress indices and a trend toward reduced HIV viral load.[8] The rationale for providing this therapy in the current era of HAART is uncertain.

Appetite Stimulants

The appetite stimulants megestrol acetate and dronabinol have been show to promote weight gain in anorexic patients. Appetite stimulation is most beneficial in the absence of local pathologic lesions affecting chewing and swallowing, malabsorption syndromes, and active systemic infections. Megestrol acetate suppresses serum testosterone concentration, which could explain its proclivity to promote weight gain via increases in body fat content, while limiting lean mass deposition. Dronabinol (delta-9-tetrahydrocannabinol [THC]) is a principal psychoactive substance present in *Cannabis sativa* (marijuana). Benefits in addition to appetite stimulation include the drug's antiemetic effect and its purported ability to improve mood. Dronabinol's effects on the composition of weight gained, i.e., fat versus lean mass, have yet to be reported. Cyproheptadine also has a mild stimulatory effect on food intake.

Enteral and Parenteral Feeding

When supplements and appetite stimulants fail to control wasting, aggressive nutritional support regimens may be required, in the form of enteral or total parenteral nutrition (TPN) feeding. Their clinical efficacy is largely determined by the underlying clinical problem. In patients with eating disorders or malabsorption syndromes, repletion of body cell mass can be achieved with TPN administration, whereas in patients with systemic infections, progressive depletion of body cell mass usually occurs despite TPN.

The relative efficacies of TPN and oral intake of a semielemental diet (SED) in AIDS patients with severe malabsorption were compared in a randomized open-label trial.[9] The TPN group had a higher mean energy intake and gained more weight and body fat than did the SED group. However, the use of TPN was fourfold more expensive and was associated with greater morbidity due to bacterial sepsis and a worsening of perceived physical functioning compared to SED. No survival differences were seen.

Formula diet administered through a percutaneous endoscopic gastrostomy (PEG) tube in patients with eating disorders and no malabsorption increases body cell mass, body fat content, serum albumin concentration, and serum iron-binding capacity, by restoring both somatic and visceral protein compartments. Of note, repletion may occur despite the persistence of systemic infection. In addition, subjective increases in cognitive function were appreciated in patients receiving nutritional support. These favorable changes may not translate into improvements of immune status. Also, the need for this therapy has fallen substantially after the introduction of HAART.

Adjunctive Therapies

Recombinant growth hormone has been shown in short-term studies (7 days to 3 months) to produce positive nitrogen balance and repletion of fat-free mass.[10] Testosterone and its conjugates also promote increases in lean mass, though adverse effects on serum lipid concentrations have been observed. In a 3-month controlled trial, thalidomide, a cytokine inhibitor, was associated with significant weight gain and increased muscle mass without adverse effects on viral burden or CD4 counts.[11] Progressive resistance exercise has been advocated as a nonpharmacological way to increase lean body mass and muscle strength. Combinations of exercise and anabolic agents have also yielded positive benefits.

Management of Lipodystrophy

Several studies have addressed the management of lipodystrophy. In general, they have concentrated on specific components of the problem such as lipoatrophy or insulin resistance. The general approach can be summarized as avoidance, switching, and treatment. Avoidance refers to strategic choices of antiretrovirals to favor those that lack the offensive side-effect. For example, the use of the reverse transcriptase inhibitors abacavir or tenofovir instead of stavudine was not associated with development of lipoatrophy. The use of atazanavir instead of nelfinavir or lopinavir/ritonavir was not associated with hyperlipidemia. When metabolic or body composition alterations develop, switching to an alternative agent may resolve the problem.

The options for treating existing lipodystrophy are more limited. Hyperlipidemia may be treated with statins or fibrates, though few patients reach targets set by the National Cholesterol Education Program. The results of several studies suggest that omega-3-fatty acid supplementation may lower serum triglyceride concentrations. Insulin-sensitizing agents increase insulin sensitivity, though not to normal values. No therapy has been shown to reliably increase subcutaneous fat, though nonorganic fillers have been approved for cosmetic use by the U.S. Food and Drug Administration. Growth hormone has been shown to reduce visceral fat content while increasing lean mass, and is being studied as a potential therapy for visceral obesity.

Conclusions

Nutritional alterations are common in HIV-infected individuals in the presence or absence of HAART therapy. The type of alteration depends on the presence or absence of HAART therapy. The influence of immune dysfunction on PEM is so strong that HAART therapy is both necessary and generally sufficient as nutritional therapy, at least on an intermediate to long-term basis. Whether or not optimal nutritional care can slow the progression of disease in the absence of antiretroviral therapy is an important global question. The management of HIV-associated lipodystrophy will depend upon the development of less toxic therapies as well as on increased attention to the problem and further developments in metabolic drug therapy.

REFERENCES

1. Akerlund B, Jarstrand C, Lindeke B, et al: Effect of N-acetylcysteine (NAC) treatment on HIV-1 infection: A double-blind placebo-controlled trial. Eur J Clin Pharmacol 50:457–461, 1996.
2. Keating J, Bjarnason I, Somasundaram S, et al: Intestinal absorptive capacity, intestinal permeability and jejunal histology in HIV and their relation to diarrhoea. Gut 37:623–629, 1995.
3. Salomon SB, Jung J, Voss T, et al: An elemental diet containing medium-chain triglycerides and enzymatically hydrolyzed protein can improve gastrointestinal tolerance in people infected with HIV. J Am Diet Assoc 98:460–462, 1998.

4. Herzlich BC, Schiano TD: Reversal of apparent AIDS dementia complex following treatment with vitamin B_{12}. J Intern Med 233: 495–497, 1993.

5. Semba RD, Lyles CM, Margolick JB, et al: Vitamin A supplementation and human immunodeficiency virus load in injection drug users. J Infect Dis 177:611–616, 1998.

6. Fawzi WW, Msamanga GI, Spiegelman D, et al: A randomized trial of multivitamin supplements and HIV disease progression and mortality. N Engl J Med 351:23–32, 2004.

7. Kanter AS, Spencer DC, Steinberg MH, et al: Supplemental vitamin B and progression to AIDS and death in black South African patients infected with HIV. J Acquir Immune Defic Syndr 21:252–253, 1999.

8. Allard JP, Aghdassi E, Chau J, et al: Effects of vitamin E and C supplementation on oxidative stress and viral load in HIV-infected subjects. AIDS 12:1653–1659, 1998.

9. Kotler DP, Fogleman L, Tierney AR: Comparison of total parenteral nutrition and an oral, semielemental diet on body composition, physical function, and nutrition-related costs in patients with malabsorption due to acquired immunodeficiency syndrome. J Parenter Enteral Nutr 22:120–126, 1998.

10. Mulligan K, Tai VW, Schambelan M: Effects of chronic growth hormone treatment on energy intake and resting energy metabolism in patients with human immunodeficiency virus associated wasting—A clinical research center study. J Clin Endocrinol Metab 83:1542–1547, 1998.

11. Kaplan G, Thomas S, Fierer DS, et al: Thalidomide for the treatment of AIDS-associated wasting. AIDS Res Hum Retroviruses 16: 1345–1355, 2000.

SUGGESTED READING

Kotler DP: HIV infection and lipodystrophy. Prog Cardiovasc Dis 45:269–284, 2003.

WEB SITES

Food Aid Management HIV Nutrition Links, http://www.foodaid.org/hiv.htm

PART IV

Appendices

Normal Laboratory Values

	Normal Values*
Hematology	
Hematocrit (Hct)	
Men	39%–49%
Women	34%–44%
Hemoglobin (Hgb)	
Men	14–17 g/dL
Women	12–15 g/dL
Children	12–14 g/dL
Newborn	14.5–24.5 g/dL
Mean cell volume (MCV)	83–99 fl
Mean cell hemoglobin (MCH)	27–32 pg
Mean cell hemoglobin concentration (MCHC)	32%–36%
Platelets	150,000–400,000/mm³
Reticulocytes	0.5%–1.5%
White blood cells (WBCs)	4,000–11,000/mm³
Differential (Diff)	
Lymphocytes	15%–52% (higher in children)
Neutrophils	35%–73% (lower in children)
Monocytes	2%–10%
Eosinophils	0–5%
Basophils	0–2%
Serum iron (Fe)	60–180 µg/dL
Transferrin	212–405 mg/dL
Iron-binding capacity	
Total (TIBC)	250–450 µg/dL
% Saturation	15%–55%
Serum ferritin	
Males 18–30 years	30–233 ng/mL
Males 31–60 years	32–284 ng/mL
Premenopausal females	6–81 ng/mL
Postmenopausal females	14–186 ng/mL
Blood Chemistry	
Alkaline phosphatase (Alk phos)	
1–3 mo	150–475 U/L
To 10 yr	120–320 U/L

Puberty	120–540 U/L
Adults	39–117 U/L
Ammonia (NH_3)	11–35 µmol/L
Bilirubin (Bili)	
Total	0–1 mg/dL
Direct	0.1–0.3 mg/dL
Calcium (Ca^{++})	8.4–10.2 mg/dL
Carbon dioxide content (HCO_3^-)	23–29 mEq/L
Carotene	79–233 µg/dL
Chloride (CI^-)	96–108 mEq/L
Creatinine	0.4–1.2 mg/dL
GGT (gamma glutamyl transpeptidase)	0–65 U/L
GOT (AST, aspartate aminotransferase)	0–31 U/L
GPT (ALT, alanine aminotransferase)	0–31 U/L
Glucose, fasting	70–105 mg/dL
LDH (lactic dehydrogenase)	120–240 U/L
Magnesium (Mg^{++})	1.7–2.2 mg/dL
Osmolality	280–305 mOsm/kg plasma
Phosphorus (Phos)	
Children	4.0–7.0 mg/dL
Adults	2.7–4.5 mg/dL
Potassium (K^+)	3.3–5.1 mEq/L
Proteins	
Total	6.5–8 g/dL
Albumin	3.5–5 g/dL
α_1 Globulin	0.15–0.4 g/dL
α_2 Globulin	0.5–0.9 g/dL
β Globulin	0.7–1.1 g/dL
γ Globulin	0.5–1.5 g/dL
Prealbumin	>15mg/dL
Sodium (Na^+)	133–145 mEq/L
Urea nitrogen (BUN)	6–19 mg/dL

Nutrients (Vitamins)   See Table 3–2

Urine Tests (24-hour excretion; varies with intake)

Calcium	100–240 mg (5–12 mEq)
Creatinine	See Tables 10–4 and 10–5
Magnesium	72–103 mg(6–8.6 mEq)
Phosphorus	0.7–1.5 g
Potassium	0.8–3.9 (20–100 mEq)
Sodium	3–8 g (130–360 mEq)
Urea nitrogen (UNN)	See Table 10–4

Stool Tests

Fat	
Total	<6 g/24 hr (with dietary fat intake >50 g/day); <30% of dry matter
Neutral	1%–5% of dry matter

Free fatty acids — 1%–10% of dry matter
  Combined fatty acids (as soap) — 1%–12% of dry matter
Nitrogen — <2 g/24 hr or 10% of urinary nitrogen

Function Tests

D-xylose absorption test: after overnight fast, 25 g xylose taken by mouth; urine collected for following 5 hr — Urine xylose 4–9 g/5 hr (or >20% of ingested dose); serum xylose 25–40 mg/dL 2 hr after oral dose

Schilling test: orally administered radio labelled vitamin B_{12} after "flushing" parenteral injection of B_{12}; intrinsic factor deficiency diagnosed with combination of pernicious anemia, gastric atrophy, and normalization of B_{12} excretion after exogenous intrinsic factor — Excretion in urine of >10% of oral dose/24 hr

*Normal ranges vary among different laboratories.

Frequently Used Equations

Equation	Reference Chapter
Energy Requirements	
Basal Energy Expenditure (Harris-Benedict Equaions)	11
Men: BEE = 66.47 + 13.75W + 5.00H − 6.76A	
Women BEE = 655.10 + 9.56W + 1.85H − 4.68A	
where	
W = weight (kg), H = height (cm), A = age (years)	

FOR OBESE PATIENTS, adjust weight as follows before
entering it into BEE equation:
Adjusted weight = [0.5 × (actual weight − ideal weight)
+ ideal weight]
Where ideal weight is calculated as:
Women: 100 lb (45.5 kg) for the first 5 feet (152 cm)
of height plus 5 lb (2.3 kg) for each additional
inch of height
Men: 106 lb (48 kg) for the first 5 feet (152 cm)
of height plus 6 lb (2.7 kg) for each additional
inch of height

FOR WEIGHT MAINTENANCE IN MOST PATIENTS, including obese patients   11
   Energy requirement = BEE × 1.1 − 1.4

FOR WEIGHT GAIN IN STABLE PATIENTS   11
   Energy goal = BEE × 2

FOR WEIGHT MAINTENANCE IN BURN PATIENTS   23
TBSA ≤40%
   Energy goal = BEE × 1.1 − 1.4
   Or energy goal (25 × Wt) + (40 × %TBSA)
   This *Modified Curreri formula* may overestimate
   requirements
TBSA >40%
   Energy goal = BEE × 2
   where
TBSA = Percent total body surface area burned (*whole
   number*, not decimal), estimated on admission and
   corrected where needed for amputation
Wt = Body weight in kilograms

Protein Loss
Urinary Urea Nitrogen
MOST PATIENTS   10

Protein catabolic rate (g/day) = [24-hour UUN (g)
   + 4] × 6.25
BURN PATIENTS   23

Protein Catabolic Rate (g/day) = (UUN + 4 + [0.2 g × %3°]
   + [0.1 g × %2°]) × 6.25
where
UUN = measured urinary urea nitrogen, in grams
% 3° = percent body surface area with 3° (full-thickness)
      burns (*whole number,* not decimal)
% 2° = percent body surface area with 2° (partial-thickness)
      burns (*whole number,* not decimal)

Urea Nitrogen Appearance for Patients with Changing
BUN and/or Body Water   10

$$UNA (g) = UUN (g) + 4 + \frac{(\Delta BUN \times 10)(W_m)(BW) + (BUN_m \times 10)(\Delta W)}{1000}$$

   where

      ΔBUN = change in BUN (mg/dL) during the urine
            collection (Final BUN − Initial BUN)

      BUN_m = mean BUN (mg/dL) during the urine collection
            [(Final BUN + Initial BUN)/2]

      ΔW = change in weight (kg) during the urine collection
            (Final weight − Initial weight)

      W_m = mean weight (kg) during the urine collection
            [(Final W + Initial W)/2]

      BW = assumed body water as a proportion of body weight
            (normal value = 0.5 for women and 0.6 for men;
            subtract 0.05 for marked obesity or dehydration;
            add 0.05 for leanness or edema)

Protein Balance   10

Protein Balance (g/day)
   = Protein intake − Protein catabolic rate

Midarm Muscle Circumference (MAMC)   10
MAMC (cm) = upper arm circumference (cm)
   − [0.314 × triceps skinfold (mm)]

Body Mass Index   17
BMI = weight (kg)/height² (m)

Relative Protein Content of Diet or Nutritional Support   11

Relative protein content (% of kcal) =
   Protein content (g) × 4 kcal/g × 100/Energy content

Desired protein intake (g) = Energy requirement $\times$
% protein desired/4 kcal/g $\times$ 100

Protein and Energy Content of Parenteral Nutrition Formulas

14

Protein content = (mL aa)[aa conc, (g/mL)]
Energy content = (protein content)(4 kcal/g) +
(mL dex)[dex conc (g/mL)](3.4 kcal/g) + (mL lipid)
(1.1 or 2.0 kcal/mL)

where

Dex = dextrose, aa = amino acids, conc = concentration
(e.g., 50% dextrose = 0.5 g/mL and 10% amino
acids = 0.10 g/mL), and 1.1 kcal/mL applies to
10% lipid and 2.0 kcal/mL to 20% lipid.

Respiratory Quotient

11, 24

RQ = moles CO_2 produced/moles O_2 consumed

The RQ for oxidation of fat = 0.7; for protein = 0.80;
for carbohydrate = 1.0

Stool Osmotic Gap

13

Stool osmotic gap = stool osmolality − 2 (stool sodium +
stool potassium)

>140 = Osmotic diarrhea (likely due to medications or
(unlikely) tube feeding)
<100 = Secretory diarrhea (possibly due to
pseudomembranous colitis or nonosmotic medications)

LDL Cholesterol Level

20

LDL cholesterol = total cholesterol − (triglycerides/5 +
HDL cholesterol)

This estimate is useful only when triglyceride levels are
below 400 mg/dL

C

Vitamin and Mineral Supplements

Because most vitamin supplements are classified by the United States Food and Drug Administration as foods rather than as drugs, they are not tightly regulated. However, vitamin preparations designated as United States Pharmacopoeia (USP) conform to established standards. It is important for clinicians to know the contents of the supplements they prescribe. A few generalizations can be made about multivitamin preparations:

1. There are no guidelines for the composition of multivitamins. Therefore, amounts of specific micronutrients such as water-soluble vitamins and minerals vary from one manufacturer to another.
2. The fat-soluble vitamin content of most multivitamins is 100% to 200% of the Recommended Daily Allowance (RDA).
3. Multivitamins containing more than 400 μg folic acid cannot be purchased without a prescription (see Chapter 26).
4. Few multivitamins contain vitamin K.
5. Multivitamins generally contain considerably less than the daily value for calcium.
6. The names of multivitamins can be deceiving. For instance, the term *stress vitamins* is a marketing tool and bears no relation to physiologic stress. In fact, these preparations are marketed mainly to normal persons with "stressful" lifestyles, without evidence that the normal stresses of daily living increase vitamin requirements or that vitamin use aids in stress management.

Multivitamins are available with or without minerals. Both of these categories can be subdivided according to the proportion of the daily value for most vitamins that they contain:

1. Replacement vitamins—up to 100% of the daily value. Pediatric multivitamins are mostly of this type, as well.

2. Therapeutic vitamins—100% to 200% of the daily value. Prenatal multivitamins fit in this category. There are no therapeutic multivitamins without minerals.

3. Super-therapeutic vitamins—200% to 1000% of the Recommended Daily Allowance (RDA). There are currently no multivitamins that strictly fit this category, since most of the "stress" multivitamins have very large amounts of some individual vitamins, RDA amounts of others, and often omit some entirely. To achieve these doses, individual vitamin supplements are often required. Levels of supplementation greater than 10 times the RDA are generally termed megadose therapy.

Indications for vitamin supplementation include the following. Recommended doses for treating deficiencies are provided in Table 3-2, and recommendations for preventing chronic diseases are provided in the Suggested Readings in Chapter 3.

1. Pregnancy and lactation (chiefly folic acid, calcium, vitamin D, iron, and zinc; see Chapter 4)

2. Newborns and infants (see Chapter 5)

3. Some high-risk situations such as low socioeconomic status, anorexia nervosa, certain very-low calorie obesity regimens, and some elderly persons and vegans (strict vegetarians)

4. Documented deficiency states

5. Conditions or medications that interfere with micronutrient intake, digestion, absorption, metabolism, or excretion, such as malabsorptive gastrointestinal disorders, heavy menses, and renal dialysis

6. Vitamin-dependent genetic disorders and diseases associated with defective vitamin transport

7. As an antidote to toxic anti-vitamins (e.g., folinic acid following high-dose methotrexate or folic acid during low-dose methotrexate therapy)

Pregnant or lactating women and infants should be given the appropriate multivitamins designed for them. Persons in group 3 should use a replacement multivitamin to achieve the RDA. Therapeutic vitamins are appropriate for treatment of deficiencies (indication 4), while doses in the super-therapeutic or megadose range may be needed for indications 5 through 7.

MULTIPLE VITAMIN PREPARATIONS

Amounts of Vitamins and

Name	Manufac-turer	Vitamin A (2997 IU)	Vitamin D (200–600 IU)	Vitamin E (15 IU)	Vitamin C (75–90 mg)	Thiamin B_1 (1.1–1.2 mg)	Riboflavin B_2 (1.1–1.3 mg)	Niacin B_3 (14–16 mg)
Replacement Vitamins								
Tab-A-Vite	Major	5000	400	30	60	1.5	1.7	20
Daily Multiple Vitamin	Rexall	5000	400	—	60	1.5	1.7	20
Therapeutic	Ivax	5000	400	30	90	3	3.4	20
Daily Value*	Freeda	5000	400	30	60	1.5	1.7	20
Multi-Day	Nature's Bounty	5000	400	10	60	1.5	1.7	20
One-A-Day Essential	Bayer	5000	400	30	60	1.5	1.7	20
Dayalets	Abbott	4500	360	27	54	1.2	1.53	18
Optilet 500	Abbott	4500	360	27	500	12.4	9	90.7
One-Tablet-Dailys	Ivax	5000	400	30	60	1.5	1.7	20
Liquid Replacement Vitamins (per 15 mL except as noted)								
Certagen	Goldline	2500	400	30	60	1.5	1.7	20
Certa Vite	Major	2500	400	30	60	1.5	1.7	20
Centrum	Wyeth	2500	400	30	60	1.5	1.7	20
Vi-Daylin†	Abbott	2250	400	13.5	54	0.842	1.08	12.2
Replacement Vitamins with Minerals								
One-Tablet-Daily with Minerals	Goldline	5000	400	30	60	1.5	1.7	20
Strovite Forte	Everett Labs	3000	400	60	500	20	20	100
FreedaVit Multivitamin with Minerals*	Freeda	5000	400	30	60	1.5	1.7	20
Theravim-M	Nature's Bounty	5000	400	30	120	3	3.4	30
Optilet-M-500	Abbott	4500	360	27	500	12.4	9	90.7
Unicap T	Pifzer	5000	400	30	500	10	10	100
Unicap Senior	Pfizer	5000	200	15	60	1.2	1.4	16
Myadec	Pfizer	5000	400	30	60	1.7	2	20
One-A-Day Maximum Formula	Bayer	5000	400	30	60	1.5	1.7	20
Unicap M	Pfizer	5000	400	30	60	1.5	1.7	20
Centrum	Wyeth	3500	400	30	60	1.5	1.7	20
Therapeutic Vitamins with or without Minerals								
Quintabs-M*	Freeda	5000	400	50	300	30	30	100
Theravim-M	Nature's Bounty	5000	400	30	90	3	3.4	20
Ultra Vita-Time	Nature's Bounty	10,000	400	12.5	150	25	25	50
CertaVite	Major	5000	400	30	60	1.5	1.7	20
Centrum Silver	Wyeth	5000	400	45	60	1.5	1.7	20
Certagen Senior	Goldline	6000	400	45	60	1.5	1.7	20

Pyridoxine D_6 (1.3-1.7 mg)	Folate (400 mcg)	B-12 (2.4 µg)	Beta carotene (IU)	Iron (8-18 mg)	Magnesium (310-420 mg)	Iodine (150 mg)	Zinc (8-11 mg)	Calcium (1000-1200 mg)	Phosphorus (700 mg)
2	0.4	6	—	18	—	—	—	—	—
1	0.4	1	—	—	—	—	—	—	—
3	0.4	9	—	—	—	—	—	66	—
2	0.4	6	—	—	—	—	—	—	—
2	0.4	6	—	—	—	—	—	—	—
2	0.4	6	—	—	—	—	—	—	—
1.8	0.36	5.4	—	—	—	—	—	—	—
3.7	—	10.8	—	—	—	—	—	—	—
2	0.4	6	—	—	—	—	—	—	—
2	—	6	—	9	—	150	3	—	—
2	—	6	—	9	—	150	3	—	—
2	—	6	—	9	—	150	3	—	—
0.945	—	4.05	—	9	—	—	—	—	—
3	0.4	6	—	18	100	150	15	130	100
25	1	50	1000	10	50	—	15	—	—
2	0.4	6	—	1.8	8	75	1.5	20	—
3	0.4	9	2500	27	—	—	15	—	—
3.7	—	10.8	—	18	72	135	1.35	—	—
6	0.4	18	—	18	—	150	15	—	—
2.2	0.4	3	—	10	30	150	15	100	77
3	0.4	6	—	18	100	150	15	162	125
2	0.4	6	—	18	100	150	15	129.6	100
2	0.4	6	—	18	—	150	15	60	45
2	0.4	6	—	18	100	150	15	162	109
30	0.4	30	—	10	15	150	7.5	30	—
3	0.4	9	—	27	100	150	15	40	31
15	0.4	50	—	5.79	0.39	100	0.66	60	24.3
2	0.4	6	—	—	100	150	15	162	109
3	0.4	25	—	4	100	150	15	200	48
3	0.2	25	—	9	100	150	15	200	48

Table continued on following page

MULTIPLE VITAMIN PREPARATIONS

Amounts of Vitamins and

Name	Manufac-turer	Vitamin A (2997 IU)	Vitamin D (200–600 IU)	Vitamin E (15 IU)	Vitamin C (75–90 mg)	Thiamin B$_1$ (1.1–1.2 mg)	Riboflavin B$_2$ (1.1–1.3 mg)	Niacin B$_3$ 16
Liquid Therapeutic Vitamins (per 15 mL except as noted)								
Thera-plus†	Hi-Tech Pharm	5000	400	—	200	10	10	100
Theravite†	Ivax	5000	400	—	200	10	10	100
Strovite Forte	Everett Labs	4000	400	30	300	15	17	100
Prenatal Vitamins								
Ultra NatalCare	Ethex	2700	400	30	120	3	3.4	20
Prenatal MR 90 Fe	Ethex	4000	400	30	120	3	3.4	20
Prenatal Vitamin	Nature's Bounty	4000	400	11	100	1.84	1.7	18
Prenatal 1-A-Day*	Freeda	4000	400	15	100	2	3	20
NatalCare Rx	Ethex	4000	400	15	80	1.5	1.6	17
NovaNatal	Novavax	—	400	30	120	3	3	20
Prenatal	Major	4000	400	11	100	1.84	1.7	18
Stuart-Prenatal	Xanodyne	4000	400	30	120	1.8	1.7	20

*Kosher, †per 5mL

Minerals (Adult RDA)

Pyridoxine B_6 (1.3–1.7 mg)	Folate (400 mcg)	B-12 (2.4 μg)	Beta carotene (IU)	Iron (8–18 mg)	Magnesium (310–420 mg)	Iodine (150 mg)	Zinc (8–11 mg)	Calcium (1000–1200 mg)	Phos-phorus (700 mg)
4.1	—	5	—	—	—	—	—	—	—
4.1	—	5	—	—	—	—	—	—	—
20	—	20	—	10	50		15	—	—
20	1	12	—	90	—	150	25	200	—
20	1	12	—	90	—	150	25	250	—
2.6	0.8	4	—	27	—	—	25	200	—
3	0.8	10	—	27	60	—	200	—	—
4	1	2.5	—	54	100	—	25	200	—
3	1	8	—	29	—	150	15	200	—
2.6	0.8	4	—	27	—	—	25	200	—
2.6	0.8	8	—	28	—	—	25	200	—

Conversion Factors for Various Minerals

Sodium (Na+)
Molecular weight = 23
1 mEq Na+ = 23 mg
1 g Na+ = 43 mEq (1000 mg × 1 mEq/23 mg)
1 g NaCl = 0.4 g Na+ (Na+ = 40% of weight of NaCl)
1 g Na+ is contained in 2.5 g NaCl

Potassium (K+)
Molecular weight = 39
1 mEq K+ = 39 mg

Calcium (Ca++)
Molecular weight = 40
1 mEq Ca++ = 20 mg (40/2)
For example, 15 mEq Ca++ in TPN = 300 mg

Magnesium (Mg++)
Molecular weight = 24
1 mEq Mg++ = 12 mg (24/2)

Phosphorus (P, phos)
Molecular weight = 31
1 mmol P = 31 mg

Index

Note: Page numbers followed by f indicate figures; those followed by t indicate tables; those followed by b indicate boxed material.